New Approaches to the Management and Diagnosis of Schizophrenia

Edited by Cicek Hocaoglu

Published in London, United Kingdom

New Approaches to the Management and Diagnosis of Schizophrenia
http://dx.doi.org/10.5772/intechopen.1001676
Edited by Cicek Hocaoglu

Contributors
Adnan Kuşman, Agota Barabassy, Aleksander Turek, Ali Irfan, Ali S. Alqahtani, Amira Bryll, António Melo, Ayesha Asghar, Cicek Hocaoglu, Darko Djuric, Dianne Smith, Elizabeth Karol, Faiza Rao, Joana Romão, Katarzyna Furman, Maciej Pilecki, Mahtab Ahmad Khan, Marta Szwajca, Natalia Śmierciak, Paulina Karcz, Paulina Mazur, Riaz Ullah, Robert Chrzan, Réka Csehi, Shazia Perveen, Shreshth Khanna, Sumaria Kanwal, Tadeusz Popiela, Tiago Duarte, Ulaş Korkmaz, Wirginia Krzyściak, Zsófia B. Dombi

First published in London, United Kingdom, 2024 by IntechOpen
IntechOpen is the global imprint of INTECHOPEN LIMITED, registered in England and Wales, registration number: 11086078, 167-169 Great Portland Street, London, W1W 5PF, United Kingdom

British Library Cataloguing-in-Publication Data
A catalogue record for this book is available from the British Library

Additional hard and PDF copies can be obtained from orders@intechopen.com

New Approaches to the Management and Diagnosis of Schizophrenia
Edited by Cicek Hocaoglu
p. cm.
Print ISBN 978-1-83769-601-7
Online ISBN 978-1-83769-600-0
eBook (PDF) ISBN 978-1-83769-602-4

For EU product safety concerns:
IN TECH d.o.o., Prolaz Marije Krucifikse Kozulić 3, 51000 Rijeka, Croatia,
info@intechopen.com or visit our website at intechopen.com.

Meet the editor

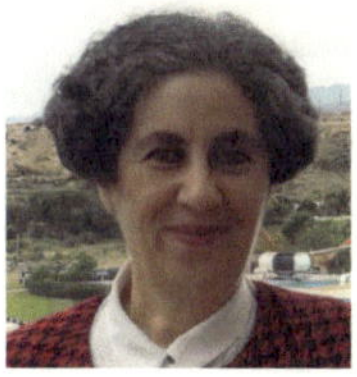

Cicek Hocaoglu obtained her medical degree from Bursa Uludag University Faculty of Medicine, Turkey. She received postgraduate training in psychiatry at the Medical School of Karadeniz Technical University, Trabzon, Turkey. She is currently a professor and head of the Department of Psychiatry, Recep Tayyip Erdogan University Medical School, Rize, Turkey.

She has published many national and international scientific articles, book chapters, and congress papers. Her interests include consultation–liaison psychiatry, suicide, schizophrenia, anxiety disorders, bipolar disorder, and psychopharmacology.

Contents

Preface

Schizophrenia is a chronic psychiatric disorder characterized by psychotic symptoms that lead to serious destructive consequences and disability. Many genetic, environmental, neurobiological, neurodevelopmental, and neurodegenerative factors are responsible for the etiology of schizophrenia. Although strong evidence has been obtained from numerous studies in this field, the etiology of schizophrenia is not fully known. The clinical appearance and prognosis of schizophrenia vary from patient to patient. Signs and symptoms may vary. Delusions, hallucinations, and cognitive dysfunction are usually at the forefront. Psychopharmacological approaches are the first choice in the treatment of schizophrenia. However, it has been reported that recovery rates have increased with psychosocial treatments in recent years.

Early initiation and long-term continuation of treatment of individuals diagnosed with schizophrenia can prevent the development of serious complications and the recurrence of symptoms. In addition, comorbid physical diseases as well as alcohol and substance-use disorders are frequently observed in individuals diagnosed with schizophrenia, especially during periods when disease symptoms increase and become more severe. However, treatment approaches initiated with appropriate therapeutic communication can help control patients' symptoms, prevent relapses, and improve the course of the disease.

A better understanding of the etiology and risk factors of schizophrenia will allow the identification of risk groups and the development of new treatment approaches. In addition, early diagnosis of the disease will be possible, and complications that may lead to disability can be prevented.

This book discusses the current literature on management and diagnosis of schizophrenia. In Chapter 1, current literature findings on the etiology and risk factors of schizophrenia are discussed. In Chapter 2, a design that activates professional boundaries to support patients with schizophrenia is discussed. Patients with schizophrenia may have difficulties in expressing and assessing pain. In Chapter 3, the role of myo-inositol in understanding pain perception in patients with schizophrenia is examined. In Chapter 4, current and new therapies in the treatment and diagnosis of schizophrenia are compared. In Chapter 5, the subject of artificial intelligence and schizophrenia is discussed. Recent developments in the diagnosis and treatment of schizophrenia with artificial intelligence applications are examined. There are still unmet needs in the treatment of schizophrenia. In Chapter 6, symptom relief and long-term needs in the treatment of schizophrenia are discussed. In Chapter 7, the role of phytochemicals in the treatment of schizophrenia is examined. Finally, in addition to psychopharmacological approaches, psychosocial therapies are important in the treatment of schizophrenia. Chapter 8 discusses current psychosocial approaches to the treatment of schizophrenia.

We would like to thank all the authors and publishers who contributed to the preparation of this book for their careful study. We hope it will be a valuable resource for our colleagues working in the field of mental health.

Cicek Hocaoglu
Recep Tayyip Erdogan University,
Rize, Turkey

Chapter 1

Aetiology and Risk Factors of Schizophrenia

Adnan Kuşman

Abstract

Schizophrenia is a disorder that begins at a young age and causes severe mortality and morbidity. The aetiology and pathophysiology of schizophrenia are still not known precisely. It is a very complex syndrome, and it is thought that more than one aetiological factor plays a role in its emergence. Genetics, epigenetics, and environmental and gene-environment interaction play a role in the aetiology of the disease. In addition, post-mortem neuropathological findings, neuroimaging findings, neurochemical studies, neuropsychological study results, and neurophysiological study results shed light on the mechanisms that cause the disease to occur. This chapter will provide an overview of the diathesis-stress, neurodegeneration, and neurodevelopmental models and summarise the work done so far in many areas.

Keywords: schizophrenia, genetics, neuroimaging, neuropathology, neurophysiology, neuropsychology, neurodevelopment, neurodegeneration

1. Introduction

In its broadest terms, psychotic disorders describe mental illnesses which involve disruption in perception, thought, and behaviour. The term psychosis describes the condition in which the mind cannot distinguish between what is real and what is unreal. Although it covers many psychopathological conditions in which the aetiology, symptoms, and course of the disease are very different, the prototype of this group of disorders is schizophrenia.

The aetiology and pathophysiology of schizophrenia are not known precisely. It is a 'syndrome' with complex symptoms, and it is thought that more than one aetiological factor plays a role in its emergence. According to the generally accepted assumption, brain development is disrupted due to genetic or environmental factors in the early life stages. This disruption creates a predisposition to the disease for the person, and symptoms of schizophrenia develop in later periods of life when the person encounters a stressful environmental effect [1]. It has been reported that subtle developmental abnormalities in the brain cause the onset of the disease before emerging clinical symptoms [2].

2. Hereditary causes

Schizophrenia is known to be a highly heritable disorder. Information on this subject is obtained from twin studies, family history, and studies with adopted persons [3–5].

2.1 Family studies

Family studies conducted in the early twentieth century showed that the rate of schizophrenia in relatives of schizophrenic patients was higher than in the general population. However, these early studies were criticised for many aspects of their study design and some other technical problems [6]. Recent studies have confirmed that the risk is higher among siblings and children than among parents and found that disease risks are not significantly different from those in older studies. As a result, family studies have revealed the high familial loading of schizophrenia, with siblings demonstrating an almost 10-fold increased risk of developing schizophrenia. This rate is greater than the increased risk reported for any other environmental factor [7]. In 2010, a Danish national register-based cohort study examined the risk of severe mental disorders. The risk of schizophrenia in the offspring of parents both affected by schizophrenia was found to be 27.3% [8].

2.2 Twin studies

Twins share many aspects of their environment. If we assume monozygotic (MZ) and dizygotic (DZ) twins share their environments to nearly an equal extent, then a higher concordance in MZ twins implies the disorder is, at least partly, genetic. A concordance of less than 100 per cent in MZ twins indicates that environmental factors are also at play [7]. Twin studies played an important role in understanding the genetic aetiology of schizophrenia. Twin studies have provided evidence that both genetic and environmental factors contribute to schizophrenia (SZ) risk. Heritability estimates of SZ in twin samples have varied methodologically. Studies between 1995 and 2000 from Europe and Japan have confirmed earlier findings. They yielded concordance rates of 41–65% in monozygotic (MZ) pairs and 0–28% in dizygotic (DZ) pairs, and heritability estimates of approximately 80–85%. Studies of discordant MZ pairs provide further insights into non-inherited factors contributing to this disorder's multifactorial aetiology [9]. Another study found that the estimated 79% heritability of SZ is congruent with previous reports. The low concordance rate of 33% in monozygotic twins demonstrates that illness vulnerability is not solely indicated by genetic factors [10]. Sullivan et al. [11] calculated heritability estimates in liability and shared and individual-specific environmental effects from the pooled twin data. They found evidence for substantial additive genetic effects. Results showed that heritability in liability to schizophrenia was 81%. Common or shared environmental influences on liability to schizophrenia were 11%. They concluded that the meta-analytic results from 12 published twin studies of schizophrenia are consistent with a view of schizophrenia as a complex trait that results from genetic and environmental aetiological influences [11].

2.3 Adoption studies

The observation that schizophrenia is more commonly observed among the relatives of individuals with schizophrenia than in the general population does not indicate the mechanism that produces such familiality occurs. Results from studies of adoptees with schizophrenia and their biological and adoptive relatives indicate that genetic factors play a highly significant role in the risk for schizophrenia. Although adoption studies have convincingly demonstrated an important role for genetic factors in schizophrenia, the necessity and specificity of such factors, their precise identity, and their interaction with environmental influences remain unknown [12].

3. Genetic studies

Many genes have been reported to be associated with schizophrenia, and these genetic features do not comply with Mendelian inheritance [13]. The first genetic studies were conducted as linkage studies, association studies, and chromosomal anomalies. As a result of linkage studies, repeated studies were carried out on chromosomes 1, 5, 8, 10, 13, and 22, and significant relationships have been demonstrated [14–19]. In chromosome anomaly studies, deletion in the 22q11 region of the 22nd chromosome and balanced translocations between the 1q42.1 and 11q14.3 regions of chromosomes 1 and 11 have been shown to be associated with schizophrenia [20]. The early studies were not fruitful. However, new technological developments have enabled the development of research methods.

3.1 Genome-wide association studies (GWAS)

GWA studies examine common alleles throughout the genome for association with a particular trait. Single-nucleotide polymorphisms (SNPs) have demonstrated that many SNPs correlate highly with neighbouring SNPs. The earliest GWA studies were not fruitful. Later studies showed dopamine receptor D2, glutamatergic neurotransmission and synaptic plasticity (GRM3, GRIN2A, SRR, GRIA1), and calcium signalling (CACNA1C, CACNB2, and CACNA1I) genes are associated with schizophrenia. Genome-wide association studies demonstrated a relationship between MHC Class 1 proteins and schizophrenia and prenatal infections [21, 22]. Supporting this finding, Aberg et al. [23] demonstrated that the major histocompatibility complex region showed a 3.7-fold overall enrichment of replication values. The replicated SNPs in TCF4, NOTCH4, POM121L2, CNNM2, AS3MT, and NT5C2 are among the most robust findings. They found that the most significant pathways involved neuronal function (axonal guidance, neuronal systems, and L1 cell adhesion molecule interaction) and the immune system (antigen processing, cell adhesion molecules relevant to T cells, and translocation to immunological synapse) [23]. In the latest and largest GWAS of schizophrenia, adding all SNPs accounts for only 7% of trait liability, which indicates additive models do not explain the risk of schizophrenia [24, 25].

3.2 Copy number variants

Copy number variants (CNVs) are deletions or duplications of chromosomes. The earliest report of a rare CNV associated with an increased risk of schizophrenia was a deletion of about 2.5 Mb on chromosome 22q11.2, which causes a congenital disorder described variably as DiGeorge syndrome. Deletion in the 22q11 region of the 22nd chromosome and balanced translocations between the 1q42.1 and 11q14.3 regions of chromosomes 1 and 11 have been shown to be associated with schizophrenia. These regions are found to be associated with the Disrupted-in-Schizophrenia-1 (DISC1) protein, which is related to disturbances in neural function and multiple disease-risk pathways [20]. Rujescu et al. [26] showed that it was the CNVs that intersected exons that increased the risk of schizophrenia. NRXN1 has been shown to be a candidate gene. NRXN1 gene codes for a cell adhesion molecule, neurexin-1. Neurexin-1 mediates interactions between pre- and postsynaptic structures. It is critical for forming, maintaining, and releasing neurotransmitters at synapses [26]. CNVs also increase the risk of developing intellectual deficits, developmental delay, autism spectrum disorders, and various congenital malformations and somatic diseases. To date schizophrenia-related CNVs found are 1q21.1 del, 1q21.1 dup, NRXN1 exonic del on chromosome 2, 3q29 del, 7q11.23 dup, 15q11.2 del, Angelman/Prader-Willi dup on chromosome 15, 15q13.3 del, 16p13.11 dup, 16p12.1 del, 16p11.2 dup, 22q11.2 del [27, 28]. The 15q11.2(BP1-BP2) deletion affects brain structure in a pattern consistent with both observed during first-episode psychosis in schizophrenia [29]. 16p11.2 duplications, 22q11.2 deletions, and 3q29 deletions are found to be related to schizophrenia. Findings suggest that multiple lines of genomic inquiry—genome-wide screens for CNVs, common variation, and exonic variation—converge on similar sets of pathways and/or genes [30]. Kirov et al. showed that 3q29, 15q11.2, 15q13.3, and 16p11.2 defects result in NMDAR postsynaptic signalling and, possibly, ARC complexes, which is an intracellular part of the synapse and plays a significant role in the pathogenesis of schizophrenia [31]. Pocklington et al. [32] showed for the first time that CNVs from individuals with schizophrenia are enriched for genes involved in GABAergic neurotransmission. Previous findings of CNV enrichment among genes involved in glutamatergic signalling are independently replicated and greatly extended [32].

3.3 Epigenetic mechanisms

It is increasingly recognised that epigenetic modifications play a role in the aetiology and pathophysiology of schizophrenia. Recent findings suggest that specific schizophrenia risk loci may influence stochastic variation in gene expression through epigenetic processes, highlighting the complex interplay between genetic and epigenetic control of neurodevelopmental trajectories. In addition, a significant part of the epigenetic changes in schizophrenia can be acquired through environmental factors, and these changes can affect brain functions [33]. Genome-scale mapping of DNA methylation, histone modifications and variants, and chromosomal loopings for promoter-enhancer interactions and other epigenetic determinants provide important clues about the dysregulated expression of synaptic and metabolic genes in schizophrenia. Epigenetic studies can also display potential links to the underlying genetic risk and environmental exposures [34]. In another study, researchers proposed that epigenetic factors and regulatory non-coding RNAs mediate the effects of environmental stressors [35]. A recent study showed that histone modifications play important roles in transcriptional regulation of the genes crucial for oligodendrocyte differentiation and myelination, specifically, histone acetylation and methylation [36].

4. Environmental factors

A relationship between the development of schizophrenia and exposure to influenza virus has been shown with data based on antibody measurements [37]. The relationship between *Toxoplasma gondii* and schizophrenia has also been demonstrated by immunoglobulin measurements. It has been shown that high maternal

IL8 levels in the second and third trimesters increase the risk of schizophrenia by twofold [38]. In another study, a relationship was found between high maternal TNF-alpha levels and the development of schizophrenia [39]. It has been shown that there is a relationship between anaemia during pregnancy, malnutrition, hyperhomocysteinemia resulting from folic acid deficiency, vitamins A and D deficiency, and increased docosahexaenoic acid levels and the child's risk of developing schizophrenia in the future [40–43]. These deficiencies or excess conditions have been shown to affect gene expressions, silencing some genes, disrupting repair mechanisms, inappropriately activating some genes, and disrupting myelination [44]. Malaspina et al. showed a relationship between advanced paternal age and schizophrenia, which was later supported by other studies [45–48]. There have been many studies showing that marijuana use is associated with schizophrenia [49]. Cannabis use, especially at the age of 18 or younger, increases the risk of developing schizophrenia [50]. Studies investigating the relationship between immigration and schizophrenia have shown that the risk of schizophrenia increases in first- and second-generation immigrants. It has been stated that the possible cause of this situation is social defeat and social exclusion and that the experience of social defeat in genetically predisposed people increases the sensitivity of the mesolimbic dopaminergic pathway, making it easier for the person to develop a psychotic disorder [51, 52]. A relationship has been found between socioeconomic level and the development of schizophrenia. Two theories have been put forward to explain this relationship: (i) social cause theory and (ii) social shift theory. According to the social cause theory, being born into a family with a low socioeconomic level increases the likelihood of exposure to environmental stresses and causes the development of schizophrenia in the predisposed individual. According to the social shift theory, the person falls to a lower socioeconomic level due to the disease. Studies on this subject have yielded contradictory results, and the person losing the social status to which he/she belongs is the result of the interaction of many factors [53–59].

5. Gene-environment interaction

The gene-environment relationship is explained as sensitivity to environmental factors determined by genes and gene expression affected by environmental conditions. This situation has been defined as the stress susceptibility model (diathesis-stress). According to this model, genetic and environmental conditions predispose the individual to the development of psychosis, with a negative and additive effect on brain development, during a critical period or more than one period of brain development [37, 60–62]. Exposure to maltreatment, especially in early life, and repetition of this exposure create a predisposition to psychosis, possibly by causing changes in dopaminergic pathways originating from the mesencephalon and projecting to higher regions [63].

6. Physiopathology

6.1 Neuropathology

Neuropathology studies have shown that neurons and glial cells exhibit different characteristics in schizophrenia cases compared to normal individuals. Although the changes were seen especially in the hippocampus and prefrontal cortex (PFC), they are not specific to these regions [64]. The first of the most consistent findings is the widespread reduction in decreased neuronal size and dendritic and axonal branching [65, 66]. The network system formed by axons, dendrites, and synaptic gaps is called 'neuropil'. The decrease in neuropils may explain the reduced brain volume at the macroscopic level and is called the 'decreased neuropil hypothesis'. In individuals with schizophrenia, the number of neurons decreases over time, and structural changes occur in dendrites and axons [67]. It has been reported that dendritic spine reduction in cortical neurons disrupts and damages information-processing processes [68, 69]. Synaptic changes observed in schizophrenia are generally decreasing, and this has been seen especially in glutamatergic neurons [65]. It has been shown that there is a selective loss of pyramidal neurons in the PFC [70]. Additionally, an increase in white matter density has been detected in the PFC, and it has been stated that this is due to the inhibition of neuronal migration during development [71–73]. In histopathological examinations of the Superior Temporal gyrus (Heschl's gyrus) and medial temporal lobe, it was observed that the pyramidal neurons in the cortical third layer were reduced in number, and the organisation of these neurons was impaired [74, 75]. It has been observed that the total number of neurons decreases in the thalamus, another most studied region, and as an indicator of this, there is a decrease in the amount of grey matter, but there is no change in cell density [76–78]. A decrease in the number of neurons and neuropils was detected, especially in the pulvinar and mediodorsal nuclei [64]. Although the number of neurons decreased in the basal ganglia, no change in neuron density was detected [79]. Immunohistochemical markers have shown a decrease in membrane density in the pre-synaptic axon terminal in the medial temporal lobe, frontal cortex, visual cortex, and cingulate cortex in schizophrenia patients [80–82]. In addition, SNAP-25, synapsin, and synaptophysin, proteins belonging to the synaptic structure, are found in the hippocampus and frontal cortex and were also found to be decreased [83].

Immunohistochemical methods could identify cortical interneurons, and it was shown that these neurons decrease by more than 10% in schizophrenia patients [84, 85]. Interneurons are marked by parvalbumin and somatostatin, and they are found in decreased amounts in the hippocampus and the parahippocampal gyrus in schizophrenia patients. Parvalbumin interneurons work in association with NMDA receptors [86, 87]. In patients with schizophrenia, neurons containing gamma amino butyric acid (GABA) and glutamic acid decarboxylase (GAD) are generally reduced compared to healthy individuals. This results in disinhibited excitatory neurons, leading to defective activation. GABA neurons have important functions, especially in the PFC, and play a critical role during executive functions. The decrease in these neurons leads to the impairment of cognitive functions [88]. Microglia cells are the source of the major pro-inflammatory cytokines of IL-6 and TNF-alpha. Increased microglia cell density has been detected in the PFC, auditory cortex, ACC, and mediodorsal thalamus in schizophrenia patients and associated with suicide in schizophrenia [89].

6.2 Neurochemical changes

The Proton Magnetic Spectroscopy method can noninvasively measure people's biochemical structures and metabolic activity states. This method has been used to measure N-acetyl aspartate (NAA), choline, creatinine, glutamine/glutamate (Glx), and myoinositol-1 molecules *in vivo* in schizophrenia patients. NAA is an indicator of neuron functionality, which is well-being at the cellular level, and Cho is an indicator of myelination [90]. Creatine (Cre) is a metabolic output whose value is relatively constant. Although the function of myo-inositol is not known, it is thought to be associated with glial cells [91]. In individuals with high genetic load for schizophrenia, NAA, Cho, and Cre were detected at low levels in the thalamus, suggesting that neuronal dysfunction in the thalamus has a role and is associated with the development of schizophrenia. It has been found that right and left mPFC NAA and left mPFC Cho levels are low in schizophrenia patients. In schizophrenia patients, NAA/Cre and NAA/Cho levels were found to be lower in the hippocampus and DLPFC compared to controls. Additionally, NAA/Cre and NAA/Cho levels were lower in the temporal cortex and thalamus in schizophrenia patients than in healthy controls [92].

6.2.1 Dopamine hypothesis

In the dopaminergic pathway, which projects from the Ventral Tegmental Area (VTA) to the limbic system, hyperactivity is defined as the oldest and most widely accepted hypothesis of the mechanism leading to psychosis. Dopamine 1R (D1R) receptors are more commonly found in the Frontal Cortex. However, this subtype, unlike D2R, shows hypoactivity and negative symptoms of schizophrenia are partially attributed to the hypoactivity of this receptor (hypofrontality) [93, 94].

6.2.2 Glutamate hypothesis

Glutamate is a neurotransmitter with both metabotropic and ionotropic receptors. The type emphasised in the pathogenesis of schizophrenia is NMDA receptors. Due to hypoactivity in NMDA receptors, since GABA neurons serving as interneurons cannot be stimulated, glutamate neurons projecting to the VTA cannot be inhibited. As a result, there is an increase in activity in the dopaminergic pathways located in the VTA and extending to the limbic system [95, 96].

6.2.3 Gamma-aminobutyric acid (GABA) hypothesis

Post-mortem studies consistently show decreased GABA levels in the PFC. An increase in the number of GABA receptors may also be observed. It has been stated that this situation may occur in response to the decrease in GABA levels. It has been suggested that GABAergic anomalies may explain working memory disorders by causing neural synchrony changes in schizophrenia patients [97, 98].

6.2.4 Serotonin hypothesis

It is a hypothesis based on the antagonism of 5HT2A receptors. The underlying mechanism of psychotic states seen especially in diseases such as Parkinson's or Alzheimer's diseases is pointed out. It has been stated that hyperactivity of 5HT2A receptors has an excitatory effect on glutamatergic neurons, and increased dopaminergic neuron activation in the VTA ultimately leads to increased DA activity in the mesolimbic pathway [99].

6.2.5 Norepinephrine hypothesis

This theory is based on various evidences revealing the anatomical and physiological properties of the locus coeruleus-norepinephrine (LC-NE) system and its involvement in brain function and cognition. Theory suggests that the phenomenology of schizophrenia, particularly cognitive symptoms, can be explained by an abnormal interaction between genetic predisposition and stress-induced LC-NE dysfunction. This dysfunction leads to an imbalance between modes of LC activity, dysfunctional regulation of brain network integration and neural acquisition, and deficits in cognitive functions [100, 101]. Catecholamine-producing midbrain and brainstem nuclei are densely connected to the PFC and dACC and contribute to cognitive control processes. It has been shown that the VTA and substantia nigra, as well as the LC, are abnormal during cognitive control in patients with schizophrenia [102].

6.2.6 Acetylcholine hypothesis

A well-known characteristic of patients with schizophrenia is that they smoke excessive amounts of cigarettes. This behaviour of patients is interpreted as a method of self-treatment to improve the positive, negative, and cognitive symptoms of schizophrenia [103]. Acetylcholine in the CNS has three sources: (i) basal forebrain nuclei, (ii) pedunculopontine tegmental nucleus and laterodorsal tegmental nucleus, and (iii) giant cholinergic interneurons in the caudate-putamen and nucleus accumbens. The cholinergic nuclei innervate the hippocampus, cortical, and subcortical regions. Acetylcholine plays a regulatory role in the dopamine, glutamate, GABA, and serotonin systems. It has also been shown to have a mutual regulatory relationship with inflammatory processes [104]. The muscarinic receptors that play a role in the aetiology of schizophrenia are thought to be M1, M4, and M5 receptors. It has been shown that M1 receptors are associated with cognitive disorders, M4 receptors with positive symptoms, and M5 receptors with prepulse inhibition. The nicotinic $\alpha 4\beta 2$ receptor is associated with attention and memory functions, and the nicotinic $\alpha 7$ nACh receptor is associated with P50 sensory transmission deficits [105–107].

7. Neuroimaging findings

7.1 Structural neuroimaging

7.1.1 Computed tomography (CT)

CT shows more significant volume reduction than expected for age in the frontal lobes, temporal lobes, caudate head, and thalamus in patients with schizophrenia. This volume decrease is progressive throughout the disease. Ventriculomegaly and cortical atrophy are also more common in patients with schizophrenia than controls. Ventriculomegaly is associated with age, impaired cognitive function, decreased response to treatment, and negative symptoms [108, 109].

7.1.2 Magnetic resonance imaging (MRI)

MRI provides high-resolution images. Increased cerebrospinal fluid (CSF) and decreased grey and white matter volume have been detected in schizophrenia. Volume reductions in the frontal lobe, temporal lobe, hippocampus, and parahippocampus have been reported, all associated with cognitive impairment [110, 111]. Auditory hallucinations have been reported to be associated with loss of superior temporal gyrus volume, and negative symptoms have been reported to be associated with loss of prefrontal lobe volume [112–114]. Many studies have shown that volume reduction in schizophrenia patients is in thalamocortical connections and prefrontal cortex grey matter [115]. Regions with decreased grey matter volume in voxel base morphometry are the frontal gyri, the temporal gyri, the parahippocampal gyri, the posterior and anterior insulae, dorsal anterior cingulate cortex (dACC), posterior cingulate cortex (PCC), bilateral angular and supramarginal gyri, bilateral thalamus, and caudate nuclei [116–118]. Although the large cava septum pellucidum is more common in patients with schizophrenia, it is not considered a causal factor [119]. However, this can be considered evidence of abnormal neurodevelopmental processes that contribute to the development of schizophrenia [120]. Histologically, this decrease in grey matter is accompanied by a decrease in dendritic and synaptic density, which leads to communication disturbances along neural circuits [69].

7.2 Functional neuroimaging

7.2.1 Single-photon emission computed tomography and positron emission tomography

Single-photon emission computed tomography (SPECT) and positron emission tomography (PET) are radionuclide neuroimaging techniques.

PET is based on the idea that people with schizophrenia have a different pattern of cerebral glucose use than normal individuals. Many researchers have noticed hypofrontality in fluorodeoxyglucose positron emission tomography (FDG PET) studies performed in schizophrenia. Decreased metabolism was observed in the frontal and temporal cortex of the patients but not in the parietal and occipital lobes [121]. However, not all studies have been able to replicate the same result [122].

SPECT detects gamma rays emitted from radionuclides. Fluorine-18 is a radionuclide that labels glucose molecules to form F18 deoxyglucose (FDG). There are two types of radionuclide studies in patients with schizophrenia: blood flow-glucose metabolism studies and neuroreceptor research. Blood flow and glucose metabolism studies are carried out in two stages: rest and active. During activation with the Wisconsin card sequencing test, patients with schizophrenia have a less significant increase in blood flow to the dorsolateral prefrontal cortices [123]. Abnormalities in blood flow to the temporolimbic pathways are associated with disorders inhibiting subcortical dopamine release and positive disease symptoms. Auditory hallucinations have been proven to be associated with increased blood flow to the medial, temporal, and limbic areas [124]. Radionuclide studies in patients with schizophrenia have shown an increase in dopamine at synapses. Each anti-psychotic drug has different receptor affinities, which PET and SPECT can demonstrate [125–128].

7.2.2 Functional magnetic resonance imaging (fMRI)

The fMRI is based on measuring locally increased cerebral blood flow of functional brain regions during a specific task called blood oxygen level-dependent (BOLD) imaging. fMRI studies in patients with schizophrenia include investigating executive and cognitive functions such as attention, memory, psychomotor function, and basic stimulus processing. In a recent meta-analysis, structural and functional studies investigated the areas of processing speed, attention, working memory, verbal learning and memory, visual learning and memory, executive function/reasoning, problem-solving, verbal fluency and verbal comprehension, emotional perception, social perception and knowledge, theory of mind, and attribution bias. The authors noted that when cognitive tasks were presented, there was a decrease in the activation of the dorsomedial prefrontal cortex, the complementary motor area, and the right lower frontal gyrus [129]. Typically, frontal hypoperfusion, anterior cingulate cortex (ACC) hypoperfusion, and medial frontal gyrus hypoperfusion are the areas and findings that have been studied the most in patients with schizophrenia [130–132]. In contrast, increased blood flow was found in the thalamus [133], putamen and inferior temporal gyrus, and unaltered blood flow in the nucleus caudatus [134]. However, some studies have shown results opposite to these findings [135]. Multiple brain networks have been discovered using resting-state fMRI, including the default mode network, central executive network, salience network, language, sensorimotor, auditory, and visual networks [136–140]. Default mode network (DMN) abnormalities, DMN abnormal activity, DMN with the severity of positive symptoms, and central executive and salience network dysconnectivity have been detected in schizophrenia [141–143]. Connections of the thalamocortical network have also been implicated in schizophrenia and psychosis, with reduced connectivity between the mediodorsal thalamus and the insula and orbitofrontal regions [144].

7.2.3 Diffusion tensor imaging (DTI)

The DTI is used in general neuroimaging to visualise the relationship of white matter, projection, or commissural fibres. Diffusion tensor imaging also allows white matter paths to be imaged in colour three-dimensional images, called tractography. Diffusion tensor imaging studies have shown that patients with schizophrenia have reduced fractional anisotropy in the cingulum and corpus callosum. The results of such studies can be biased, as these findings may also be influenced by various characteristics of the subject's age, gender, and hand dominance [145, 146]. The uncinate fascicle is particularly interesting, as it connects the amygdala to regions of executive function (medial and orbitofrontal cortices). Decreased fractional anisotropy and decreased structural integrity were detected in this circuit [147]. In terms of specificity, four of the neuropsychiatric disorders studied, obsessive-compulsive disorder, major depressive disorder, bipolar disorder, and schizophrenia, had abnormal DTI measurements of varying degrees in the corpus callosum and superior longitudinal fascicle [148].

7.2.4 Magnetic resonance spectroscopy (MRS)

With MRS, concentrations of different chemical species can be analysed *in vivo*. N-acetyl aspartate (NAA), creatinine (Cre), choline (Cho), myoinositol (mI), and glutamate-glutamine (Glx) are frequently analysed markers in MRS studies. NAA is a marker of neuronal integrity, and its low concentration indicates neuronal or axonal damage. Cho is part of the cell membrane and reflects cell membrane turnover rates. The increase in Cho levels reflects cellular hyperplasia. Cre is a marker of energy metabolism functioning, and Cre levels decrease in hypermetabolic states. Glutamine and glutamate are components of the neurotransmitter system, and their concentrations can be measured as two separate peaks. Lactate, acetate, aspartate, and lipid molecules are indicators of pathological conditions at the cellular level. Changes at the molecular level in the internal environment are evident even before morphological changes are observed [149, 150].

In schizophrenia, lower levels of glutamate in the ACC and higher levels in the centrum semiovale were noted. Others have found decreases in GABA, NAA, mI, and total Cho in the ACC in first-episode psychosis patients [151]. In general, the most consistent finding in most studies is that NAA is reduced in schizophrenia and first-episode psychosis. This finding suggests the possibility of neuronal damage/dysfunction early in the disease. There is a negative correlation between NAA levels in the dorsolateral prefrontal cortex and negative symptoms in schizophrenia [152]. A higher glutamate/creatine ratio in the medial frontal cortex was (i) positively associated with overall symptom severity, (ii) positively associated with schizophrenia symptomatology severity, and (iii) negatively associated with overall functioning [153].

7.2.5 Magnetoencephalography (MEG)

The MEG is an electrophysiological measuring device that measures the magnetic fields emitted by postsynaptic neuronal activity in the brain. MEG measures brain function with millisecond temporal resolution. When combined with the patient's brain anatomical structure on MRI, MEG can show the 3D location of brain activity (spontaneous or evoked) in real time with millisecond temporal resolution [154]. In the resting state, the most robust finding of MEG is an increase in slow-wave activity in the delta (1–4 Hz) and theta (4–8 Hz) bands localised in the frontotemporal and parietal regions in patients with schizophrenia. Zeev-Wolf et al. found that patients with high positive symptoms commonly had low alpha power, and more beta power was seen in the left hemisphere of patients with high negative symptoms [155]. Due to MEG's ability to precisely measure neural oscillation processes and its good spatial localisation using advanced resource reconstruction algorithms, MEG is a valuable technique for assessing whole brain functional activity.

7.2.6 Functional neur-infrared spectroscopy (fNIRS)

The fNIRS is a non-invasive imaging method for measuring cortical activity *in vivo*. The measurement of fNIRS is based on the different absorption properties of infrared light by oxy (Oxy-Hb) and deoxy (Hb) haemoglobin [156]. Compared to fMRI, the fNIRS environment is much more natural and resembles real-world environments. It is comparatively less sensitive to head movements. It is easy to use and noiseless. These advantages allow the monitoring of cortical activity during complex tasks. fNIRS has a high temporal resolution, provides a representative experimental environment, and can contribute highly to social cognitive neuroscience, especially neuroimaging [157, 158].

8. Neurophysiological study findings

When schizophrenic patients follow an object with their eyes, a pendulum-like movement is observed. It is also seen more frequently in the first-degree relatives of patients than in the normal population. In twin studies, eye movement disorders were found to be a highly heritable biological marker [159, 160]. The recovery of eye movement disorder similar to the P50 gating disorder by using nicotinic stimulation suggests that in both cases, it results from a common mechanism that depends on the failure of hippocampal inhibitory interneurons to be stimulated by nicotinic cholinergic receptors [161].

8.1 EEG findings

The P300 response measures the neural activity underlying the processes of immediate memory and attention orientation. While its amplitude is related to the attentional resources directed to the task, its latency reflects the speed at which the stimulus is classified [162]. Although amplitude reduction is a relatively constant finding, a prolongation of P300 latency has been reported in schizophrenia [163]. Additionally, it has been reported that as the disease progresses, the latency is prolonged in parallel with the progressive volume decrease in the frontal, temporal, and hippocampal regions [164–166]. It has been shown that there is a hierarchical sequence between schizophrenia patients, healthy relatives of schizophrenia patients, and healthy controls according to the amplitude of the P300 wave, and these findings together have been interpreted as P300 anomalies may be a hereditary marker in schizophrenia [167].

9. Neuropsychological study findings

It was determined that schizophrenia patients performed lower than healthy individuals in tests evaluating attention, learning and memory, executive functions, working memory, language functions, and social cognitive functions. Low cognitive skills performance is an essential reason for a person's decreased functionality [168–170].

10. Psychological approach to psychotic disorders

The leading cognitive model of psychotic disorders is the Theory of Mind (ToM). ToM is based on understanding the differences between one's own and others' mental states. Premack and Woodruff first proposed the theory (1978), and then the works of Baron-Cohen and Frith came to the fore [171–173]. Garety et al. described probabilistic inference, that is, Jumping to Conclusion Bias (JTC) [174]. Accordingly, a person with psychotic thought content makes a judgement without collecting sufficient data. The probabilistic inference proposed by Garety et al. was used at a high rate in later studies. They have shown consistency and have been designed to include different probabilities and conditions [175–177]. Higgins [178], on the other hand, created a model based on the inconsistency in self-value (the self that actually exists, the self that one wants, and the one that society wants). These inconsistencies determine the person's perception of himself/herself, and he stated that depressed people emerge with a difference between the person they are and the person they want to be [178]. Bentall et al. stated that psychotic patients make attributional biases and develop delusions [179]. To evaluate patients' attribution, they invented the Internal, Personal, and Situational Attributions Questionnaire (IPSAQ) to evaluate attributional biases and errors [180]. Kinderman et al. discussed a possible relationship between ToM deficits and attributional biases and errors [181].

11. Diathesis-stress model of schizophrenia

The diathesis-stress model explains schizophrenia as the result of the interaction between genetic predisposition (diathesis) and environmental stressors.

This model suggests that a person may have a genetic predisposition to schizophrenia, but the combination of this predisposition and stressful life experiences triggers the onset of the disorder. Many neuropsychiatric disorders and schizophrenia are thought to develop concerning hypothalamic-pituitary-adrenal (HPA) axis dysfunction, neurodevelopmental characteristics, epigenetic regulation, neurotransmitter systems, inflammatory processes, and brain structure and function. The events or 'stressors' can be psychological (e.g. social rejection) or biological (e.g. physical injury or illness) [182]. The activation of the stress system causes a series of integrated physiological responses. This response consists of the HPA axis and the secretion of adrenal stress hormones, which trigger a fight or flight response, prompting the organism to use coping strategies. Therefore, it has been hypothesised that adverse events early in life may shape the maturation of the neuroendocrine systems and corticolimbic circuits, leading to increased stress responses in adulthood.

Several theories have been proposed to explain how stressors can become 'built-in' in brain physiology. One of the best known is the 'cumulative stress' hypothesis. Stress affects the developmental program of an organism, leading to specific functional and structural changes in the brain (e.g. hippocampal damage, ventricular expansion, altered cell architecture, migration of neurons) and disruptions in neurochemical parameters (dopamine (DA), glutamate, γ-amino butyric acid (GABA), serotonin) [183]. In response to stress, CRH is synthesised, which causes ACTH to be released from the pituitary glands, and then, glucocorticoids (GCs) are released from the adrenal glands. This system is controlled by the feedback system in the brain. CRH directly affects the brain, including the locus coeruleus, the periventricular nucleus of the hypothalamus, the bed nucleus stria terminalis (BNST), and the central nucleus of the amygdala. The interaction of CRH with the noradrenergic system in these regions can lead to significant changes in homeostasis, that is feedforward activation, which can lead to psychopathology. Neurotoxicity in the hippocampus and PFC causes disruptions in the negative feedback system that reduce HPA axis activation [184].

Epigenetic mechanisms, which affect the management of DNA function without changing the DNA structure due to environmental factors, stand out as an essential issue. It plays a role in reshaping brain circuits during the developmental process. The most affected regions are the temporal and prefrontal cortical-thalamic-ventral striatal pathways [183]. A primary irregularity in the executive functions of the prefrontal cortex can lead to abnormal regulation of stress-induced circuitry in regions downstream of the prefrontal cortex, such as the amygdala, ventral striatum, and hippocampus [184]. The synaptic pruning hypothesis is one of the leading models for the development of symptoms in schizophrenia. Synaptic pathology can occur in sensitive adolescents due to an abnormal process of neuromodulation, which can be amplified by environmental factors such as genetic predisposition or early life stress exposure. In schizophrenia, dendritic pathology consistently has been found with stress-induced changes in both the hippocampal formation and the prefrontal cortex [183]. Howes [185] emphasised the importance of microglia and inflammatory processes in brain development. Microglia have a central role in the inflammatory response and are involved in synaptic pruning and neuronal restructuring. Microglial activation occurs in response to psychosocial stress. Perinatal activation of microglia may sensitise them to stressors later in life. Genetic research has shown that variations in the complement system are associated with schizophrenia and that this system also regulates microglial synaptic pruning [185].

To summarise the possible risk factors:

Prenatal stress: prenatal stress leads to cognitive impairments, neuromotor abnormalities, and hyperreactivity to stress. Maternal biopsychosocial stress, death of the father during pregnancy, unwanted pregnancy, and exposure to war and natural disasters cause a prolonged increase in HPA axis activity and changes in GC receptor density. Several maternal complications are associated with adverse foetal development, including low birth weight, cognitive deficits, depression, schizophrenia, anxiety, attention-deficit/hyperactivity disorder, antisocial behaviours, depression, diabetes, infection/inflammation, and obesity. The enzyme 11β-hydroxysteroid dehydrogenase type 2 (HSD2) acts as a shield, ensuring rapid inactivation of GCs in the mother. Controlled fluctuations in the expression levels and functionality of HSD2 are necessary to ensure that GCs reach the foetus in the right amount and at the right time for the maturation of the organs. Many factors, including hypoxia, catecholamines, and proinflammatory cytokines, can downregulate placental HSD2 activity, increasing GC transport to the foetus [183, 184].

Postnatal stress: early stressors can cause long-term changes in neuroendocrine responses to brain morphology and emotional and behavioural regulation. Neuroendocrine activity can reprogram the nucleus accumbens to increase dopamine release due to stress. Studies on genetically high-risk populations show that stress in childhood increases the risk of schizophrenia. In addition, childhood abuse predicts the development of psychotic disorders [184]. Tetrahydrocannabinol and amphetamines have been observed to increase cortisol levels in both schizophrenia patients and control cases. Opiates, on the other hand, have been found to suppress cortisol secretion [186].

12. Neurodegeneration model of schizophrenia

The neurodegeneration model of schizophrenia suggests that the disorder involves progressive neurostructural changes, particularly in grey matter content and ventricular size. This model considers schizophrenia as a disorder that has neurodevelopmental antecedents but is characterised by the course of neurodegeneration. Brain gliosis is indicative of neuronal degeneration. Glial cells respond to specific neuron injuries and are seen in brains with neurodegenerative disorders. Post-mortem examinations show that patients with schizophrenia do not have gliosis, which contradicts the hypothesis that schizophrenia is a neurodegenerative disorder [187]. On the other hand, some studies have shown histopathological findings and evidence that schizophrenia is a limited neurodegenerative disease. Reports of neuropathological abnormalities in the brains of post-mortem schizophrenia patients have shown that they are present in almost all areas of the brain [188]. In post-mortem studies completed by Schnieder et al., it has been stated that differences in astrocytosis and microgliosis have been observed in the brains of schizophrenia patients, although not conclusively [189]. Oligodendrocytes, on the other hand, presented remarkable new findings. This type of gliosis is thought to be observed in schizophrenia and can be interpreted as an altered response to a pathological process in the brain [190]. Some researchers suggested that the altered mechanism observed in the myelination process in schizophrenia may be the trigger for white matter loss in the prefrontal cortex. These researchers also noted that inhibitory synapse formation decreases during the disease, and excitatory synapses are excessively shortened [191, 192]. Since shortening is a form of axonal degeneration, retraction or excessive excretion supports the neurodegeneration hypothesis [193]. Neuroplasticity has been proposed as another mechanism to explain progressive degeneration in schizophrenia [194]. Other variables that support the neurodegeneration hypothesis are based on the presence of chemical alterations. Dopamine, glutamate, and GABA are associated with neurodegenerative processes [195–197]. In addition, it has been stated that apoptotic hyperfunction may support degenerative processes in schizophrenia [198]. High levels of Bax/Bcl-2 are indicative of susceptibility to apoptosis, and patients with chronic schizophrenia exhibit a 50% higher Bax/Bcl-2 ratio than the non-psychiatric population [199]. Despite the findings mentioned here, more studies are needed in this area.

13. Neurodevelopmental model of schizophrenia

The neurodevelopmental model of schizophrenia suggests that the disorder develops over time because of abnormal neurodevelopmental processes that begin early in life, potentially during prenatal development. According to this hypothesis, disorders in neuronal developmental processes, such as migration and arborisation in the prenatal period, lead to abnormal brain maturation [200]. Over time, the individual interacts with environmental factors and the disease is triggered. In this process, the person is influenced by external and internal factors [201, 202]. According to this theory, biological variants of the disorder are present long before the development of pathological symptoms in the individual. However, by interacting with many external factors, clinical impairment will not occur until obvious symptoms appear [203–207]. Genetics, neurodevelopmental processes, and schizophrenia are inextricably linked. All molecules that influence neural development are controlled by specific genes involved in brain development and pre- and postnatal maturation. Numerous links have been discovered between schizophrenia and genes-encoding proteins such as neuroregulin 1 (NRG1), dysbindin, DISC-1, regulatory of G protein signalling 4 (RGS4), COMT, and proline dehydrogenase [208–211]. Deficiency in reelin expression has been observed in patients with schizophrenia after death. Reelin is a protein that directs the migrations of certain groups of neurons and is released extensively in this process [212, 213]. In addition, a decrease in polysialic acid (PSA) expression on neural cell adhesion molecules (NCAM) has been observed in patients with schizophrenia. This molecule is involved in axonal growth, synaptogenesis of interneurons, and the formation of inhibitory circuits [214, 215]. It has also been stated that proteins such as brain-derived growth factor (BDNF), glial cell-derived neurotrophic factor (GDNF), and epidermal growth factor (EGF) are also involved in this process [216–218]. The presence of several minor physical abnormalities in patients with schizophrenia supports the hypothesis of abnormal neurodevelopment. These abnormalities occur during the first trimester of pregnancy and early in the second trimester. Researchers have found that the smaller circumference of the head at birth, delayed brain development, droopy ears, palate arch anomalies, epicanthus, cleft palate, telecanthus, craniofacial minor physical abnormalities and a large gap between the first two toes have a relationship with schizophrenia [219–221]. Given that hereditary factors alone cannot explain the aetiology of schizophrenia, research has been conducted on the role of environmental factors. Infections, delivery time, obstetric complications, substance use, childhood and adolescent traumas, social exclusion and social defeat, children of mothers who had influenza in the second trimester of pregnancy and mothers who had rubella infection during pregnancy, the place of birth, and the size of cities can predispose to psychosis in sensitive individuals [222–228]. Meta-analytic studies on cognition before and in the early stages of the disease have revealed that attention, memory, and executive functions worsen in patients with schizophrenia than controls [229, 230]. One of the most consistent findings in schizophrenia is dysfunction in motor skills. It has been stated that it can be considered a predictive finding in children and adolescents who develop schizophrenia in the future [231, 232]. Notwithstanding, the available data are far from reaching a definitive conclusion.

14. Conclusions

Schizophrenia was identified at the end of the nineteenth century and the beginning of the twentieth century. Immediately afterwards, scientists began to conduct studies to understand the nature of schizophrenia. At the beginning of the twentieth century, studies were carried out to understand whether schizophrenia was a familial disorder. However, these studies were found inadequate in many respects, and their validity was questioned. New studies have been conducted since the second half of the twentieth century.

Results from family, twin, and adoption studies have made significant contributions to our understanding of schizophrenia. As a result of these studies, it was shown that the risk of schizophrenia increases as the degree of kinship gets closer and decreases as the degree of kinship gets farther away. Data obtained from twin studies indicate that schizophrenia is not only a genetically inherited disorder, but environmental factors also play a role in the development of the disease. Adoption studies have found that the risk of the disease is higher in adoptees whose biological parents have a history of schizophrenia.

In later periods, genetic studies were carried out along with technological developments. The results of genome-wide association studies, copy number variant studies, sequencing studies, and epigenetic studies have significantly contributed to our understanding of the molecular genetic aetiology of schizophrenia. However, none of these studies could reveal a specific genetic abnormality or disturbance for schizophrenia. The results were generally interpreted as suggesting that many genetic abnormalities contribute to the development of schizophrenia through additive influence and dynamic interaction.

During this process, many researchers tried to identify environmental factors that contribute to the development of schizophrenia and conducted studies in this field. Repeated studies have consistently shown that factors such as infections during the intrauterine period, immune system activation, nutritional disorders, advanced paternal age, cannabis use at an early age, and immigration are risk factors for the development of schizophrenia. Immune system dysfunctions show a remarkable feature at this point. Genetic studies show that the MHC Class 1 gene region plays a role in the development of schizophrenia. Likewise, the demonstration that immune dysfunctions in the mother during pregnancy increase the risk of developing schizophrenia for the child in the future. This situation constitutes an excellent example of gene-environment interaction.

In post-mortem neuropathological examinations, thinning of the cortical grey matter was detected in patients with schizophrenia. The first of the most consistent findings is the widespread reduction in neuronal size with accompanying reduced dendritic and axonal branching. Another important finding is that a decrease in the number of neurons was detected, especially in regions such as the prefrontal cortex, temporal cortex, hippocampus, and insula. Synaptic changes observed in schizophrenia are generally decreasing, and this is especially seen in glutamatergic neurons. Additionally, an increase in white matter density was detected in the PFC, and it was stated that this was due to the inhibition of neuronal migration during development. Data regarding the anterior cingulate cortex and orbitofrontal cortex are inconsistent. It has been reported that although there is a decrease in total number of neurons in the thalamus and basal ganglia, the neuron density does not change. Another neuropathological finding is the relatively consistent occurrence of ventricular dilatation. In neuropathological studies, pyramidal cell loss was detected in prefrontal and temporal cortices. Additionally, a decrease in GABAergic interneurons was detected in the prefrontal cortex. A decrease in Purkinje cells was also detected in the cerebellum.

Dysfunction of several neurotransmitter systems has been proposed to explain schizophrenia neurochemically. The dopamine hypothesis was first put forward. It has been suggested that psychotic symptoms result from hyperactivity of dopamine D2 receptors or excess dopamine in synapses in mesolimbic dopaminergic pathways. It has been suggested that negative symptoms in schizophrenia are related to the hypoactivity of dopamine D1 receptors in the prefrontal cortex. Although this theory was supported, it was insufficient to explain the pathophysiology of schizophrenia. The glutamate hypothesis, which was put forward later, suggested that GABAergic pathways control dopaminergic pathways originating from the ventral tegmental area. This GABAergic pathway is controlled by glutamate, and in glutamate deficiency, the GABAergic system cannot be stimulated and cannot control the dopaminergic system. In theories based on GABAergic system disorder, it has been suggested that loss of cortical GABAergic neurons disrupts information processing and top-down control processes. Theories based on the serotonin system have been put forward with the understanding that psychotic symptoms seen in Parkinson's disease and Alzheimer's disease are related to serotonin 5HT2A receptor activity. It has been stated that the hyperactivity of 5HT2A receptors has an excitatory effect on glutamatergic neurons, and the increase in dopaminergic neuron activation in the VTA of glutamatergic neurons ultimately leads to an increase in dopaminergic activity in the mesolimbic pathway. In addition, the fact that the activity of second-generation antipsychotics affects both the dopamine and serotonin systems supports this idea. Theories about acetylcholine have generally been associated with nicotinic alpha7 receptor activity located in the hippocampus, and it has been stated that some symptoms of schizophrenia are the result of this receptor dysfunction. In addition to alpha receptors, muscarinic acetylcholine receptors, especially M1, M4, and M5 receptors, also have a role emerging of psychosis. Additionally, some researchers put forward that norepinephrine has a significant role in the development of psychosis and the deterioration of cognitive functions based on HPA axis dysfunction.

Imaging methods have also been used extensively in the aetiology of schizophrenia. In structural neuroimaging studies, dilatation in the brain ventricles and cortical thinning have emerged as the most consistent findings with computed tomography. In MRI studies, thinning was detected in the prefrontal and orbitofrontal cortex. Results regarding the anterior cingulate cortex are inconsistent. Some studies reported that the amount of grey matter increased in the caudate nucleus, while others reported a decrease. It has been observed that there is a decrease in the amount of grey matter in the thalamus. Additionally, thinning was detected in the cerebellar cortex. Diffusion tensor examinations revealed increased white matter density, but organisational disorder exists. These results are interpreted as a supportive finding for neuronal migration defects. In conclusion, this finding supports the idea that schizophrenia is a neurodevelopmental disorder. fMRI studies are the most studied method when functional neuroimaging studies are examined. Accordingly, the most common findings in fMRI studies were a decrease in prefrontal cortex activity, a decrease in temporal cortex activity, and an increase in activity in the mesolimbic regions during psychotic exacerbation. Anterior cingulate cortex, insula and cerebellum activity patterns gave variable results. Functional near-infrared spectroscopy studies are relatively new and have advantages and disadvantages compared to fMRI studies. In fNIRS studies, abnormal activity patterns have been consistently observed in the prefrontal, temporoparietal, and temporal cortex. These findings support neuropsychological theories such as cognitive impairments and theory of mind deficits seen in schizophrenia. Methods such as positron emission tomography and single-photon emission tomography have low practical applicability. These methods are primarily used in determining molecular structures and drug development studies.

EEG is the leading study method in neurophysiological studies. The literature reports P300 gating dysfunction as an endophenotype. Another finding is related to the P50 response. Neuropsychological studies have found impairments in attention, working memory, semantic memory, executive functions, language functions, learning, motor function speed, and changing setup. However, none of these tasks were specific to schizophrenia, and each function was affected to varying degrees.

In the psychological approach to schizophrenia, an attempt has been made to explain especially the delusional thought development processes. In this regard, the theory of mind deficits, self-discrepancy theory, attributional bias, and judgmental bias (jumping to conclusion bias) have emerged. Theory of mind has mainly taken up room in autism studies. Self-discrepancy studies have not yielded consistent results. Attributional bias and reasoning bias theories are still being studied, and they stand out as the two theories that provide the most comprehensive explanations for the development of delusional thoughts.

Authorship

Adnan Kuşman completed the literature search, designed the study, and wrote the protocol and the manuscript. The author has seen and agreed with the manuscript's content and guarantees the references' accuracy.

Conflict of interest

The author declares no conflict of interest.

Author details

Adnan Kuşman
Medical Faculty, Department of Psychiatry, Bahçeşehir University, İstanbul, Turkey

*Address all correspondence to: adnan.kusman@bau.edu.tr

References

[1] Meehl PE. Primary and secondary hypohedonia. Journal of Abnormal Psychology. 2001;**110**:188-193. DOI: 10.1037/0021-843X.110.1.188

[2] Rossi A, De Cataldo S, Di Michele V, Manna V, Ceccoli S, Stratta P, et al. Neurological soft signs in schizophrenia. British Journal of Psychiatry. 1990;**157**:735-739. DOI: 10.1192/bjp.157.5.735

[3] Lowing PA, Mirsky AF, Pereira R. The inheritance of schizophrenia spectrum disorders: A reanalysis of the Danish adoptee study data. American Journal of Psychiatry. 1983;**140**:1167-1171. DOI: 10.1176/ajp.140.9.1167

[4] Reiss D. The family and schizophrenia. The American Journal of Psychiatry. 1976;**133**:181-185. DOI: 10.1176/ajp.133.2.181

[5] Tienari P, Lahti I, Sorri A, Naarala M, Moring J, Wahlberg KE, et al. The Finnish adoptive family study of schizophrenia. Journal of Psychiatric Research. 1987;**21**:437-445. DOI: 10.1016/0022-3956(87)90091-4

[6] Henriksen MG, Nordgaard J, Jansson LB. Genetics of schizophrenia: Overview of methods, findings and limitations. Frontiers in Human Neuroscience. 2017;**11**:250542. DOI: 10.3389/FNHUM.2017.00322/BIBTEX

[7] Sadock J, Sadock A, Ruiz P, Akiskal S, Jeste DV, Krystal JH, et al. Comprehensive Textbook of Psychiatry. 10th ed. Hong-Kong: Wolters Kluwer; 2017

[8] Gottesman II, Laursen TM, Bertelsen A, Mortensen PB. Severe mental disorders in offspring with 2 psychiatrically ill parents. Archives of General Psychiatry. 2010;**67**:252. DOI: 10.1001/archgenpsychiatry.2010.1

[9] Cardno AG, Gottesman II. Twin studies of schizophrenia: From bow-and-arrow concordances to star wars mx and functional genomics. American Journal of Medical Genetics. 2000;**97**:12-17. DOI: 10.1002/(SICI)1096-8628(200021)97:1%3C12::AID-AJMG3%3E3.0.CO;2-U

[10] Hilker R, Helenius D, Fagerlund B, Skytthe A, Christensen K, Werge TM, et al. Heritability of schizophrenia and schizophrenia spectrum based on the Nationwide Danish Twin Register. Biological Psychiatry. 2018;**83**:492-498. DOI: 10.1016/j.biopsych.2017.08.017

[11] Sullivan PF, Kendler KS, Neale MC. Schizophrenia as a complex trait: Evidence from a meta-analysis of twin studies. Archives of General Psychiatry. 2003;**60**:1187-1192. DOI: 10.1001/archpsyc.60.12.1187

[12] Ingraham LJ, Kety SS. Adoption studies of schizophrenia. American Journal of Medical Genetics. 2000;**97**:18-22. DOI: 10.1002/(sici)1096-8628(200021)97:1<18::aid-ajmg4>3.0.co;2-l

[13] McGuffin P, Owen MJ, Farmer AE. Genetic basis of schizophrenia. The Lancet. 1995;**346**:678-682. DOI: 10.1016/S0140-6736(95)92285-7

[14] Blaveri E, Kalsi G, Lawrence J, Quested D, Moorey H, Lamb G, et al. Genetic association studies of schizophrenia using the 8p21-22 genes: Prepronociceptin (PNOC), neuronal nicotinic cholinergic receptor alpha

polypeptide 2 (CNRNA2) and arylamine N-acetyltransferase 1 (NAT1). European Journal of Human Genetics. 2001;**9**:469-472. DOI: 10.1038/sj.ejhg.5200646

[15] Brzustowicz LM, Honer WG, Chow EWC, Little D, Hogan J, Hodgkinson K, et al. Linkage of familial schizophrenia to chromosome 13q32. American Journal of Human Genetics. 1999;**65**:1096-1103. DOI: 10.1086/302579

[16] Faraone SV, Matise T, Svrakic D, Pepple J, Malaspina D, Suarez B, et al. Genome scan of European-American schizophrenia pedigrees: Results of the NIMH genetics initiative and millennium consortium. American Journal of Medical Genetics - Neuropsychiatric Genetics. 1998;**81**:290-295. DOI: 10.1002/(SICI)1096-8628(19980710)81:4<290::AID-AJMG3>3.0.CO;2-Y

[17] Faraone SV, Meyer J, Matise T, Svrakic D, Pepple J, Malaspina D, et al. Suggestive linkage of chromosome 10p to schizophrenia is not due to transmission ratio distortion. American Journal of Medical Genetics. 1999;**88**:607-608. DOI: 10.1002/(sici)1096-8628(19991215)88:6<607::aid-ajmg6>3.0.co;2-q

[18] Levinson DF, Levinson MD, Segurado R, Lewis CM. Genome scan meta-analysis of schizophrenia and bipolar disorder, part I: Methods and power analysis. American Journal of Human Genetics. 2003;**73**:17-33. DOI: 10.1086/376548

[19] Pulver AE, Wolyniec PS, Housman D, Kazazian HH, Antonarakis SE, Nestadt G, et al. The Johns Hopkins University collaborative schizophrenia study: An epidemiologic-genetic approach to test the heterogeneity hypothesis and identify schizophrenia susceptibility genes. Cold Spring Harbor Symposia on Quantitative Biology. 1996;**61**:797-814. DOI: 10.1101/sqb.1996.061.01.079

[20] Shao L, Lu B, Wen Z, Teng S, Wang L, Zhao Y, et al. Disrupted-in-Schizophrenia-1 (DISC1) protein disturbs neural function in multiple disease-risk pathways. Human Molecular Genetics. 2017;**26**:2634-2648. DOI: 10.1093/hmg/ddx147

[21] McAllister AK. Major histocompatibility complex I in brain development and schizophrenia. Biological Psychiatry. 2014;**75**:262-268. DOI: 10.1016/J.BIOPSYCH.2013.10.003

[22] Walters JTR, Rujescu D, Franke B, Giegling I, Vásquez AA, Hargreaves A, et al. The role of the major histocompatibility complex region in cognition and brain structure: A schizophrenia GWAS follow-up. American Journal of Psychiatry. 2013;**170**:877-885. DOI: 10.1176/appi.ajp.2013.12020226

[23] Aberg KA, Liu Y, Bukszár J, McClay JL, Khachane AN, Andreassen OA, et al. A comprehensive family-based replication study of schizophrenia genes. JAMA Psychiatry. 2013;**70**:573-581. DOI: 10.1001/jamapsychiatry.2013.288

[24] Weinberger DR. Epistasis in schizophrenia genetics: What's missing is not heritability. Schizophrenia Research. 2014;**160**:e2-e3. DOI: 10.1016/j.schres.2014.09.063

[25] Schizophrenia Working Group of the Psychiatric Genomics Consortium, Ripke S, Neale BM, Corvin A, Walters JTR, Farh KH, et al. Biological insights from 108 schizophrenia-associated genetic loci. Nature. 2014;**511**:421-427. DOI: 10.1038/nature13595

[26] Rujescu D, Ingason A, Cichon S, Pietiläinen OPH, Barnes MR, Toulopoulou T, et al. Disruption of the neurexin 1 gene is associated with schizophrenia. Human Molecular Genetics. 2009;**18**:988-996. DOI: 10.1093/HMG/DDN351

[27] Rees E, O'Donovan MC, Owen MJ. Genetics of schizophrenia. Current Opinion in Behavioral Sciences. 2015;**2**:8-14. DOI: 10.1016/J.COBEHA.2014.07.001

[28] Rees E, Kendall K, Pardiñas AF, Legge SE, Pocklington A, Escott-Price V, et al. Analysis of intellectual disability copy number variants for association with schizophrenia. JAMA Psychiatry. 2016;**73**:963. DOI: 10.1001/jamapsychiatry.2016.1831

[29] Stefansson H, Meyer-Lindenberg A, Steinberg S, Magnusdottir B, Morgen K, Arnarsdottir S, et al. CNVs conferring risk of autism or schizophrenia affect cognition in controls. Nature. 2014;**505**:361-366. DOI: 10.1038/NATURE12818

[30] Szatkiewicz JP, O'Dushlaine C, Chen G, Chambert K, Moran JL, Neale BM, et al. Copy number variation in schizophrenia in Sweden. Molecular Psychiatry. 2014;**19**:762. DOI: 10.1038/MP.2014.40

[31] Kirov G, Pocklington AJ, Holmans P, Ivanov D, Ikeda M, Ruderfer D, et al. De novo CNV analysis implicates specific abnormalities of postsynaptic signalling complexes in the pathogenesis of schizophrenia. Molecular Psychiatry. 2012;**17**:142-153. DOI: 10.1038/MP.2011.154

[32] Pocklington AJ, Rees E, Walters JTR, Han J, Kavanagh DH, Chambert KD, et al. Novel findings from CNVs implicate inhibitory and excitatory signaling complexes in schizophrenia. Neuron. 2015;**86**:1203-1214. DOI: 10.1016/j.neuron.2015.04.022

[33] Richetto J, Meyer U. Epigenetic modifications in schizophrenia and related disorders: Molecular scars of environmental exposures and source of phenotypic variability. Biological Psychiatry. 2021;**89**:215-226. DOI: 10.1016/J.BIOPSYCH.2020.03.008

[34] Akbarian S. Epigenetic mechanisms in schizophrenia. Dialogues in Clinical Neuroscience. 2014;**16**:405-417. DOI: 10.31887/dcns.2014.16.3/sakbarian

[35] Khavari B, Cairns MJ. Epigenomic dysregulation in schizophrenia: In search of disease etiology and biomarkers. Cells. 2020;**9**:1837. DOI: 10.3390/CELLS9081837

[36] Li M, Xiao L, Chen X. Histone acetylation and methylation underlie oligodendroglial and myelin susceptibility in schizophrenia. Frontiers in Cellular Neuroscience. 2022;**16**:1-7. DOI: 10.3389/FNCEL.2022.823708

[37] Brown AS, Derkits EJ. Prenatal infection and schizophrenia: A review of epidemiologic and translational studies. American Journal of Psychiatry. 2010;**167**:261-280. DOI: 10.1176/APPI.AJP.2009.09030361/ASSET/IMAGES/LARGE/0361TBL6.JPEG

[38] Brown AS, Schaefer CA, Quesenberry CP, Liu L, Babulas VP, Susser ES. Maternal exposure to toxoplasmosis and risk of schizophrenia in adult offspring. American Journal of Psychiatry. 2005;**162**:767-773. DOI: 10.1176/appi.ajp.162.4.767

[39] Buka SL, Tsuang MT, Torrey EF, Klebanoff MA, Wagner RL, Yolken RH. Maternal cytokine levels during pregnancy and adult psychosis. Brain, Behavior, and Immunity.

2001;**15**:411-420. DOI: 10.1006/brbi.2001.0644

[40] Brown AS, Bottiglieri T, Schaefer CA, Quesenberry CP, Liu L, Bresnahan M, et al. Elevated prenatal homocysteine levels as a risk factor for schizophrenia. Archives of General Psychiatry. 2007;**64**:31-39. DOI: 10.1001/archpsyc.64.1.31

[41] Bao Y, Ibram G, Blaner WS, Quesenberry CP, Shen L, McKeague IW, et al. Low maternal retinol as a risk factor for schizophrenia in adult offspring. Schizophrenia Research. 2012;**137**:159-165. DOI: 10.1016/j.schres.2012.02.004

[42] HarperKN, HibbelnJR, DeckelbaumR, Quesenberry CP, Schaefer CA, Brown AS. Maternal serum docosahexaenoic acid and schizophrenia spectrum disorders in adult offspring. Schizophrenia Research. 2011;**128**:30-36. DOI: 10.1016/j.schres.2011.01.009

[43] Picker JD, Coyle JT. Do maternal folate and homocysteine levels play a role in neurodevelopmental processes that increase risk for schizophrenia? Harvard Review of Psychiatry. 2005;**13**:197-205. DOI: 10.1080/10673220500243372

[44] Wu C, Wei J, Tian D, Feng Y, Miller RH, Wang Y. Molecular probes for imaging myelinated white matter in CNS. Journal of Medicinal Chemistry. 2008;**51**:6682-6688. DOI: 10.1021/jm8003637

[45] Malaspina D, Harlap S, Fennig S, Heiman D, Nahon D, Feldman D, et al. Advancing paternal age and the risk of schizophrenia. Archives of General Psychiatry. 2001;**58**:361-367. DOI: 10.1001/archpsyc.58.4.361

[46] Brown AS, Schaefer CA, Wyatt RJ, Begg MD, Goetz R, Bresnahan MA, et al. Paternal age and risk of schizophrenia in adult offspring. American Journal of Psychiatry. 2002;**159**:1528-1533. DOI: 10.1176/appi.ajp.159.9.1528

[47] Dalman C, Allebeck P. Paternal age and schizophrenia: Further support for an association. American Journal of Psychiatry. 2002;**159**:1591-1592. DOI: 10.1176/appi.ajp.159.9.1591

[48] Tsuchiya KJ, Takagai S, Kawai M, Matsumoto H, Nakamura K, Minabe Y, et al. Advanced paternal age associated with an elevated risk for schizophrenia in offspring in a Japanese population. Schizophrenia Research. 2005;**76**:337-342. DOI: 10.1016/j.schres.2005.03.004

[49] Zammit S, Allebeck P, Andreasson S, Lundberg I, Lewis G. Self reported cannabis use as a risk factor for schizophrenia in Swedish conscripts of 1969: Historical cohort study. British Medical Journal. 2002;**325**:1199-1201. DOI: 10.1136/bmj.325.7374.1199

[50] Epstein KA, Kumra S. Executive attention impairment in adolescents with schizophrenia who have used cannabis. Schizophrenia Research. 2014;**157**:48-54. DOI: 10.1016/j.schres.2014.04.035

[51] Cantor-Graae E, Selten JP. Schizophrenia and migration: A meta-analysis and review. American Journal of Psychiatry. 2005;**162**:12-24. DOI: 10.1176/appi.ajp.162.1.12

[52] Selten JP, Cantor-Graae E, Kahn RS. Migration and schizophrenia. Current Opinion in Psychiatry. 2007;**20**:111-115. DOI: 10.1097/YCO.0b013e328017f68e

[53] Dohrenwend BP, Levav I, Shrout PE, Schwartz S, Naveh G, Link BG, et al. Socioeconomic status and psychiatric disorders: The causation-selection issue. Science. 1979;**1992**(255):946-952. DOI: 10.1126/science.1546291

[54] Hare EH, Price JS, Slater E. Parenthal social class in psychiatric patients. The British Journal of Psychiatry. 1972;**121**:515-534. DOI: 10.1192/bjp.121.5.515

[55] Mäkikyrö T, Isohanni M, Moring J, Oja H, Hakko H, Jones P, et al. Is a child's risk of early onset schizophrenia increased in the highest social class? Schizophrenia Research. 1997;**23**:245-252. DOI: 10.1016/s0920-9964(96)00119-3

[56] Mulvany F, O'Callaghan E, Takei N, Byrne M, Fearon P, Larkin C. Effect of social class at birth on risk and presentation of schizophrenia: Case-control study. British Medical Journal. 2001;**323**:1398-1401. DOI: 10.1136/bmj.323.7326.1398

[57] Timms D. Gender, social mobility and psychiatric diagnoses. Social Science & Medicine. 1998;**46**:1235-1247. DOI: 10.1016/S0277-9536(97)10052-1

[58] Wicks S, Hjern A, Gunnell D, Lewis G, Dalman C. Social adversity in childhood and the risk of developing psychosis: A national cohort study. The American Journal of Psychiatry. 2005;**162**:1652-1657. DOI: 10.1176/APPI.AJP.162.9.1652

[59] Wicks S, Hjern A, Dalman C. Social risk or genetic liability for psychosis? A study of children born in Sweden and reared by adoptive parents. American Journal of Psychiatry. 2010;**167**:1240-1246. DOI: 10.1176/appi.ajp.2010.09010114

[60] Arnsten AFT. Stress signalling pathways that impair prefrontal cortex structure and function. Nature Reviews. Neuroscience. 2009;**10**:410-422. DOI: 10.1038/nrn2648

[61] Brown AS. The environment and susceptibility to schizophrenia. Progress in Neurobiology. 2011;**93**:23-58. DOI: 10.1016/j.pneurobio.2010.09.003

[62] Van Os J, Kenis G, Rutten BPF. The environment and schizophrenia. Nature. 2010;**468**:203-212. DOI: 10.1038/nature09563

[63] Glaser J-P, van Os J, Portegijs PJM, Myin-Germeys I. Childhood trauma and emotional reactivity to daily life stress in adult frequent attenders of general practitioners. Journal of Psychosomatic Research. 2006;**61**:229-236. DOI: 10.1016/j.jpsychores.2006.04.014

[64] Harrison PJ. Neuropathology of schizophrenia. Psychiatry. 2008;**7**:421-424. DOI: 10.1016/j.mppsy.2008.07.013

[65] Garey L. When cortical development goes wrong: Schizophrenia as a neurodevelopmental disease of microcircuits. Journal of Anatomy. 2010;**217**:324. DOI: 10.1111/J.1469-7580.2010.01231.X

[66] Roeske MJ, Konradi C, Heckers S, Lewis AS. Hippocampal volume and hippocampal neuron density, number and size in schizophrenia: A systematic review and meta-analysis of postmortem studies. Molecular Psychiatry. 2020;**26**:3524-3535. DOI: 10.1038/s41380-020-0853-y

[67] Selemon LD, Goldman-Rakic PS. The reduced neuropil hypothesis: A circuit based model of schizophrenia. Biological Psychiatry. 1999;**45**:17-25. DOI: 10.1016/S0006-3223(98)00281-9

[68] Garey LJ, Ong WY, Patel TS, Kanani M, Davis A, Mortimer AM, et al. Reduced dendritic spine density on cerebral cortical pyramidal neurons in schizophrenia. Journal of Neurology, Neurosurgery, and Psychiatry. 1998;**65**:446-453. DOI: 10.1136/jnnp.65.4.446

[69] Glantz LA, Lewis DA. Decreased dendritic spine density on prefrontal cortical pyramidal neurons in schizophrenia. Archives of General Psychiatry. 2000;**57**:65-73. DOI: 10.1001/ARCHPSYC.57.1.65

[70] Rajkowska G, Selemon LD, Goldman-Rakic PS. Neuronal and glial somal size in the prefrontal cortex: A postmortem morphometric study of schizophrenia and Huntington disease. Archives of General Psychiatry. 1998;**55**:215-224. DOI: 10.1001/archpsyc.55.3.215

[71] Beasley CL, Reynolds GP. Parvalbumin-immunoreactive neurons are reduced in the prefrontal cortex of schizophrenics. Schizophrenia Research. 1997;**24**:349-355. DOI: 10.1016/S0920-9964(96)00122-3

[72] Eastwood SL, Harrison PJ. Interstitial white matter neuron density in the dorsolateral prefrontal cortex and parahippocampal gyrus in schizophrenia. Schizophrenia Research. 2005;**79**:181-188. DOI: 10.1016/j.schres.2005.07.001

[73] Joshi D, Fung SJ, Rothwell A, Weickert CS. Higher gamma-aminobutyric acid neuron density in the white matter of orbital frontal cortex in schizophrenia. Biological Psychiatry. 2012;**72**:725-733. DOI: 10.1016/j.biopsych.2012.06.021

[74] Beasley CL, Chana G, Honavar M, Landau S, Everall IP, Cotter D. Evidence for altered neuronal organisation within the planum temporale in major psychiatric disorders. Schizophrenia Research. 2005;**73**:69-78. DOI: 10.1016/j.schres.2004.08.011

[75] Sweet RA, Pierri JN, Auh S, Sampson AR, Lewis DA. Reduced pyramidal cell somal volume in auditory association cortex of subjects with schizophrenia. Neuropsychopharmacology. 2003;**28**:599-609. DOI: 10.1038/sj.npp.1300120

[76] Pakkenberg B. Pronounced reduction of total neuron number in mediodorsal thalamic nucleus and nucleus accumbens in schizophrenics. Archives of General Psychiatry. 1990;**47**:1023-1028. DOI: 10.1001/archpsyc.1990.01810230039007

[77] Popken GJ, Bunney WE, Potkin SG, Jones EG. Subnucleus-specific loss of neurons in medial thalamus of schizophrenics. Proceedings of the National Academy of Sciences of the United States of America. 2000;**97**:9276-9280. DOI: 10.1073/pnas.150243397

[78] Young KA, Manaye KF, Liang CL, Hicks PB, German DC. Reduced number of mediodorsal and anterior thalamic neurons in schizophrenia. Biological Psychiatry. 2000;**47**:944-953. DOI: 10.1016/S0006-3223(00)00826-X

[79] Kreczmanski P, Heinsen H, Mantua V, Woltersdorf F, Masson T, Ulfig N, et al. Volume, neuron density and total neuron number in five subcortical regions in schizophrenia. Brain. 2007;**130**:678-692. DOI: 10.1093/brain/awl386

[80] Eastwood SL, Harrison PJ. Decreased synaptophysin in the medial temporal lobe in schizophrenia demonstrated using immunoautoradiography. Neuroscience. 1995;**69**:339-343. DOI: 10.1016/0306-4522(95)00324-C

[81] Perrone-Bizzozero NI, Sower AC, Bird ED, Benowitz LI, Ivins KJ, Neve RL. Levels of the growth-associated protein GAP-43 are selectively increased in association cortices in schizophrenia. Proceedings of the National Academy of Sciences of the United States of America. 1996;**93**:14182-14187. DOI: 10.1073/pnas.93.24.14182

[82] Honer WG, Falkai P, Bayer TA, Xie J, Hu L, Li H-Y, et al. Abnormalities of SNARE mechanism proteins in anterior frontal cortex in severe mental illness. Cerebral Cortex. 2002;**12**:349-356. DOI: 10.1093/cercor/12.4.349

[83] Honer WG, Young CE. Presynaptic proteins and schizophrenia. International Review of Neurobiology. 2004;**59**:175-199. DOI: 10.1016/S0074-7742(04)59007-4

[84] Wang AY, Lohmann KM, Yang CK, Zimmerman EI, Pantazopoulos H, Herring N, et al. Bipolar disorder type 1 and schizophrenia are accompanied by decreased density of parvalbumin- and somatostatin-positive interneurons in the parahippocampal region. Acta Neuropathologica. 2011;**122**:615-626. DOI: 10.1007/s00401-011-0881-4

[85] Zhang ZJ, Reynolds GP. A selective decrease in the relative density of parvalbumin-immunoreactive neurons in the hippocampus in schizophrenia. Schizophrenia Research. 2002;**55**:1-10. DOI: 10.1016/S0920-9964(01)00188-8

[86] Beneyto M, Lewis DA. Insights into the neurodevelopmental origin of schizophrenia from postmortem studies of prefrontal cortical circuitry. International Journal of Developmental Neuroscience. 2011;**29**:295-304. DOI: 10.1016/j.ijdevneu.2010.08.003

[87] Gonzalez-Burgos G, Hashimoto T, Lewis DA. Alterations of cortical GABA neurons and network oscillations in schizophrenia. Current Psychiatry Reports. 2010;**12**:335-344. DOI: 10.1007/s11920-010-0124-8

[88] Tse MT, Piantadosi PT, Floresco SB. Prefrontal cortical gamma-aminobutyric acid transmission and cognitive function: Drawing links to schizophrenia from preclinical research. Biological Psychiatry. 2015;**77**:929-939. DOI: 10.1016/J.BIOPSYCH.2014.09.007

[89] Steiner J, Bielau H, Brisch R, Danos P, Ullrich O, Mawrin C, et al. Immunological aspects in the neurobiology of suicide: Elevated microglial density in schizophrenia and depression is associated with suicide. Journal of Psychiatric Research. 2008;**42**:151-157. DOI: 10.1016/J.JPSYCHIRES.2006.10.013

[90] Yoo SY, Yeon S, Choi C-H, Kang D-H, Lee J-M, Shin NY, et al. Proton magnetic resonance spectroscopy in subjects with high genetic risk of schizophrenia: Investigation of anterior cingulate, dorsolateral prefrontal cortex and thalamus. Schizophrenia Research. 2009;**111**:86-93. DOI: 10.1016/j.schres.2009.03.036

[91] Kalayci D, Ozdel O, Prof A, Sozeri-Varma G. Medial prefrontal cortex neurochemical metabolites in schizophrenia and schizoaffective disorder: A proton magnetic resonance spectroscopy study. Bulletin of Clinical Psychopharmacology. 2013;**23**:215-223. DOI: 10.5455/bcp.20130713094216

[92] Başoğlu C, Çetin M, Ömer Ö, Ebrinç S, Başer Ü, Kandilcioğlu H, et al. Comparison of right thalamus and temporal cortex metabolite levels of drug-naive first episode psychotic and chronic schizophrenia in patients. Turk Psikiyatri Dergisi. 2006;**17**:85-91

[93] Howes OD, Kapur S. The dopamine hypothesis of schizophrenia: Version III--The final common pathway. Schizophrenia Bulletin. 2009;**35**:549-562. DOI: 10.1093/schbul/sbp006

[94] Tost H, Alam T, Meyer-Lindenberg A. Dopamine and psychosis: Theory, pathomechanisms and intermediate phenotypes. Neuroscience

and Biobehavioral Reviews. 2010;**34**:689. DOI: 10.1016/J.NEUBIOREV.2009.06.005

[95] Lewis DA, Hashimoto T, Volk DW. Cortical inhibitory neurons and schizophrenia. Nature Reviews. Neuroscience. 2005;**6**:312-324. DOI: 10.1038/nrn1648

[96] Hu W, Macdonald ML, Elswick DE, Sweet RA. The glutamate hypothesis of schizophrenia: Evidence from human brain tissue studies. Annals of the New York Academy of Sciences. 2015;**1338**:38-57. DOI: 10.1111/NYAS.12547

[97] de Jonge JC, Vinkers CH, Hulshoff Pol HE, Marsman A. GABAergic mechanisms in schizophrenia: Linking postmortem and in vivo studies. Frontiers in Psychiatry. 2017;**8**:118. DOI: 10.3389/FPSYT.2017.00118

[98] Radhu N, Garcia Dominguez L, Farzan F, Richter MA, Semeralul MO, Chen R, et al. Evidence for inhibitory deficits in the prefrontal cortex in schizophrenia. Brain. 2015;**138**:483-497. DOI: 10.1093/brain/awu360

[99] Eggers AE. A serotonin hypothesis of schizophrenia. Medical Hypotheses. 2013;**80**:791-794. DOI: 10.1016/j.mehy.2013.03.013

[100] Mäki-Marttunen V, Andreassen OA, Espeseth T. The role of norepinephrine in the pathophysiology of schizophrenia. Neuroscience and Biobehavioral Reviews. 2020;**118**:298-314. DOI: 10.1016/J.NEUBIOREV.2020.07.038

[101] Maletic V, Eramo A, Gwin K, Offord SJ, Duffy RA. The role of norepinephrine and its α-adrenergic receptors in the pathophysiology and treatment of major depressive disorder and schizophrenia: A systematic review. Frontiers in Psychiatry. 2017;**8**:249925. DOI: 10.3389/FPSYT.2017.00042/BIBTEX

[102] Köhler S, Wagner G, Bär KJ. Activation of brainstem and midbrain nuclei during cognitive control in medicated patients with schizophrenia. Human Brain Mapping. 2019;**40**:202. DOI: 10.1002/HBM.24365

[103] Manzella F, Maloney SE, Taylor GT. Smoking in schizophrenic patients: A critique of the self-medication hypothesis. World Journal of Psychiatry. 2015;**5**:35-46. DOI: 10.5498/wjp.v5.i1.35

[104] Scarr E, Gibbons AS, Neo J, Udawela M, Dean B. Cholinergic connectivity: It's implications for psychiatric disorders. Frontiers in Cellular Neuroscience. 2013;7:43748. DOI: 10.3389/FNCEL.2013.00055/BIBTEX

[105] Freedman R, Adams CE, Leonard S. The α7-nicotinic acetylcholine receptor and the pathology of hippocampal interneurons in schizophrenia. Journal of Chemical Neuroanatomy. 2000;**20**:299-306. DOI: 10.1016/S0891-0618(00)00109-5

[106] Young JW, Geyer MA. Evaluating the role of the alpha-7 nicotinic acetylcholine receptor in the pathophysiology and treatment of schizophrenia. Biochemical Pharmacology. 2013;**86**:1122-1132. DOI: 10.1016/j.bcp.2013.06.031

[107] Foster DJ, Jones CK, Conn PJ. Emerging approaches for treatment of schizophrenia: Modulation of cholinergic signaling. Discovery Medicine. 2012;**14**:413

[108] Malla AK, Mittal C, Lee M, Scholten DJ, Assis L, Norman RMG. Computed tomography of the brain morphology of patients with

first-episode schizophrenic psychosis. Journal of Psychiatry and Neuroscience. 2002;**27**:350

[109] Dabiri M, Dehghani Firouzabadi F, Yang K, Barker PB, Lee RR, Yousem DM. Neuroimaging in schizophrenia: A review article. Frontiers in Neuroscience. 2022;**16**:1-22. DOI: 10.3389/fnins.2022.1042814

[110] Sadeghi D, Shoeibi A, Ghassemi N, Moridian P, Khadem A, Alizadehsani R, et al. An overview of artificial intelligence techniques for diagnosis of schizophrenia based on magnetic resonance imaging modalities: Methods, challenges, and future works. Computers in Biology and Medicine. 2022;**146**. DOI: 10.1016/J.COMPBIOMED.2022.105554

[111] Nestor PG, O'Donnell BF, McCarley RW, Niznikiewicz M, Barnard J, Shen ZJ, et al. A new statistical method for testing hypotheses of neuropsychological/MRI relationships in schizophrenia: Partial least squares analysis. Schizophrenia Research. 2002;**53**:57-66. DOI: 10.1016/S0920-9964(00)00171-7

[112] Fuentes-Claramonte P, Ramiro N, Torres L, Argila-Plaza I, Salgado-Pineda P, Soler-Vidal J, et al. Negative schizophrenic symptoms as prefrontal cortex dysfunction: Examination using a task measuring goal neglect. NeuroImage: Clinical. 2022;**35**:103119. DOI: 10.1016/J.NICL.2022.103119

[113] Rajarethinam R, DeQuardo JR, Miedler J, Arndt S, Kirbat RA, Brunberg J, et al. Hippocampus and amygdala in schizophrenia: Assessment of the relationship of neuroanatomy to psychopathology. Psychiatry Research: Neuroimaging. 2001;**108**:79-87. DOI: 10.1016/S0925-4927(01)00120-2

[114] Barta PE, Pearlson GD, Powers RE, Richards SS, Tune LE. Auditory hallucinations and smaller superior temporal gyral volume in schizophrenia. The American Journal of Psychiatry. 1990;**147**:1457-1462. DOI: 10.1176/AJP.147.11.1457

[115] Radua J, Vieta E, Shinohara R, Kochunov P, Quidé Y, Green MJ, et al. Increased power by harmonizing structural MRI site differences with the ComBat batch adjustment method in ENIGMA. NeuroImage. 2020;**218**. DOI: 10.1016/J.NEUROIMAGE.2020.116956

[116] McCarley RW, Wible CG, Frumin M, Hirayasu Y, Levitt JJ, Fischer IA, et al. MRI anatomy of schizophrenia. Biological Psychiatry. 1999;**45**:1099. DOI: 10.1016/S0006-3223(99)00018-9

[117] Ellison-Wright I, Glahn DC, Laird AR, Thelen SM, Bullmore E. The anatomy of first-episode and chronic schizophrenia: An anatomical likelihood estimation meta-analysis. American Journal of Psychiatry. 2008;**165**:1015-1023. DOI: 10.1176/appi.ajp.2008.07101562

[118] Fornito A, Yücel M, Patti J, Wood SJ, Pantelis C. Mapping grey matter reductions in schizophrenia: An anatomical likelihood estimation analysis of voxel-based morphometry studies. Schizophrenia Research. 2009;**108**:104-113. DOI: 10.1016/j.schres.2008.12.011

[119] Kasai K, McCarley RW, Salisbury DF, Onitsuka T, Demeo S, Yurgelun-Todd D, et al. Cavum septi pellucidi in first-episode schizophrenia and first-episode affective psychosis: An MRI study. Schizophrenia Research. 2004;**71**:65. DOI: 10.1016/J.SCHRES.2003.12.010

[120] Lubman DI, Velakoulis D, McGorry PD, Smith DJ, Brewer W,

Stuart G, et al. Incidental radiological findings on brain magnetic resonance imaging in first-episode psychosis and chronic schizophrenia. Acta Psychiatrica Scandinavica. 2002;**106**:331-336. DOI: 10.1034/J.1600-0447.2002.02217.X

[121] Buchsbaum MS, Buchsbaum BR, Hazlett EA, Haznedar MM, Newmark R, Tang CY, et al. Relative glucose metabolic rate higher in white matter in patients with schizophrenia. The American Journal of Psychiatry. 2007;**164**:1072-1081. DOI: 10.1176/AJP.2007.164.7.1072

[122] Whitehurst TS, Osugo M, Townsend L, Shatalina E, Vava R, Onwordi EC, et al. Proton magnetic resonance spectroscopy of N-acetyl aspartate in chronic schizophrenia, first episode of psychosis and high-risk of psychosis: A systematic review and meta-analysis. Neuroscience and Biobehavioral Reviews. 2020;**119**:255-267. DOI: 10.1016/J.NEUBIOREV.2020.10.001

[123] Parellada E, Catafau AM, Bernardo M, Lomeña F, Catarineu S, González-Monclús E. The resting and activation issue of hypofrontality: A single photon emission computed tomography study in neuroleptic-naive and neuroleptic-free schizophrenic female patients. Biological Psychiatry. 1998;**44**:787-790. DOI: 10.1016/S0006-3223(98)00057-2

[124] Erritzoe D, Talbot P, Frankle WG, Abi-Dargham A. Positron emission tomography and single photon emission CT molecular imaging in schizophrenia. Neuroimaging Clinics of North America. 2003;**13**:817-832. DOI: 10.1016/S1052-5149(03)00089-3

[125] Woolley J, McGuire P. Neuroimaging in schizophrenia: What does it tell the clinician? Advances in Psychiatric Treatment. 2005;**11**:195-202. DOI: 10.1192/APT.11.3.195

[126] Kapur S, Seeman P. Does fast dissociation from the dopamine d(2) receptor explain the action of atypical antipsychotics?: A new hypothesis. The American Journal of Psychiatry. 2001;**158**:360-369. DOI: 10.1176/APPI.AJP.158.3.360

[127] Abi-Dargham A, Laruelle M. Mechanisms of action of second generation antipsychotic drugs in schizophrenia: Insights from brain imaging studies. European Psychiatry. 2005;**20**:15-27. DOI: 10.1016/J.EURPSY.2004.11.003

[128] Zipursky RB, Meyer JH, Verhoeff NP. PET and SPECT imaging in psychiatric disorders. Canadian Journal of Psychiatry. 2007;**52**:146-157. DOI: 10.1177/070674370705200303

[129] Picó-Pérez M, Vieira R, Fernández-Rodríguez M, De Barros MAP, Radua J, Morgado P. Multimodal meta-analysis of structural gray matter, neurocognitive and social cognitive fMRI findings in schizophrenia patients. Psychological Medicine. 2022;**52**:614-624. DOI: 10.1017/S0033291721005523

[130] Pinkham A, Loughead J, Ruparel K, Wu WC, Overton E, Gur R, et al. Resting quantitative cerebral blood flow in schizophrenia measured by pulsed arterial spin labeling perfusion MRI. Psychiatry Research. 2011;**194**:64-72. DOI: 10.1016/J.PSCYCHRESNS.2011.06.013

[131] Walther S, Federspiel A, Horn H, Razavi N, Wiest R, Dierks T, et al. Resting state cerebral blood flow and objective motor activity reveal basal ganglia dysfunction in schizophrenia. Psychiatry Research. 2011;**192**:117-124. DOI: 10.1016/J.PSCYCHRESNS.2010.12.002

[132] Kindler J, Jann K, Homan P, Hauf M, Walther S, Strik W, et al. Static and

dynamic characteristics of cerebral blood flow during the resting state in schizophrenia. Schizophrenia Bulletin. 2015;**41**:163-170. DOI: 10.1093/SCHBUL/SBT180

[133] Scheef L, Manka C, Daamen M, Kühn KU, Maier W, Schild HH, et al. Resting-state perfusion in nonmedicated schizophrenic patients: A continuous arterial spin-labeling 3.0-T MR study. Radiology. 2010;**256**:253-260. DOI: 10.1148/RADIOL.10091224

[134] Zhu J, Zhuo C, Qin W, Xu Y, Xu L, Liu X, et al. Altered resting-state cerebral blood flow and its connectivity in schizophrenia. Journal of Psychiatric Research. 2015;**63**:28-35. DOI: 10.1016/j.jpsychires.2015.03.002

[135] Liu J, Qiu M, Constable RT, Wexler BE. Does baseline cerebral blood flow affect task-related blood oxygenation level dependent response in schizophrenia? Schizophrenia Research. 2012;**140**:143-148. DOI: 10.1016/J.SCHRES.2012.06.028

[136] Raichle ME, MacLeod AM, Snyder AZ, Powers WJ, Gusnard DA, Shulman GL. A default mode of brain function. Proceedings of the National Academy of Sciences of the United States of America. 2001;**98**:676-682. DOI: 10.1073/PNAS.98.2.676

[137] Fox MD, Snyder AZ, Vincent JL, Corbetta M, Van Essen DC, Raichle ME. The human brain is intrinsically organized into dynamic, anticorrelated functional networks. Proceedings of the National Academy of Sciences of the United States of America. 2005;**102**:9673-9678. DOI: 10.1073/PNAS.0504136102

[138] Seeley WW, Menon V, Schatzberg AF, Keller J, Glover GH, Kenna H, et al. Dissociable intrinsic connectivity networks for salience processing and executive control. The Journal of Neuroscience. 2007;**27**:2349-2356. DOI: 10.1523/JNEUROSCI.5587-06.2007

[139] Bressler SL, Menon V. Large-scale brain networks in cognition: Emerging methods and principles. Trends in Cognitive Sciences. 2010;**14**:277-290. DOI: 10.1016/J.TICS.2010.04.004

[140] Cabral J, Kringelbach ML, Deco G. Exploring the network dynamics underlying brain activity during rest. Progress in Neurobiology. 2014;**114**:102-131. DOI: 10.1016/J.PNEUROBIO.2013.12.005

[141] Fan F, Tan S, Huang J, Chen S, Fan H, Wang Z, et al. Functional disconnection between subsystems of the default mode network in schizophrenia. Psychological Medicine. 2022;**52**:2270-2280. DOI: 10.1017/S003329172000416X

[142] Woodward ND, Rogers B, Heckers S. Functional resting-state networks are differentially affected in schizophrenia. Schizophrenia Research. 2011;**130**:86-93. DOI: 10.1016/J.SCHRES.2011.03.010

[143] Palaniyappan L, White TP, Liddle PF. The concept of salience network dysfunction in schizophrenia: From neuroimaging observations to therapeutic opportunities. Current Topics in Medicinal Chemistry. 2013;**12**:2324-2338. DOI: 10.2174/156802612805289881

[144] Ramsay IS, Mueller B, Ma Y, Shen C, Sponheim SR. Thalamocortical connectivity and its relationship with symptoms and cognition across the psychosis continuum. Psychological Medicine. 2023;**53**:5582-5591. DOI: 10.1017/S0033291722002793

[145] Kanaan RAA, Kim JS, Kaufmann WE, Pearlson GD, Barker GJ,

McGuire PK. Diffusion tensor imaging in schizophrenia. Biological Psychiatry. 2005;**58**:921-929. DOI: 10.1016/J.BIOPSYCH.2005.05.015

[146] Kubicki M, McCarley R, Westin CF, Park HJ, Maier S, Kikinis R, et al. A review of diffusion tensor imaging studies in schizophrenia. Journal of Psychiatric Research. 2007;**41**:15-30. DOI: 10.1016/J.JPSYCHIRES.2005.05.005

[147] Ho NF, Chong PLH, Lee DR, Chew QH, Chen G, Sim K. The amygdala in schizophrenia and bipolar disorder: A synthesis of structural MRI, diffusion tensor imaging, and resting-state functional connectivity findings. Harvard Review of Psychiatry. 2019;**27**:150-164. DOI: 10.1097/HRP.0000000000000207

[148] Luttenbacher I, Phillips A, Kazemi R, Hadipour AL, Sanghvi I, Martinez J, et al. Transdiagnostic role of glutamate and white matter damage in neuropsychiatric disorders: A systematic review. Journal of Psychiatric Research. 2022;**147**:324-348. DOI: 10.1016/J.JPSYCHIRES.2021.12.042

[149] Steen RG, Hamer RM, Lieberman JA. Measurement of brain metabolites by 1H magnetic resonance spectroscopy in patients with schizophrenia: A systematic review and meta-analysis. Neuropsychopharmacology. 2005;**30**:1949-1962. DOI: 10.1038/sj.npp.1300850

[150] Abbott C, Bustillo J. What have we learned from proton magnetic resonance spectroscopy about schizophrenia? A critical update. Current Opinion in Psychiatry. 2006;**19**:135-139. DOI: 10.1097/01.YCO.0000214337.29378.CD

[151] Wang M, Barker PB, Cascella NG, Coughlin JM, Nestadt G, Nucifora FC, et al. Longitudinal changes in brain metabolites in healthy controls and patients with first episode psychosis: A 7-Tesla MRS study. Molecular Psychiatry. 2023;**28**:2018-2029. DOI: 10.1038/s41380-023-01969-5

[152] Smucny J, Carter CS, Maddock RJ. Magnetic resonance spectroscopic evidence of increased choline in the dorsolateral prefrontal and visual cortices in recent onset schizophrenia. Neuroscience Letters. 2022;**770**. DOI: 10.1016/J.NEULET.2021.136410

[153] Merritt K, McGuire PK, Egerton A, Aleman A, Block W, Bloemen OJN, et al. Association of age, antipsychotic medication, and symptom severity in schizophrenia with proton magnetic resonance spectroscopy brain glutamate level: A mega-analysis of individual participant-level data. JAMA Psychiatry. 2021;**78**:667-681. DOI: 10.1001/JAMAPSYCHIATRY.2021.0380

[154] Hämäläinen M, Huang M, Bowyer SM. Magnetoencephalography signal processing, forward modeling, magnetoencephalography inverse source imaging, and coherence analysis. Neuroimaging Clinics of North America. 2020;**30**:125-143. DOI: 10.1016/J.NIC.2020.02.001

[155] Zeev-Wolf M, Levy J, Jahshan C, Peled A, Levkovitz Y, Grinshpoon A, et al. MEG resting-state oscillations and their relationship to clinical symptoms in schizophrenia. Neuroimage Clinical. 2018;**20**:753-761. DOI: 10.1016/j.nicl.2018.09.007

[156] Franceschini MA, Boas DA. Noninvasive measurement of neuronal activity with near-infrared optical imaging. NeuroImage. 2004;**21**:372-386. DOI: 10.1016/j.neuroimage.2003.09.040

[157] Ehlis A-C, Schneider S, Dresler T, Fallgatter AJ. Application of functional near-infrared spectroscopy in psychiatry. NeuroImage. 2014;**85**(Pt 1):478-488. DOI: 10.1016/j.neuroimage.2013.03.067

[158] Hoshi Y. Functional near-infrared spectroscopy: Potential and limitations in neuroimaging studies. International Review of Neurobiology. 2005;**66**:237-266. DOI: 10.1016/S0074-7742(05)66008-4

[159] Bell BB, Abel LA, Li W, Christian JC, Yee RD. Concordance of smooth pursuit and saccadic measures in normal monozygotic twin pairs. Biological Psychiatry. 1994;**36**:522-526. DOI: 10.1016/0006-3223(94)90616-5

[160] Keefe RSE, Siever LJ, Mohs RC, Peterson AE, Mahon TR, Bergman RL, et al. Eye tracking, schizophrenic symptoms, and schizotypal personality disorder. European Archives of Psychiatry and Neurological Sciences. 1989;**239**:39-42. DOI: 10.1007/BF01739742

[161] Onitsuka T, Oribe N, Nakamura I, Kanba S. Review of neurophysiological findings in patients with schizophrenia. Psychiatry and Clinical Neurosciences. 2013;**67**:461-470. DOI: 10.1111/pcn.12090

[162] Mathalon DH, Ford JM, Pfefferbaum A. Trait and state aspects of p300 amplitude reduction in schizophrenia: A retrospective longitudinal study. Biological Psychiatry. 2000;**47**:434-449. DOI: 10.1016/S0006-3223(99)00277-2

[163] Turetsky BI, Dress EM, Braff DL, Calkins ME, Green MF, Greenwood TA, et al. The utility of P300 as a schizophrenia endophenotype and predictive biomarker: Clinical and socio-demographic modulators in COGS-2. Schizophrenia Research. 2015;**163**:53-62. DOI: 10.1016/j.schres.2014.09.024

[164] Martín-Loeches M, Molina V, Muñoz F, Hinojosa JA, Reig S, Desco M, et al. P300 amplitude as a possible correlate of frontal degeneration in schizophrenia. Schizophrenia Research. 2001;**49**:121-128. DOI: 10.1016/S0920-9964(00)00125-0

[165] O'Donnell BF, Faux SF, McCarley RW, Kimble MO, Salisbury DF, Nestor PG, et al. Increased rate of P300 latency prolongation with age in schizophrenia: Electrophysiological evidence for a neurodegenerative process. Archives of General Psychiatry. 1995;**52**:544-549. DOI: 10.1001/ARCHPSYC.1995.03950190026004

[166] Dutt A, Ganguly T, Shaikh M, Walshe M, Schulze K, Marshall N, et al. Association between hippocampal volume and P300 event related potential in psychosis: Support for the Kraepelinian divide. NeuroImage. 2012;**59**:997-1003. DOI: 10.1016/J.NEUROIMAGE.2011.08.067

[167] Hamilton HK, Mathalon DH, Ford JM. P300 in schizophrenia: Then and now. Biological Psychology. 2024;**187**:108757. DOI: 10.1016/j.biopsycho.2024.108757

[168] Yu M, Tang XW, Wang X, Zhang XR, Bin ZX, Sha WW, et al. Neurocognitive impairments in deficit and non-deficit schizophrenia and their relationships with symptom dimensions and other clinical variables. PLoS One. 2015;**10**(9). DOI: 10.1371/journal.pone.0138357

[169] Zhu Y, Womer FY, Leng H, Chang M, Yin Z, Wei Y, et al. The relationship between cognitive dysfunction and symptom dimensions across schizophrenia, bipolar disorder, and major depressive disorder. Frontiers in Psychiatry. 2019;**10**. DOI: 10.3389/fpsyt.2019.00253

[170] Huang YC, Lee Y, Lee CY, Lin PY, Hung CF, Lee SY, et al. Defining

cognitive and functional profiles in schizophrenia and affective disorders. BMC Psychiatry. 2020;**20**(1). DOI: 10.1186/s12888-020-2459-y

[171] Premack D, Woodruff G. Does the chimpanzee have a theory of mind? Behavioral and Brain Sciences. 1978;**1**:515-526. DOI: 10.1017/S0140525X00076512

[172] Frith CD. Schizophrenia and theory of mind. Psychological Medicine. 2004;**34**:385-389. DOI: 10.1017/S0033291703001326

[173] Baron-Cohen S, Leslie AM, Frith U. Does the autistic child have a "theory of mind"? Cognition. 1985;**21**:37-46. DOI: 10.1016/0010-0277(85)90022-8

[174] Garety PA, Hemsley DR, Wessely S. Reasoning in deluded schizophrenic and paranoid patients. Biases in performance on a probabilistic inference task. The Journal of Nervous and Mental Disease. 1991;**179**:194-201. DOI: 10.1097/00005053-199104000-00003

[175] Garety PA, Freeman D. Cognitive approaches to delusions: A critical review of theories and evidence. The British Journal of Clinical Psychology. 1999;**38**:113-154. DOI: 10.1348/014466599162700

[176] Huq SF, Garety PA, Hemsley DR. Probabilistic judgements in deluded and non-deluded subjects. The Quarterly Journal of Experimental Psychology. A, Human Experimental Psychology. 1988;**40**:801-812. DOI: 10.1080/14640748808402300

[177] Young HF, Bentall RP. Probabilistic reasoning in deluded, depressed and normal subjects: Effects of task difficulty and meaningful versus non-meaningful material. Psychological Medicine. 1997;**27**:455-465. DOI: 10.1017/S0033291796004540

[178] Higgins ET. Self-discrepancy: A theory relating self and affect. Psychological Review. 1987;**94**:319-340. DOI: 10.1037/0033-295X.94.3.319

[179] Bentall RP, Kinderman P, Kaney S. The self, attributional processes and abnormal beliefs: Towards a model of persecutory delusions. Behaviour Research and Therapy. 1994;**32**:331-341. DOI: 10.1016/0005-7967(94)90131-7

[180] Kinderman P, Bentall RP. A new measure of causal locus: The internal, personal, and situational attributions questionnaire. Personality and Individual Differences. 1996;**20**:261-264

[181] Kinderman P, Dunbar R, Bentall RP. Theory-of-mind deficits and causal attributions. British Journal of Psychology. 1998;**89**:191-204. DOI: 10.1111/j.2044-8295.1998.tb02680.x

[182] Pruessner M, Cullen AE, Aas M, Walker EF. The neural diathesis-stress model of schizophrenia revisited: An update on recent findings considering illness stage and neurobiological and methodological complexities. Neuroscience and Biobehavioral Reviews. 2017;**73**:191-218. DOI: 10.1016/j.neubiorev.2016.12.013

[183] Berry A, Cirulli F. Toward a diathesis-stress model of schizophrenia in a neurodevelopmental perspective. In: Handbook of Behavioral Neuroscience, Vol. 23. San Diego, CA, US: Elsevier B.V.; 2016. pp. 209-224. DOI: 10.1016/B978-0-12-800981-9.00013-4

[184] Corcoran C, Walker E, Huot R, Mittal V, Tessner K, Kestler L, et al. The stress cascade and schizophrenia: Etiology and onset. Schizophrenia Bulletin.

2003;**29**:671-692. Available from: https://psycnet.apa.org/doi/10.1093/oxfordjournals.schbul.a007038

[185] Howes OD, McCutcheon R. Inflammation and the neural diathesis-stress hypothesis of schizophrenia: A reconceptualization. Translational Psychiatry. 2017;**7**(2). DOI: 10.1038/TP.2016.278

[186] Walker E, Mittal V, Tessner K. Stress and the hypothalamic pituitary adrenal axis in the developmental course of schizophrenia. Annual Review of Clinical Psychology. 2008;**4**:189-216. DOI: 10.1146/annurev.clinpsy.4.022007.141248

[187] Falkai P, Honer WG, David S, Bogerts B, Majtenyi C, Bayer TA. No evidence for astrogliosis in brains of schizophrenic patients. A post-mortem study. Neuropathology and Applied Neurobiology. 1999;**25**:47-52. DOI: 10.1046/J.1365-2990.1999.00162.X

[188] Iritani S. Neuropathology of schizophrenia: A mini review. Neuropathology. 2007;**27**:604-608. DOI: 10.1111/j.1440-1789.2007.00798.x

[189] Schnieder TP, Dwork AJ. Searching for neuropathology: Gliosis in schizophrenia. Biological Psychiatry. 2011;**69**:134-139. DOI: 10.1016/J.BIOPSYCH.2010.08.027

[190] Dwork AJ, Mancevski B, Rosoklija G. White matter and cognitive function in schizophrenia. The International Journal of Neuropsychopharmacology. 2007;**10**:513-536. DOI: 10.1017/S1461145707007638

[191] Bartzokis G, Lu PH, Amar CP, Raven EP, Detore NR, Altshuler LL, et al. Long acting injection versus oral risperidone in first-episode schizophrenia: Differential impact on white matter myelination trajectory. Schizophrenia Research. 2011;**132**:35-41. DOI: 10.1016/J.SCHRES.2011.06.029

[192] Bartzokis G, Lu PH, Raven EP, Amar CP, Detore NR, Couvrette AJ, et al. Impact on intracortical myelination trajectory of long acting injection versus oral risperidone in first-episode schizophrenia. Schizophrenia Research. 2012;**140**:122-128. DOI: 10.1016/j.schres.2012.06.036

[193] Insel TR. Rethinking schizophrenia. Nature. 2010;**468**:187-193. DOI: 10.1038/nature09552

[194] Black JE, Kodish IM, Grossman AW, Klintsova AY, Orlovskaya D, Vostrikov V, et al. Pathology of layer V pyramidal neurons in the prefrontal cortex of patients with schizophrenia. The American Journal of Psychiatry. 2004;**161**:742-744. DOI: 10.1176/APPI.AJP.161.4.742

[195] Gaur N, Gautam S, Gaur M, Sharma P, Dadheech G, Mishra S. The biochemical womb of schizophrenia: A review. Indian Journal of Clinical Biochemistry. 2008;**23**:307. DOI: 10.1007/S12291-008-0071-X

[196] Flores-Soto ME, Chaparro-Huerta V, Escoto-Delgadillo M, Vazquez-Valls E, González-Castañeda RE, Beas-Zarate C. Structure and function of NMDA-type glutamate receptor subunits. Neurología. 2012;**27**:301-310. DOI: 10.1016/J.NRL.2011.10.014

[197] Lewis DA. Neuroplasticity of excitatory and inhibitory cortical circuits in schizophrenia. Dialogues in Clinical Neuroscience. 2009;**11**:269. DOI: 10.31887/DCNS.2009.11.3/DALEWIS

[198] Boyajyan AS, Chavushyan AS, Zakharyan RV, Mkrtchyan GM. Markers of apoptotic dysfunctions in schizophrenia. Molecular Biology. 2013;**47**:587-591. DOI: 10.1134/S002689331304002X/METRICS

[199] Lawrie SM, Whalley HC, Abukmeil SS, Kestelman JN, Miller P, Best JJK, et al. Temporal lobe volume changes in people at high risk of schizophrenia with psychotic symptoms. The British Journal of Psychiatry. 2002;**181**:138-143. DOI: 10.1017/S0007125000161860

[200] Zhang Z, Zheng F, You Y, Ma Y, Lu T, Yue W, et al. Growth arrest specific gene 7 is associated with schizophrenia and regulates neuronal migration and morphogenesis. Molecular Brain. 2016;**9**(1). DOI: 10.1186/s13041-016-0238-y

[201] Fatemi SH, Folsom TD. The neurodevelopmental hypothesis of schizophrenia, revisited. Schizophrenia Bulletin. 2009;**35**:528-548. DOI: 10.1093/SCHBUL/SBN187

[202] Rapoport JL, Giedd JN, Gogtay N. Neurodevelopmental model of schizophrenia: Update 2012. Molecular Psychiatry. 2012;**17**:1228-1238. DOI: 10.1038/MP.2012.23

[203] McGrath JJ, Féron FP, Burne THJ, Mackay-Sim A, Eyles DW. The neurodevelopmental hypothesis of schizophrenia: A review of recent developments. Annals of Medicine. 2003;**35**:86-93. DOI: 10.1080/07853890310010005

[204] Maynard TM, Sikich L, Lieberman JA, LaMantia AS. Neural development, cell-cell signaling, and the "two-hit" hypothesis of schizophrenia. Schizophrenia Bulletin. 2001;**27**:457-476. DOI: 10.1093/oxfordjournals.schbul.a006887

[205] Guma E, Cupo L, Chakravarty MM. Cannabis, Neurodevelopment, and the "Two-Hit" Hypothesis. Cannabis Use, Neurobiology, Psychology, and Treatment. San Diego, CA, US: Elsevier; 2023. pp. 457-472. DOI: 10.1016/B978-0-323-89862-1.00022-2

[206] Guma E, Cupo L, Ma W, Gallino D, Moquin L, Gratton A, et al. Investigating the "two-hit hypothesis": Effects of prenatal maternal immune activation and adolescent cannabis use on neurodevelopment in mice. Progress in Neuro-Psychopharmacology & Biological Psychiatry. 2023;**120**:110642. DOI: 10.1016/j.pnpbp.2022.110642

[207] Bayer TA, Falkai P, Maier W. Genetic and non-genetic vulnerability factors in schizophrenia: The basis of the "Two hit hypothesis". Journal of Psychiatric Research. 1999;**33**:543-548. DOI: 10.1016/S0022-3956(99)00039-4

[208] Jaaro-Peled H, Hayashi-Takagi A, Seshadri S, Kamiya A, Brandon NJ, Sawa A. Neurodevelopmental mechanisms of schizophrenia: Understanding disturbed postnatal brain maturation through neuregulin-1-ErbB4 and DISC1. Trends in Neurosciences. 2009;**32**:485-495. DOI: 10.1016/J.TINS.2009.05.007

[209] Fan JB, Zhang CS, Gu NF, Li XW, Sun WW, Wang HY, et al. Catechol-O-methyltransferase gene Val/Met functional polymorphism and risk of schizophrenia: A large-scale association study plus meta-analysis. Biological Psychiatry. 2005;**57**:139-144. DOI: 10.1016/J.BIOPSYCH.2004.10.018

[210] Guo X, Tang P, Yang C, Li R. Proline dehydrogenase gene (PRODH) polymorphisms and schizophrenia susceptibility: A meta-analysis. Metabolic Brain Disease. 2018;**33**:89-97. DOI: 10.1007/S11011-017-0128-8/METRICS

[211] Mirnics K, Middleton FA, Stanwood GD, Lewis DA, Levitt P. Disease-specific changes in regulator of G-protein signaling 4 (RGS4) expression in schizophrenia. Molecular Psychiatry. 2001;**6**:293-301. DOI: 10.1038/SJ.MP.4000866

[212] Abdolmaleky HM, Cheng KH, Russo A, Smith CL, Faraone SV, Wilcox M, et al. Hypermethylation of the reelin (RELN) promoter in the brain of schizophrenic patients: A preliminary report. American Journal of Medical Genetics. Part B, Neuropsychiatric Genetics. 2005;**134B**:60-66. DOI: 10.1002/AJMG.B.30140

[213] Impagnatiello F, Guidotti AR, Pesold C, Dwivedi Y, Caruncho H, Pisu MG, et al. A decrease of reelin expression as a putative vulnerability factor in schizophrenia. Proceedings of the National Academy of Sciences of the United States of America. 1998;**95**:15718-15723. DOI: 10.1073/PNAS.95.26.15718

[214] Gómez-Climent MÁ, Guirado R, Castillo-Gómez E, Varea E, Gutierrez-Mecinas M, Gilabert-Juan J, et al. The polysialylated form of the neural cell adhesion molecule (PSA-NCAM) is expressed in a subpopulation of mature cortical interneurons characterized by reduced structural features and connectivity. Cerebral Cortex. 2011;**21**:1028-1041. DOI: 10.1093/CERCOR/BHQ177

[215] Guirado R, Perez-Rando M, Sanchez-Matarredona D, Castillo-Gómez E, Liberia T, Rovira-Esteban L, et al. The dendritic spines of interneurons are dynamic structures influenced by PSA-NCAM expression. Cerebral Cortex. 2014;**24**:3014-3024. DOI: 10.1093/CERCOR/BHT156

[216] Green MJ, Matheson SL, Shepherd A, Weickert CS, Carr VJ. Brain-derived neurotrophic factor levels in schizophrenia: A systematic review with meta-analysis. Molecular Psychiatry. 2011;**16**:960-972. DOI: 10.1038/MP.2010.88

[217] Lee KB, Kunugi H, Nanko S. Glial cell line-derived neurotrophic factor (GDNF) gene and schizophrenia: Polymorphism screening and association analysis. Psychiatry Research. 2001;**104**:11-17. DOI: 10.1016/S0165-1781(01)00294-3

[218] Futamura T, Toyooka K, Iritani S, Niizato K, Nakamura R, Tsuchiya K, et al. Abnormal expression of epidermal growth factor and its receptor in the forebrain and serum of schizophrenic patients. Molecular Psychiatry. 2002;**7**:673-682. DOI: 10.1038/SJ.MP.4001081

[219] Weinberg SM, Jenkins EA, Marazita ML, Maher BS. Minor physical anomalies in schizophrenia: A meta-analysis. Schizophrenia Research. 2007;**89**:72-85. DOI: 10.1016/J.SCHRES.2006.09.002

[220] Xu T, Chan RCK, Compton MT. Minor physical anomalies in patients with schizophrenia, unaffected first-degree relatives, and healthy controls: A meta-analysis. PLoS One. 2011;**6**(9). DOI: 10.1371/JOURNAL.PONE.0024129

[221] Kusman A, Yalçınkaya B, Kır Y, Aksoy UM, Özdemir BN, Dilek ZG, et al. The association of minor physical anomalies with clinical and subclinical psychotic symptoms. Journal of Ankara University Faculty of Medicine. 2020;**73**:216-223. DOI: 10.4274/atfm.galenos.2020.79553

[222] Gottesman II, Erlenmeyer-Kimling L. Family and twin strategies as a head start in defining prodromes and endophenotypes for hypothetical early-interventions in schizophrenia. Schizophrenia Research. 2001;**51**:93-102. DOI: 10.1016/S0920-9964(01)00245-6

[223] Brown AS. Prenatal infection as a risk factor for schizophrenia. Schizophrenia Bulletin. 2006;**32**:200-202. DOI: 10.1093/SCHBUL/SBJ052

[224] Monk C, Lugo-Candelas C, Trumpff C. Prenatal developmental

origins of future psychopathology: Mechanisms and pathways. Annual Reviews. 2019;**15**:317-344. DOI: 10.1146/annurev-clinpsy-050718

[225] Hambrecht M, Häfner H. Substance abuse and the onset of schizophrenia. Biological Psychiatry. 1996;**40**:1155-1163. DOI: 10.1016/S0006-3223(95)00609-5

[226] Thornicroft G, Salvia DDE, Tansella M, Tansella M. Urban-rural differences in the associations between social deprivation and psychiatric service utilization in schizophrenia and all diagnoses: A case-register study in Northern Italy. Psychological Medicine. 1993;**23**:487-496. DOI: 10.1017/S0033291700028579

[227] Geddes JR, Lawrie SM. Obstetric complications and schizophrenia: A meta-analysis. The British Journal of Psychiatry. 1995;**167**:786-793. DOI: 10.1192/BJP.167.6.786

[228] Selten JP, Van Der Ven E, Rutten BPF, Cantor-Graae E. The social defeat hypothesis of schizophrenia: An update. Schizophrenia Bulletin. 2013;**39**:1180. DOI: 10.1093/SCHBUL/SBT134

[229] Mesholam-Gately RI, Giuliano AJ, Goff KP, Faraone SV, Seidman LJ. Neurocognition in first-episode schizophrenia: A meta-analytic review. Neuropsychology. 2009;**23**:315-336. DOI: 10.1037/A0014708

[230] Fusar-Poli P, Deste G, Smieskova R, Barlati S, Yung AR, Howes O, et al. Cognitive functioning in prodromal psychosis: A meta-analysis. Archives of General Psychiatry. 2012;**69**:562-571. DOI: 10.1001/ARCHGENPSYCHIATRY.2011.1592

[231] Clarke MC, Tanskanen A, Huttunen M, Leon DA, Murray RM, Jones PB, et al. Increased risk of schizophrenia from additive interaction between infant motor developmental delay and obstetric complications: Evidence from a population-based longitudinal study. The American Journal of Psychiatry. 2011;**168**:1295-1302. DOI: 10.1176/APPI.AJP.2011.11010011

[232] Dickson H, Laurens KR, Cullen AE, Hodgins S. Meta-analyses of cognitive and motor function in youth aged 16 years and younger who subsequently develop schizophrenia. Psychological Medicine. 2012;**42**:743-755. DOI: 10.1017/S0033291711001693

Chapter 2

Design to Support People with Schizophrenia: Activating Professional Boundaries

Dianne Smith and Elizabeth Karol

Abstract

For people with schizophrenia, home environments that are readily understandable, easily managed, provide opportunities for self-expression and support psychosocial needs can enhance their wellbeing. Importantly, symptoms of schizophrenia (including agitation, anxiety, helplessness, perceptual distortion) can potentially be reduced through responsive accommodation design. The embedded potential of design of homes to offer support or create hindrances for people with schizophrenia has been poorly explored. Cues as to what things are and how to function in a space can be designed to provide support. This chapter records a multi-prong action research approach to develop a resource to assist designers and service providers create responsive residential environments for people with impeded cognitive functioning. Research from such fields as environmental psychology, sociology and design, together with discussions with people with schizophrenia, indicates that quality of life for people with schizophrenia can be enhanced through design. A key outcome is a Framework that enables the user to both understand the reason why a person with schizophrenia may respond to the environment in a particular way and how to design to acknowledge that potential response.

Keywords: design, home, accommodation, schizophrenia, design process, wellbeing at home, enabling housing, architecture, person environment relationship

1. Introduction

Placed within a collection of chapters that cover a broad field of topics connected to schizophrenia, our work is a nonmedical approach to the subject of schizophrenia. Our backgrounds, based in architecture, interiors, building science, art therapy as well as research, influence this approach. Over our careers we have become intensely aware that environments can assist or inhibit the way people live; and consequently, that those responsible for the commissioning, design, construction, and management of accommodation have a responsibility to attend to these potential environmental influences through the projects they undertake. Our work has evolved to study home environments for those who live with schizophrenia.

When seeking insights into issues such as poor mental health, cognitive impairment or schizophrenia, people naturally are drawn to medical sources. The role of the creative arts, such as building design, does not immediately come to mind as a source of insight. However, as practitioners in this field we have come to realise the embedded potential in this area. By drawing on the theories of the sociologist, Bourdieu [1], it is evident that the body of knowledge from architecture and design can broaden and enrich the discussion and encourage new knowledge to emerge [2].

Consequently, we have taken a place 'on the field' as we join 'the game'. Bourdieu's concepts of 'field' and 'habitus' can inform propositions about design that can complement medical disciplines in achieving a common goal of improving quality of life for people with schizophrenia. In a 'field', disciplines have practices of thoughts and modes of operating that those within understand (initially through education and the like). However, these areas can become 'struggles for legitimisation' of one's knowledge and practices in relation to its distinctiveness from other disciplines [1]. In this chapter, we present building design as a discipline that can potentially impact on the symptoms associated with cognitive difficulties (including poor mental health, cognitive impairment (CI) or schizophrenia) through responsive accommodation design.

Bourdieu referenced our unconscious perception of our position or place in the world as our 'habitus'; and it is this which influences our actions and relations [3]. At an individual level, the habitus exists and provides the 'sense' of what action we are inclined to take; and we use the symbols available to us according to our habitus [1, 4]. The environment then not only provides the context, it holds 'implicit rules that regulate transactions' [5]; and are integral to the cultural system [6].

This is linked to discrimination, as 'field' and 'habitus' underpin meaning-making in respect to 'discriminatory practices' that may be embedded in our interpretations of others [7]. In the general community, people with impeded cognitive functioning (ICF)[1] are often regarded as distinct from others. In the context of Bourdieu, this raises the notions of social capital and symbolic capital. Both reflect how people accidently or deliberately project their value or role on to the community; it is a means to identify distinction and differences [8]. It is acknowledged that architecture creates a field laden with social values [9] with symbols embedded within an environment. These symbols reflect societal standards, attitudes toward occupants, as well as economic, political, and educative values and associated worth (or not). This raises three questions. Does accommodation for those with ICF reflect a common understanding held by the society it is embedded in? Does the architectural profession apply the same common understanding? Is accommodation having a high social standing or rich social capital available to people with ICF?

In Australia, although many people with mental illnesses reside with family or in group houses, others (including those with schizophrenia) are dependent on social

[1] Throughout the chapter various terms and acronyms are used to describe these people's condition. They include cognitive impairment (CI), impeded cognitive functioning (ICF), impaired cognitive functioning and impaired cognitive abilities. The reason is that over the past couple of decades terminology describing conditions (or the collection of people experiencing the condition) has evolved. As this chapter captures a series of projects that occurred over time, the terms of the day are used here as well as in the reporting of the published outcomes.

housing or low-cost housing [10]. This accommodation is often basic compared to the surrounding housing stock. Thus designers 'create the aesthetics and the ideas that reinforce distinctions between groups' [11]. Judgements are, in turn, made by and about the occupant of the accommodation. There is a social cost in making these judgements: firstly, for the resident and secondly, for families, organisations and/or society through the costs of care.

Having established the place of design in this conversation, we will describe our research in developing a Practice Document that can guide the development of good quality accommodation that potentially improves the quality of life for people with ICF. The core of the Practice Document is a Framework that informs the practice of responsive accommodation design for people with ICF.

This chapter outlines a series of projects that enabled us to achieve this end. Our process reflects both *action research* and *design practice*, where a situation is diagnosed to reveal the issue or problem; staged research carried out; actions proposed, undertaken, monitored, and evaluated prior to commencing the next stage of research. This continues until reaching a potential resolution; with each step bringing new understandings as well as cautionary notes.

2. Architects join 'the game'

In 2015, a provider of services and accommodation for people with disability, poor mental health and/or who were homeless in Perth, Western Australia approached us (as architects and academics). They requested our expertise to help them better understand the impact of accommodation design on their clients: an increasing number of whom had impaired cognitive abilities. The provider was expressly interested in aspects of design that reduce the amount of building damage wrought by clients when they were agitated, frustrated or generally unwell because of poor mental health. At that time therapeutic design in accommodation largely referred to universal design principles, which made accommodation accessible and manageable for those with mobility issues.

Our initial research showed that there were additional aspects of design that played a part in improving wellbeing for everyone, but particularly for those who are marginalised with ICF. These additional aspects revolved around what Pallasmaa, a highly acclaimed Finnish architect/academic referred to as "the process of living" [12]. He argued that for people to care about their accommodation they needed to think of it as 'home'. Our research showed that for accommodation to become home it must allow for individualised expression of personality, patterns of life, rituals and routines. Ioannidou, an architectural researcher and designer, refers to "home as an intangible concept. It is the emotional and meaningful relationship between people and their familiar environment" [13].

We adapted this idea of intangibles to identify such aspects of the home environment that subtly create opportunities for wellbeing through opportunities for self-determination, a setting for personal possessions, spatial diversity and spatial delight. Thus, started our journey to discover how designers (including architects, interior designers, landscape architects) and service providers could commission, design, construct and manage accommodation for people with ICF, so it was better able to support this growing sector of our community.

By using design thinking as a reflective and evolutionary process over a series of projects we developed a generic Framework for designers and service providers. One that would help them foster health and wellbeing in the home for people with ICF. We used the generic Framework to establish design details for one particular condition, schizophrenia, thereby providing a demonstration case for how some symptoms of a mental health condition could be addressed through integration of certain design considerations. These design considerations are regarded as part of a package of support for people with schizophrenia.

In order to clarify the field of this study—particularly for those with limited knowledge of architectural and design theory—an overview is provided of three areas: the person-environment relationship (PER), accommodation design for people with ICF and action research.

2.1 Person-environment relationship

Many authors across environmental psychology and sociology as well as the design fields have described the impact of the person-environment relationship (PER) including how people feel and behave: see [14–16]. PER is well documented and various forms have been identified. Three forms of PER were described by Smith [7]. These ranged from a relationship where the environment was completely separate to the person to those where the environment and person were completely interdependent. Returning to Bourdieu's concept of habitus, a person is said to have a 'sense of the game'; knowing what is happening, what is expected and what to do [1]. That person may develop a strong sense of control, sense of identity or self-worth as the environmental setting reflects who they are and fosters self-expression as part everyday living.

So functional, emotional, psychological, and social aspects of a person's life are all impacted by how they feel about their accommodation [17]. When translated to people with ICF, including those with schizophrenia, it is noted that a person may not be able to overcome negative environmental aspects, due to their cognitive attributes [17], and consequently may have their quality of life severely and detrimentally impacted. Although there is a broad and growing cross section of literature that relates physical places with impacts on people with ICF, in-depth knowledge of how this occurs and how design facilitates positive impacts is still scarce. Our work sought to navigate this field and explore the PER for people with schizophrenia.

2.2 Accommodation design for people with impeded cognitive functioning

The aim of architects and designers should be to not cause harm to the occupants of the buildings they design [18]. Our literature review [17] showed that the majority of houses designed and built in Australia meet functional needs. However, the intangible qualities of a home environment that address emotional, psychological, and/or social needs are rarely addressed. The building itself was generally considered as a 'disembodied commodity' [19], with no recognition that it is in fact "at the helm of a major force of neural functional dynamics" [20].

From the review of psychology and environmental psychology sources [15, 16, 21–25] the possible human responses which would indicate that a person at home felt emotionally, psychologically, and/or socially supported were identified. These responses included:

- emotional and spiritual enhancement (including delight),
- sense of belonging and control (including connectedness and privacy),

- sense of self, self-esteem, and identity,
- sense of dignity, homeliness, comfort, and affordance.

Sociologist and academic, Aaron Antonovsky [26] posited the concept of a sense of coherence. He identified physical, soulful, and spiritual coherence as being fundamental to health and wellbeing. Further to coherence, Lockard [25] references engagement with both space and community as being critical for well-being.

However, current housing stock in Western Australia shows little attention to the needs of people with an ongoing impairment in comprehension, reason, adaptive functioning, judgement, learning, or memory. There is little indication that designers are aware that by treating the home as a 'disembodied commodity' it may trigger significant responses and curtail a sense of wellbeing for people with ICF. From the literature there is minimal evidence, even from designers who professionally claim this space in their expertise, that detailed knowledge of how to incorporate appropriate intangible characteristics in a design is available.

For a person with ICF and limited choice in where they live, it seems to be particularly important that the home environment is designed to be both functionally and emotionally enabling. What is unclear is how designer-controlled elements can be extended to include intangible characteristics, so that a person with ICF feels nurtured and supported at home. We identified a need for evidence-based qualitative design research at the individual level and at a group level. Firstly, this was to analyse affordable home designs occupied by people with ICF in order to identify specifically what emotionally, psychologically and socially enabling intangible aspects exist. Secondly, to identify what people with CI value in their homes and what gives them a sense of well-being and emotional, psychological and social support.

An integrated approach is needed for holistic understanding of what it is to be at home as a person with ICF. This is complex, as people who have ICF have a wide variety of needs and are implicitly or explicitly conceptualised by researchers in each discipline in a variety of ways.

2.3 Action research

The Practice Document has been built from an ongoing process that involved continuous reflection and extrapolation to generate each subsequent step. This process is captured by an action research approach [27]. Such an approach is not linear, rather it is dynamic 'where research, action, participation and evaluation interact' [27] and strives to link practice and theory. Action research has traditionally been described as a repeated cycle involving planning, acting, observing and reflecting; and as such, mirrors the design process where the outcome emerges from a series of propositions, creations, tests against emergent criteria and reflection cycles toward each consequent proposition.

The involvement of those implicated is also part of action research – in this case accommodation providers, people from the target resident group, and researchers. The driver of action research is to generate change. In this case we aimed to challenge the accepted accommodation generated through current design practice and typical procurement strategies. It was recognised that this sector often has restricted budgets and opportunities to experiment with new ways of 'doing architecture'. The involvement of a breadth of committees and funding bodies may mean that challenging everyday ways of doing is put to one side. However, improvement to accommodation design was worth exploring to ameliorate costs in terms of quality of life for residents, and financially for the providers and support workers.

The markers of success of an action research program are described by McTaggart [28] as being defensible, educative, politically effectual, and morally appropriate. The main aspects of action research that are common across the breadth of the various approaches described in the literature [29] are captured in **Table 1**. The seven aspects, summarised in **Table 1**, have been addressed in the development of the Practice Document.

Aspect of Action Research	Application to development of the Practice Document
Problem-focused, context specific, future oriented	Addressed real life issues and explored the need for change through literature reviews, conversations with providers, and interviews with people with schizophrenia.
Change intervention (change experiment)	A wide cross section of strategies of research were involved that led to a range of actions and propositions
Aims toward improvement	Improvement is targeted toward improved quality of life and wellbeing for future occupants with schizophrenia.
Cyclical process	Each step revealed relevant aspects that were then considered as part of the subsequent step/s.
Research relationship	Researchers are also designers, who developed a relationship with provider organisations, who in turn, provided access to properties and/or residents with ICF.
Educative	Designers, service providers, people with schizophrenia educated the researchers and will have open access to the findings.
Individuals are seen as members of social group	Service providers and accommodation providers for people with schizophrenia participated. People with schizophrenia are potential residents.

Table 1.
Summary of use of action research to develop practice document.

3. Building the foundations: a reflective process

A multi-prong approach was required to develop a resource, a Practice Document, to assist designers and providers to create suitable environments for people with ICF. This approach evolved through a series of projects over many years. Each project arose through observations and reflections on the preceding activities. Collectively, they provide a pluralistic interrogation of what is going on.

3.1 Action research

Figure 1 depicts the cycles of research over the decade. Each adds to providing an overall sense of the systematic expansion of our understanding. We also have noted any articles or reports produced en route and publicly available so that readers can explore the process and outcomes identified. The cycles did not necessarily occur in a neat linear manner as some investigations overlapped at times.

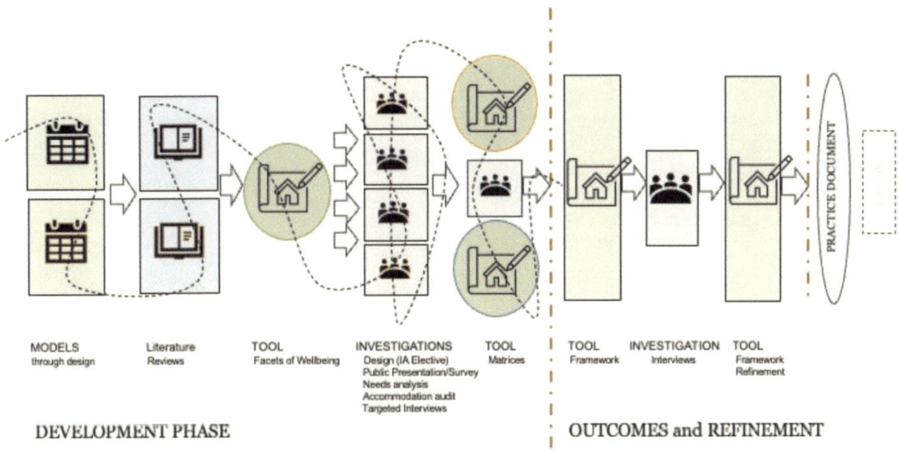

Figure 1.
Action embedded in research.

As noted in **Figure 1** the process can be divided into two overarching phases: The Development Phase and the Outcomes and Refinement phase. The tool that emerged, called a Framework, is a comprehensive way of capturing the cycles of research and presenting the parameters that may influence design practice whilst including reference to the user's (resident) condition (such as schizophrenia). The Framework was then contextualised within a Practice Document for those designing and investing in affordable housing for people with ICF. The hope is that others will build on this research by applying the Practice Document to the construction of accommodation for people with schizophrenia.

3.2 Cycles of research

Each cycle in the Development Phase is summarised in **Tables 2–14**. To succinctly explain the research, the activity and the outcome generated are stated, as well as a summary of our reflections. The Outcomes and Refinement Phase is then summarised.

3.2.1 The development phase

There were 13 cycles of research in the development phase, culminating in the Framework and Practice Document. We started by using design thinking to assist service provider managers to rethink ways of looking at the design of a day facility for homeless people (**Table 2**). We went on to develop a model that enabled better collaboration between all stakeholders when designing for marginalised people (**Table 3**). This was followed by literature reviews (**Tables 4** and 5), creative design practice (**Table 6**), and an examination of language that captured the essence of the impact of intangible qualities of space (**Table 9**). Eventually we developed a design tool matrix that could assist designers and service providers to improve the PER in accommodation for people with ICF (**Table 14**).

Initially we were approached by a service provider to assist in the design of a day centre for homeless people. To achieve the best results within a very limited budget it was necessary to reframe the thinking of the service provider staff and collaboratively

Activity:	**Reflection**
To explore visual tools to create new insights into the design of places for marginalised people. **Generated:** 7 step Wellbeing Management Model.	Complex contemporary issues require new ways of tackling recurring issues. Creative processes can enable the discovery of alternative outcomes. Business/management were challenged while being open to new conceptualisations of available options.

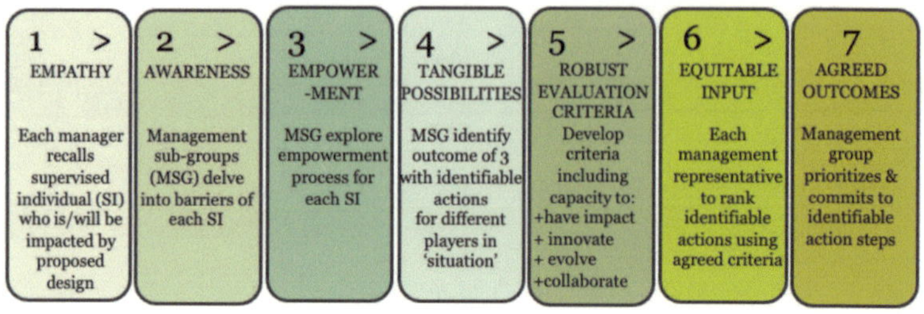

Table 2.
Wellbeing management model [30].

reconceptualize the situation and explore ways of tackling it. **Table 2** summarises the project.

The proposed action resulting from the first project was to utilise creative practice processes on future projects at the brief and design development phases. We set out to apply this when considering alternative ways of approaching design for a supportive day centre for homeless people that integrates end-users as collaborators (**Table 3**).

Activity:	**Reflection**	
Establish principles and test them through design practice. **Generated:** SEDM that integrates theory, design thinking, and creative practice.	The process did challenge the traditional approach to designing facilities for marginalised people. Although principles are very person-centred, an ecological perspective also highlights the interdependency of the PER in context. All stakeholders (service providers, managers and clients) indicated open engagement was increased and the outcome had a positive impact on staff and clients.	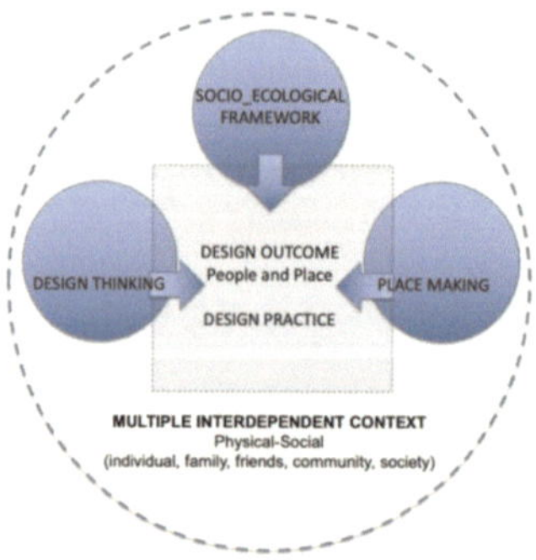

Table 3.
Socio-ecological design model (SEDM) [31].

It was recognised that design solutions to cater for people with ICF was needed. To start this process we initially needed to identify what was already known about the characteristics of domestic settings that support well-being for those with ICF. A literature review was carried out as summarised in **Table 4**.

Activity:	**Reflection**
Literature review: home design and its impact on emotional, psychological, or social well-being for people with CI. **Generated:** Six Implications for Practice.	Researchers understand that pragmatic design inputs alone may not be sufficient. Others have shown or surmise that there are other "intangible" designer-controlled elements that have beneficial impacts. Information is sparse, and the degree of quality of life improvement for a person with CIP is not well understood.

	Identified aspects of the environment: (FE) Functionally enabling (FS) Functionally supportive (EPSE) Emotionally, psychologically, and/or socially enabling (EPSS) Emotionally, psychologically, and/or socially supportive (PER) Aspects of environment combined with resident's particular attributes.

Table 4.
Literature review: Round 1.

The initial literature review identified an absence of research involving the nuanced qualities of the physical environment. We, therefore, proposed to revisit the literature to target these intangible qualities. In addition, we proposed it would also be of value to analyse affordable home designs to identify what emotionally, psychologically, and/or socially enabling intangible aspects exist; identify what people with CI value in their homes; and what gives them a sense of wellbeing and being emotionally, psychologically, and/or socially supportive (**Table 5**).

Activity:	**Reflection**
Literature Review **Generated:** An understanding of intangible qualities and their impacts.	Addressing intangible qualities has the potential to change the approach to environmental design and the user-experiences.

Table 5.
Literature review: Round 2 [32].

By identifying what the intangible qualities could be and their potential link to the built environment, we proposed that intangible qualities could be integrated into environmental design strategies to support the end users (in this case, residents).

To explore this proposal a project was developed for a small group of interior architecture students. Three university students were each to redesign an existing house for

Activity:	**Reflection**
Creative practice (design) was used as a vehicle to introduce new ideas/extend current understandings about accommodation for people with disabilities (ICF). **Generated:** At least 17 environmentally based intangible attributes can be considered when designing accommodation.	It is possible to integrate intangible qualities with tangible requirements for people with disabilities in residential design. An overarching design concept embracing the impact of built environment on the person was significant in all schemes. *Image: example of part project* 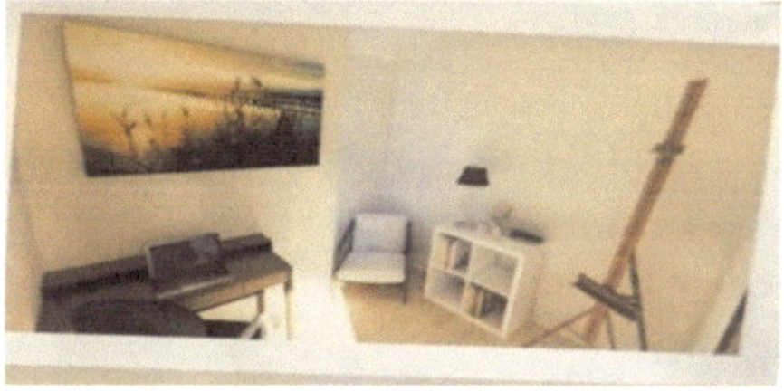

Table 6.
Design schemes suggested by interior architecture students.

one of three hypothetical clients who each had ICF. They utilised the knowledge gained from the literature reviews but were not limited by what already existed as we aimed to generate ideas to stimulate new or alternative ways of looking at current design practice.

The resultant designs proved very useful in exploring intangible qualities and extending accommodation design ideas. The ideas were presented to the accommodation provider and their affiliates (**Table 7**) to educate them on future possibilities and to gain feedback on feasibilities of the ideas generated. In addition, we hoped to generate further discussion and stimulate new ideas to share.

Activity:	**Reflection**
A public presentation of design schemes. Attendees and post-presentation visitors were surveyed. **Generated:** A public forum. A random sample of visitors commented via the survey.	15 areas where ideas for improvements of existing accommodation were identified. Response was positive to the process and ideas at the forum. As only a small number responded to the survey further investigation is required.

Table 7.
Assessment by service provider and affiliates.

Through the discussions, we identified several ideas to explore further, particularly in the details embedded in suggestions. This also reinforced the value of integrating the intangible aspects in future designs. We, therefore, targeted those constructed architectural projects, noted as best-practice, to ascertain if intangible qualities were noted and considered. This was done via a desktop audit (**Table 8**).

Activity:	**Reflection**
A desk-top search to identify recognised projects where the designers /clients/stakeholders claiming to cater for users' needs/aspirations beyond pragmatic requirements. **Generated:** Realisation that the impact of intangible design elements are not well understood.	The most informative projects state and depict significant intangibles as contributing to mental health of the occupants. Intangible features mentioned: • supporting dignity • quality of light • the views and connectedness to outside. • social dignity and socialising • a sense of comfort Only three of the projects clearly included an element of delight.

Table 8.
Desktop audit [33].

As a result of the audit and our previous work, we identified there was a need to develop a common language to identify the intangible features. In addition, we aimed to include the intangibles into all housing experimentation to improve wellbeing for occupants' with ICF.

It was proposed that local accommodation, controlled by the provider, would be audited to gain an in-depth knowledge of the physical environment of the accommodation. Eight single homes plus one group home for 12 people were audited

DOI: http://dx.doi.org/10.5772/intechopen.1004807

Activity:	**Reflection**
Literature survey and generation of tool. **Generated:** Facets of Wellbeing. These are explained on the website [33].	Concepts are difficult to define but are essential to this work. Designers need to grasp these terms. 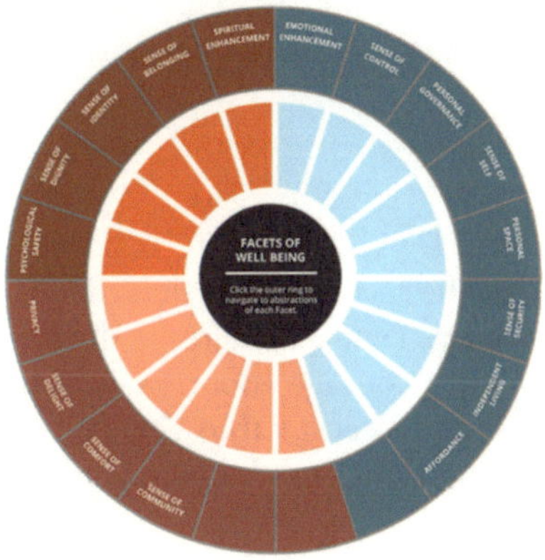

Table 9.
Facets of wellbeing [34].

(**Table 10**). This involved mapping the current design attributes, identifying those attributes that target the therapeutic needs identified in the literature, and ascertaining the tangible and intangible qualities of homes (**Table 10**).

Activity:	**Reflection**
Visit, record and analyse the physical attributes of the provider's homes. **Generated:** Four general principles were identified.	As the physical settings were fully recorded, the qualities of the spaces could be analysed for such intangible qualities as location, orientation, lighting and noise. However, the occupants were not interviewed. Personal items used by the occupant were only considered if indicating adequate storage or adequate space for typical furniture layouts and the like. The four general principles were based on the identified design elements or environmental attributes, which can influence the level of sensory overload and/or social participation. Limitations of accommodation included size and layouts, access and external areas in relation to climate, as well as quality of building services.

Table 10.
Accommodation audit [35].

It was evident from the accommodation audit that the potential of services (lighting, air temperature, air quality) and technologies for improving quality of life for people with ICF needed to be updated considering currently available technology. The sector was contacted to ascertain if they considered there was a need to adopt alternative housing designs to improve the residents' wellbeing (**Table 11**).

Activity:	**Reflection**
A telephone and email survey of local providers.	There was lack of clarity in 2015 regarding the need for change across the sector; although it was noted that accommodation was not being tailored to particular people with special needs.

Generated: Little useable information was available.	Principles of Universal Design are integrated; yet distinctions between people with cognitive and physical disabilities were not made. Some organisations have their own guidelines for general adaptable designs; and although not available, the National Disability Insurance Agency was thought to be developing their own guidelines at the time.

Table 11.
Needs analysis.

The lack of clarity across the sector means that the likely adoption of this research by the sector needs monitoring. That will increase the likelihood of uptake and environmental improvements. To encourage adoption, a comprehensive tool to assist designers and providers was proposed (**Table 12**). The researchers' aim was to develop a tool to assist designers and providers to generate supportive environments for those with ICF.

Activity: Generation of a tool based on what is known to date. **Generated:** A Matrix consisting of: Indicators of a Supportive Environment axis and Design Directives axis.	**Reflection** Lesson learned: Home (building and interior) and setting (garden) have the potential to impact on an occupant with reduced cognitive functioning by: 1. providing a setting, which affords certain ways of perceiving, using and experiencing it. 2. the qualities of the physical setting can induce a sense of coherence. 3. a sense-of-wellbeing can be fostered. The intersection of a person's CI with indicators for supportive environments is proposed as a point to start to improve residential environments.

Table 12.
Design tool matrix 01 [35].

The resultant Matrix was a forerunner to resident interviews to enable an in-depth understanding of the PER relationship, as well as informing the refinement of the Matrix. Research was proposed to understand the relationship between a particular condition and the physical environment and to build on what was already known about such relationships (**Table 13**). A list of considerations to increase the environmental affordance toward a supportive environment for those with ICF unfolded.

Activity: Interview three residents who live in accommodation that was previously audited. **Generated:** A set of considerations to inform the development of a design tool for designers and providers.	**Reflection** Some understandings were challenged or extended by interviews. Observations and telling of first-hand experiences were critical to understanding the opportunities and limitations of current homes and future strategies.

Table 13.
Interviews with residents who have schizophrenia.

Our initial understandings developed by listening to the first-hand experiences of people with schizophrenia. Further research showed that the intangible qualities of design and their impact on a person with ICF can be examined by assessing if a person with ICF is better able to cope with activities of daily living when they are able to comprehend, manage and find meaningfulness in their home. Collectively these three aspects of support are referred to as enabling a sense of coherence [36, 37]. Our research and reflections identified an additional aspect of the PER, the emotional aspect. This relates to a person feeling that their abilities are accepted, they are supported to participate in their community and can get involved. We refer to this as emotional affordance: a concept that complements the work of others [20, 25]. Collectively these four aspects of support in this chapter are referred to as enabling a sense of coherence (SoC). Although the person-environment relationship is complex as discussed previously, in our work were able to relate the four aspects of SoC to some foregrounded designing qualities as shown in **Figure 2**.

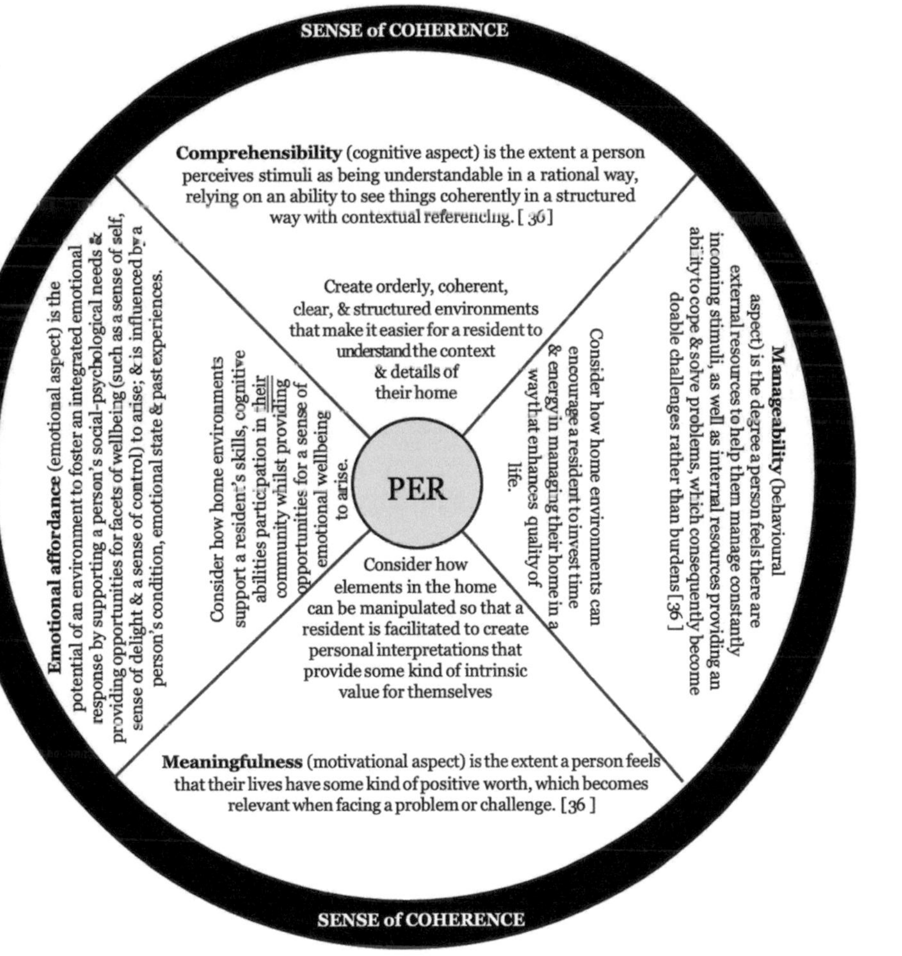

Figure 2.
Aspects of SoC related to PER.

It became clear that SoC needed to be integrated into the tools being developed. This led to a more refined Matrix (**Table 14**).

Activity: Refine the Matrix based on what is known to date including principles of Salutogenic Design [36] **Generated:** A tool providing a practical way of enhancing the design of a physical home environment to help reduce negative impacts and increase supportive qualities.	**Reflection** The homes of the interviewees achieved differing degrees of SoC. They catered for daily requirements, interaction/socialisation, non-sedentary activities within common forms of accommodation and were comprehensible. The overall SoC should include what is emotionally afforded through the PER. This adds another dimension to developing a design model. This dimension aligns with the previously generated Facets of Wellbeing. Overall the development of a new multidimensional tool to embrace the complex and competing demands of provider, designer, and resident is required while not sacrificing the non-functional for the functional.

Table 14.
Design tool matrix 02 [34].

To further refine the proposed strategy (and resultant tools) that was emerging, further research was required across various aspects including more interviews and observations that involved people with schizophrenia. In particular, areas requiring additional study included links between meaningfulness and environmental contexts; fine-grain understanding and links between specific environmental elements and the four dimensions of SoC. The theoretical basis reflecting these developments was also integrated. These realisations brought the project to a point where clear principles needed to be communicated to enable design practitioners to embrace the findings to inform their approach to designing accommodation for people with schizophrenia.

3.2.2 Refinement of outcomes

There were three cycles of research in the Outcomes and Refinement Phase. All related to creating an easily accessible way for designers, architects and service and accommodation providers to understand the impact of the home environment on their clients with ICF. Initially, we produced a generic Framework through which to tackle the design of accommodation for those with ICF. The generic Framework evolved to explicitly address the requirements of accommodation for people with schizophrenia. Schizophrenia was addressed rather than another condition of ICF for the following reasons. Our literature review indicated an initial depth of knowledge that we could build on. The provider of services and accommodation who initially approached us, advised that a large percentage of the clients presenting to them were people with schizophrenia and we had been able to interview some of them. In addition, we were able to procure further interviews with people with schizophrenia through another service provider.

Having contextualised the parameters that influence design practice such as the user (resident) and the condition (such as schizophrenia), we aimed to reflect upon the development of the Framework and test its application. The final DEKS Practice Document [38], which includes the Framework, contextualises the users' condition (schizophrenia). The Practice Document enables a reader to move from understanding the reasons why a person with ICF may respond to the environment in particular ways to examine the design aspects to be considered to positively influence the wellbeing of a person with ICF. Details of the Framework are described in detail below.

4. Framework in action: a demonstration case

The Framework suggests incorporating specific design features in an environment so that the wellbeing of a person with schizophrenia can be impacted positively (and avoid negative impacts). This section summarises critical aspects of the Framework, describes two applications which continued our action research approach and analyses the educative value of the process as well as the challenges in applying the Framework in practice.

4.1 The framework

The overall intent of the Framework is to enable a practitioner to appreciate the reason why a person with ICF may respond to the environment in particular ways and to examine design aspects that impact on SoC to positively influence wellbeing. The Framework itself consists of 3 parts: Guiding Parameters, Design Considerations and Potential Overall Impact on Wellbeing. The Guiding Parameters include two sets of principles. The first principle provides explicit descriptions of symptoms of a specific condition that may influence how a person responds to the environment. The second principle identifies in sweeping terms what is needed to create a positive supportive physical environment. One that creates a sense of coherence and thus can be responsive to the needs of a resident. The second part of the Framework essentially provides the designing cues. The Design Considerations establish how each of the four aspects of SoC can be met to help a person better cope with everyday living. The Design Considerations include general design instructions and detailed design strategies to explain the environmental requirements necessary to facilitate an integrated approach to accommodation design. The final part of the Framework describes the potential overall impact on wellbeing resulting from addressing the Design Considerations. **Table 15** summarises the generic Framework.

Guiding parameters		**Design considerations**		**Potential overall impact on well-being**
ICF Principles	**Designing Principles**	**Design Intentions**	**Design Provisions**	
A designer is required to understand: ICF may include 'an ongoing impairment in comprehension, reason, adaptive functioning, judgement, learning or memory' [39]. The symptoms a person may exhibit when they have a particular condition of ICF.	Establish how the four SoC dimensions (cognitive, behavioural, motivational and emotional affordance) can be fostered in the home for a person's particular condition.	Provide instructions for a designer to enable them to address each dimension of SoC for the target group.	Establish a series of design strategies that contribute to fulfilling the Design Intentions	Establish expected beneficial experiences for the home occupant.

Table 15.
The generic framework.

The generic Framework was populated to address the needs of people with schizophrenia. This resulted in a total of 12 general Design Intentions and 25 detailed Design Provisions. **Table 16** shows the first part of the Framework relating to providing the cognitive aspect of support to contribute to a SoC.

Designing Principles	Design Intentions	Design Provisions	Potential overall impact on wellbeing
COMPREHENSION Create orderly, coherent, clear, and structured environments that make it easier for a resident to understand the context and details of their home.	A. Create an uncomplicated comprehensible home environment for activities of daily living; B. Reduce likelihood of negative perceptions of ordinary spaces or amplifications of perceptions of non-existing dangers.	1. Simple (uncomplicated) orderly design solutions; 2. Home layout that provides intuitive way-finding based on recognisable spatial clues and focal points; 3. Clear sight lines and straightforward entry points;	*Increase a resident's ability to function and perform activities of daily living; *Reduce anxiety levels; *Assist replenishment of cognitive energy; *Reduce depression; *Reduce feelings of helplessness; *Reduce mental load on functioning;

Table 16.
Part of framework related to supporting comprehension for people with schizophrenia.

4.2 Applying the framework

We utilised the Framework on two test projects. The first project was a virtual redesign of a home occupied by a person with schizophrenia and the second was to review design development drawings for a new home where one of the occupants has schizophrenia.

4.2.1 Virtual redesign with resident feedback

One of the volunteers, who had participated in the interviews as we were refining the Framework (Section 3.2.2), agreed that we could redesign his home using it. He was prepared to comment on the result. This person had lived in his accommodation for 25 years and was an avid collector of books, records and CDs. Three designer-researchers independently set about redesigning the existing 62 square metres two-bedroom home for him, within practical limits, using all 25 of the Design Provisions incorporated in the Framework. The three designer-researchers came together to assess their design proposals and, after reviewing and discussing the proposals, agreed on a final design that best met the Design Intentions and Design Provisions. A document was prepared to record the designer-researcher's commentary on how each of the Design Provisions had been met in the final design. It is acknowledged that some of the Design Provisions could not be fully achieved due to the inherent nature of the building; the home is within a complex of home units, so orientation of windows is predetermined. However, most of the Design Provisions could be met.

The final design was digitised into a three-minute video that enabled a viewer to move virtually through the home [40]. **Figure 3** shows a view of the living space. The indicative sketch of the original space is on the left, while a screen save from the video is on the right.

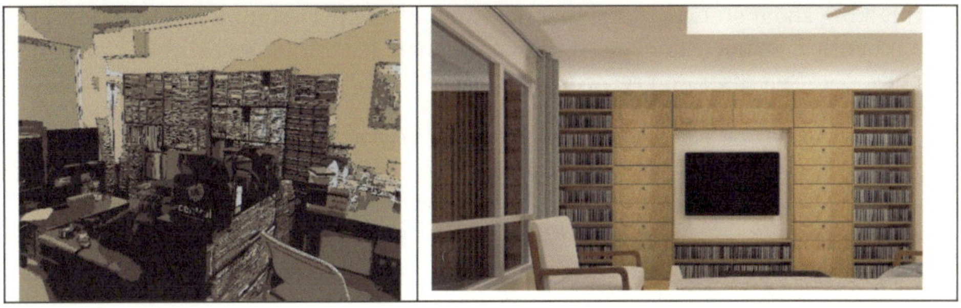

Figure 3.
Abstracted existing living space (left); screen save of living space from the video (right).

The occupant viewed the video with the three designer-researchers. His comments are discussed below. The occupant said he liked the proposal saying:

> *I love it. I mean it's really clever use of space ... There are some aspects of it that are really good.*

However, he had some general reservations saying:

> *A person with schizophrenia might find it a little bit too organised ... A lot of people I hang around with are generally disorganised in how they live ... have stuff everywhere.*

Another reservation related to how light the space looked. Although he seemed to appreciate the additional light he said:

> *the space, the light ... it's a lot lighter ... I'd feel kind of exposed or vulnerable in such a light, bright environment. I'd have to get used to it. I might have chosen, with the colour of the storage, something slightly darker. Even the dining room table ... because I'm so used to this place ... A dark environment for me makes me kind of feel more cosy ... I would not kind of feel as exposed or vulnerable as in such a light, bright environment.*

It is not uncommon for people to express trepidation to a change in a familiar setting and imagining their possessions set in unfamiliar surroundings. Foremost in a person's mind are associations with memories of the current or previous home [41] and the emotional relationship they have with the familiar environment they call home [14].

The comment relating to a darker environment feeling more cosy may be about nostalgia or could be about hiding/not wanting to be seen/being suspicious of the outside world/feeling secluded when feeling unwell. In our interviews with numerous people with schizophrenia, a number talked about choosing to live in darker environments and keeping curtains and blinds drawn during the day.

Therefore, in order to enable the resident to control their environment during the day as their emotions and requirements shifted, strategies needed to be integrated. In the redesign, curtains or blinds were provided on all glazing. Also, dimmer switches were proposed on living area lights. However, on reflection, a darker finish on the storage units may have made for a more mellow environment. The Designing Principles of coherence and manageability are both at play here.

In talking about storage units, that are integral to the Designing Principles of comprehension, manageability and meaningfulness for this person with his collections of books, compact discs and records, he said:

> *I would use it, but I do not know if somebody else would ... I'm not talking about everyone with a mental illness, I'm talking about people I know ... And how they kind of, they have storage but they do not use it ... So it depends how organised their thinking is – or obsessive – and how they do things when they are actually using what they have got in their flat ... Not just using the storage but using what they have collected.*

In our conversations with people with schizophrenia, appropriate storage was raised as a means of decreasing anxiety and agitation. One person talked about the calming effect of being able to put away kitchen condiments in a shallow cupboard that enabled her to see the contents at a glance. Another person in rental accommodation with no doors on her wardrobe talked about how upsetting this was whilst a third person, who liked to paint had to go to great lengths to arrange his home so that he could store his paintings.

Another of the reservations expressed related to the notion of 'discriminatory practices' where society projects onto a person with schizophrenia certain expectations. In addition, the resident has an embodied construct about their place in society (and what built forms are appropriate for a person complying with that construct). The 'habitus' is reflected in the transcript below; that is, they are not worthy of living in a carefully designed home. This relates to one of the Designing Principles identified in our Framework, emotional affordance. The occupant said:

> *I'd have a bit of trouble living in this space that was a little bit - too designed ... so I'm kind of living in this space but I'm feeling I'd be living beyond my means in a sense ... and also I'd be a bit worried about spoiling it.*

In conclusion, in talking about the appropriateness of the redesign for others with schizophrenia, the interviewee said:

> *I can see they would like the design ... how useful it would be to them I do not know – they would be impressed as a place they'd like to live – but whether they would actually use it the way it's designed – maybe – maybe not ... the problem with schizophrenia is that some of the negative symptoms are that kind of lack of living skills - lack of motivation – general apathy and things like that ... So people like that cannot really get it together to do something in their own space .... Their minds are elsewhere.*

Statements such as these complement others made in our earlier user interviews. They challenge designers to reconceptualise what is required and how to resolve the issues. Spaces and furniture may have to be rethought and move beyond the taken-for-granted resolutions to address the issues at hand that surround, for example, storage. The intangible needs as well as the pragmatic requirements need to be integrated purposefully.

4.2.2 Review design development drawings

A local designer, with a large client base, was working with a client where one senior member of the family had schizophrenia (referred to as H in this chapter). The designer agreed to apply the Framework to his design and have it evaluated by the researchers. To this end the designer and his team were briefed on the Practice Document and were given the document to study. During the briefing, the researchers used a number of the designer's previous projects to demonstrate how the Framework could have been incorporated. The designer prepared a preliminary design of a 2-storey house based on his client's brief and on his understanding of the Framework.

Two designer-researchers independently evaluated that preliminary design in relation to the brief, the family needs, the needs of the family member having schizophrenia and the four Designing Principles of comprehension, manageability, meaningfulness and emotional affordance. They both identified similar inadequacies but came up with different design suggestions to better address the Designing Principles. Major limitations revolved around confusing circulation spaces and contorted access to H's room, poor sight lines to major spaces and lack of daylight in critical circulation areas. These design limitations could impact on H's wellbeing by decreasing her ability to function, increase agitation and anxiety, disturb circadian rhythms, create high demand on cognitive energy and suppress her identity.

The researchers advised the designer of the limitations identified. The designer recognised that the design had some limitations and agreed to try to integrate some of the points raised by the researchers. However, from the point of view of a wholehearted commitment to working toward achieving the Design Provisions in the Framework, Bourdieu's concept habitus may be implicated. The designer's 'sense of the game' or unspoken rules may be overriding the opportunity to delve into the issues from different perspectives. The pragmatics of a speedy and cost effective design was the designer's mode of practice. With the agreement of the designer, the researchers attempted to meet independently with the client to better understand the needs of H. This did not eventuate so this review project was terminated.

Questions regarding some common myths about designing for people with ICF were raised. These myths include that:

- designing for people with ICF is essentially about universal design and functionality,
- architecture is of minor value to improving a residents' quality of life and wellbeing,
- ICF is irrelevant if a 'humanistic' approach to design is adopted (i.e. generic 'good design' will always encompass attributes to cater for the needs of people with ICF).

Further reflection on our work with the designer highlighted another consideration when using the Framework to evaluate a design. As the evaluation is confined to addressing the 12 Design Intentions which are all connected with creating a sense of coherence, no other aspects of 'good design' are addressed. The assumption is that the 12 Design Intentions will be used to enhance a 'good design'.[2] If a design does not have the qualities of 'good design' (and it is recognised that this is a contestable space) will

[2] In the only treatise on architecture to survive from antiquity, *De Architectura*, the Roman architect and engineer, Vitruvius, defined three characteristics of good design. They are:

- Durability–It should stand up robustly and remain in good condition
- Utility–It should be useful and function well for the people using it
- Beauty–It should delight people and raise their spirits [42].

the application of our Framework still be able to create a sense of coherence for the occupant of the home? By raising this question we are also implying that good design is a deep understanding known and practiced by all of those associated with the design disciplines, including architecture. Through enculturation and experience accepted ways of practicing and who belongs due to their social capital – and in this case architectural cultural capital—determine or map 'the field'. Therefore, assessing good design when creating environments for positive support and wellbeing raises further issues for discussion.

5. Discussion

As stated throughout this chapter, the Framework is a tool to assist designers and providers to create informed accommodation designs to support those with schizophrenia. The underlying principles acknowledge (in keeping with salutogenic design) [37] that having a sense of coherence enables a person to adapt to a situation and lead a desirable lifestyle for themself. The environment potentially reflects who the resident is in the eyes of others as well as to the individual themselves. It supports the functional requirements and has the potential to also do so for the emotional requirements.

As people do live somewhere, ignoring the physical environment assumes that its role is minimal or insignificant. However, it is well documented that an environment can facilitate functional needs, influence the atmosphere, construct a person's identity, influence judgements made about the resident and add to or reduce the level of stigmatisation. Everyday examples indicate how environmental qualities can influence actions and behaviours; lighting levels, glare levels, temperatures, noise levels, or boundary design can add to insecurities, agitation, anxiety, and the like.

When designing we have proposed that designers and providers need to commence by understanding any conditions that a person from the target-resident group are likely to have, and how it will influence their experience of their day-to-day life at home. And how in turn the environment may play a role, impacting on their quality of life. In summary: Schizophrenia is a condition that some people acquire/have. When designing for such people it is important to consider not only the functional aspects of home, but also how they experience their world emotionally, socially and culturally as well through the PER.

Designers need to be reflective practitioners [43]. Firstly, by being aware that if the person is defined only in terms of their condition, then the functional aspects will dominate the thinking and the outcomes. Also, by being aware that cultural hegemonies infiltrate what people generally believe, everyday myths can be assessed; for example, the proposition that a person with schizophrenia is typically dangerous or violent. Such assumptions influence how the person is integrated into the community, neighbourhood, street, or housing complex—and environmental design is an important component of these situations.

Secondly, as a designer (or provider), it is imperative that they become aware of the assumptions of what the accommodation should be like and what the target-resident will be like. The design process allows the designer to offer innovation through exploration. The innovation will be influenced by the limits of possibilities we set, without reflecting upon where the boundary-construct has come from. In this case, how the collective body of professionals and society conceptualise people with schizophrenia, generates the tacit beliefs that underpin the accommodation typology and its resolution.

With the increasing numbers of people with ICF in our societies across the world it seems timely to look at design and how we assist marginalised groups through our practices. We seek to invite designers and providers to reconsider their practices. At the core of this is the person environment relationship; particularly where the person is part of an interdependent relationship as one defines and influences the other; or in the extreme case where the relationship is no longer noticed. This is where ones habitus may reside [7]. The environment is not just objectified or a removed entity, rather it can be much more integral to a person's being and lifestyle.

Therefore, by designers joining this multidisciplinary 'field', maybe more existing players will develop a greater awareness of the relationship between home and the wellbeing of people with ICF. Perhaps preconceptions of the sort of homes that people with schizophrenia (or other conditions relating to impeded cognitive functioning) deserve can be reconsidered.

6. What of the future

Will the Framework be useful? We envisage that this tool will continually evolve. Firstly, as medical knowledge concerning ICF evolves, so will the knowledge of the condition and the impacts identified. Secondly, as building and digital technologies change, likewise opportunities for sensitive designs will evolve. And thirdly, sociological theories and new understandings of practice may also inform and challenge concepts such as disabilities and mental health. Consequently, the taken-for-granted beliefs and practices may be thrown into relief. Importantly, we established that design-based interventions, for people with cognitive impairment, in domestic situations are low risk and potentially high benefit. The Framework, therefore, has the potential to remain relevant to designers and providers. This comment supports our premise that design considerations can only ever be part of a comprehensive package of support for people with schizophrenia.

We envisage that the process embedded in the Practice Document, including the Framework, will be tested further through its application to constructed projects (houses, units). Testing is complex due to the length of time and cost of construction, the multitude of procurement variables involved and the mix of experiential qualitative aspects with functional and measurable attributes therein. Through assessing the experiences of people living in those homes, the Framework can potentially become more sensitive to the target-resident requirements. Both their daily experiences and the resultant impacts need to be ascertained rather than focusing purely on the pragmatic and functional dimensions. Once again, gauging shifts in peoples' experiences of place and their wellbeing suggest the benefits in marrying disciplines. With all players on the field, opportunities for new understandings at the disciplinary boundaries arise.

Acknowledgements

We acknowledge the assistance of two service providers, Rise and Neami National, including their role in enabling us to contact interviewees who have schizophrenia. We also acknowledge Gaia Sebastiani for her informed input into several of the projects.

Author details

Dianne Smith and Elizabeth Karol*
DEKS Design and Research Consultancy, Curtin University, Perth, West Australia

*Address all correspondence to: elizabeth@deksdesignresearch.com.au

References

[1] Swartz D. Culture and Power: The Sociology of Pierre Bourdieu. Chicago: University of Chicago Press; 1997

[2] Owen C, Lorrimar-Shanks J. Framing the field: The award for sustainable architecture. Art. 2015;**4**(2):34-48. DOI: 10.3390/arts4020034

[3] Bourdieu P, Wacquant L. An Invitation to Reflexive Sociology. London: University of Chicago Press; 1992

[4] Miller D, Branson J. Pierre Bourdieu: Culture and Praxis. In: Austin-Broos D, editor. Creating Culture: Profiles in the Study of Culture. Sydney, NSW: Allen and Unwin; 1987. pp. 210-225

[5] Minami H, Tanaka K. Social and environmental psychology: Transaction between physical space and group-dynamic processes. Environment and Behavior. 1995;**27**(1):43-55

[6] Potter FM. Constructing Trust in Acute Inpatient Mental Healthcare Facilities: The Role of Physical, Social and Symbolic Environments of Care in Supporting Therapeutic Safety [Thesis]. Sydney: UTS; 2017

[7] Smith D. Architectural Experience: A Composition of Viewpoints [Thesis]. Brisbane: Queensland University of Technology; 2000

[8] Malone P. Bourdieu in London. The Journal of Architecture. 2020;**25**(6): 679-696. DOI: 10.1080/13602365.2020.1800792

[9] Matthewson G, Stead N, Burns K. Women and leadership in the Australian architecture profession: Prelude to a research project. In: Seizing the Initiative: Australian Women Leaders in Politics, Workplaces and Communities. Melbourne: eScholarship Research Centre, The University of Melbourne; 2012. p. 10

[10] Australian Bureau of Statistics. Housing Circumstances of People Using Mental Health Services and Prescription Medications [Internet]. Canberra: ABS; 2011 . Available from: https://www.abs.gov.au/statistics/health/mental-health/housing-circumstances-people-using-mental-health-services-and-prescription-medications/latest-release [Accessed: February 1, 2024]

[11] Tehve K, Furgiuele A. Taste and the modern interior, a seminar. In: Proceedings of Interior Design Educators Council; 24–27 March 2010. Atlanta, GA: IDEC; 2010. p. 584

[12] Pallasmaa J. The Eyes of the Skin: Architecture and the Senses. New York: John Wiley; 2005

[13] Ioannidou E. Home no. 7 (a sample of). Interiors. 2021;**11**(1):1-16. DOI: 10.1080/20419112.2020.1836804

[14] Gibson J. The Ecological Approach to Visual Perception. Boston, MA: Houghton Mifflin; 1979

[15] Gifford R. Environmental Psychology: Principles and Practice. Colville, WA: Optimal Books; 2002

[16] Bechtel R, Churchman A, editors. Handbook of Environmental Psychology. New York: Wiley; 2002

[17] Karol E, Smith D. Impact of design on emotional, psychological, or social well-being for people with cognitive impairment. Health Environments Research & Design Journal. 2019;**12**(3): 220-232

[18] Chrysikou E. Why we need new architectural and design paradigms to meet the needs of vulnerable people. Palgrave Communications. 2018;**4**(1):6. DOI: 10.1057/s41599-018-0171-z

[19] Erwine B. Creating Sensory Spaces: The Architecture of the Invisible. New York, NY: Routledge; 2017

[20] Golembiewski J. The designed environment and how it affects the brain. Health Environments Research & Design Journal. 2016;**9**(2):161-171. DOI: 10.1177/1937586715609562

[21] Rivlin L, Moore J. Home-making: Supports and barriers to the process of home. Journal of Social Distress and the Homeless. 2001;**10**(4):323-336

[22] Diener E, Chan M. Happy people live longer: Subjective well-being contributes to health and longevity. Applied Psychology Health Well-Being. 2011; **3**(1):1-43

[23] Lyons G. Quality of life for persons with intellectual disabilities: A review of the literature. In: Kober R, editor. Enhancing the Quality of Life of People with Intellectual Disabilities: From Theory to Practice. Dordrecht: Springer; 2011. pp. 73-126

[24] Saruwono M. Shouting in silence: Expression of self in private homes. Procedia. Social and Behavioral Sciences. 2012;**42**:34-41

[25] Lockard E. Human Migration to Space: Alternative Technological Approaches for Long-Term Adaptation to Extraterrestrial Environments. New York: Springer eBooks; 2014. p. 2014

[26] Hudson K. Salutogenesis: The origin of health. Nursing Management. 2013; **44**(11):12-30. DOI: 10.1097/01. NUMA.0000436369.45139.81

[27] Breakwell G, Hammond S, Fife-Schaw C, Smith J. Research Methods in Psychology. 3rd ed. London: Sage Publications; 2006. p. 311

[28] McTaggart R. Is validity really an issue for participatory action research. Studies in Cultures, Organizations & Societies. 2005;**4**(2):10245286

[29] Hart E, Bond M. Action Research for Health and Social Care: A Guide to Practice. Buckingham: Open University Press; 1995. ISBN 0 335 19262 9

[30] Karol E, Smith D. Using creative practice to re-conceptualize provision of services in intractable situations. The International Journal of Design in Society. 2015;**8**(3/4):15-25. DOI: 10.18848/2325-1328/CGP/v08i3-4/38567

[31] Smith D, Karol E. Improving chances? A design strategy to improve health and wellbeing for marginalised people. Australasian Medical Journal. 2017;**10**(6):478-488. DOI: 10.21767/AMJ.2017.2993

[32] Karol E, Smith D. Impact of design on emotional, psychological, or social well-being for people with cognitive impairment. HERD: Health Environments Research & Design Journal. 2018;**12**(3): 220-232. Advanced online publication. DOI: 10.1177/1937586718813194

[33] Smith D, Karol E. Beyond the Tangible [Internet]. 2017. Available from: https://beyondtangible.wixsite.com/beyondtangibledesign [Accessed: January 30, 2024]

[34] Karol E, Smith D. Expanding design approaches to create supportive home environments for people with impeded cognitive functioning. Design for Health. 2020;**4**(1):43-62. DOI: 10.1080/24735132.2020.1732730

[35] Smith D, Karol E. An accommodation design matrix to assist the provision of supportive accommodation for people with altered cognitive functioning. Design for Health. 2019;**3**(2):261-282. DOI: 10.1080/24735132.2019.1641398

[36] Riopel L. What does it mean to have a sense of coherence? (+ Scale) [Internet]. 2020. Available from: https://positivepsychology.com/sense-of-coherence-scale/ [Accessed: February 21, 2024]

[37] Dilani A. Psychosocially supportive design: A salutogenic approach to the design of the physical environment. Design and Health Scientific Review. 2008;**1**(2):47-55

[38] Karol E, Smith D. Beyond the Tangible-DEKS Practice Document [Internet]. 2017. Available from: https://beyondtangible.wixsite.com/beyondtangibledesign [Accessed: January 30, 2024]

[39] NSW Law Reform Commission. People with Cognitive and Mental Health Impairments in the Criminal Justice System – Diversion. Sydney, Australia: NSW Law Reform Commission. Report No. 135 June 2012. 2012. Available from: https://lawreform.nsw.gov.au/documents/Publications/Reports/Report-135.pdf [Accessed: February 21, 2024]

[40] Smith D, Karol E. Beyond the Tangible-Testing the Framework: Virtual redesign [Internet]. 2024. Available from: https://beyondtangible.wixsite.com/beyondtangibledesign. [Accessed: January 30, 2024]

[41] Rybczynski W. Home: Á Short History of an Idea. New York: Penguin Books; 1987

[42] Vitruvius M. The 10 Books of Architecture. New York: Dover Publications; 1960

[43] Schon D. The Reflective Practitioner: How Professionals Think in Action. New York: Basic Books; 1983

Chapter 3

Myo-inositol's Role in Understanding the Pain Perception in Patients with Schizophrenia

Wirginia Krzyściak, Marta Szwajca, Paulina Karcz, Aleksander Turek, Natalia Śmierciak, Amira Bryll, Paulina Mazur, Robert Chrzan, Katarzyna Furman, Maciej Pilecki and Tadeusz Popiela

Abstract

The molecular explanation for the changes in pain perception in schizophrenia lies in nerve inflammation. The decrease in inositol, mainly localized in glial cells, can support these changes. There are also significant alterations in the viability and functioning of neurons, which are linked to a significant reduction of N-acetyl-aspartate (NAA). Our study demonstrates significantly increased myo-inositol levels in the anterior and posterior cingulate cortex. An increase in the myo-inositol/sum of the creatinine and phosphocreatinine (Cr + PCr) ratio and NAA levels additionally supports the notion of inositol's beneficial impact on brain metabolism and neuronal integrity, which is particularly relevant to schizophrenia's neurodegenerative changes. However, varying NAA/Cr + PCr ratios indicate a complex interaction between the brain's inositol level and energy metabolism or neurochemical balance. These findings highlight inositol's potential role in modulating neurochemical profiles in schizophrenia. Furthermore, high inositol levels are linked to significant reductions in trauma-related symptoms in schizophrenia, as indicated by the International Trauma Questionnaire and the Child Trauma Questionnaire. Inositol's potential to mitigate trauma effects, and enhance social functioning and its multifaceted role in schizophrenia, offers a promising avenue for further research into its therapeutic applications.

Keywords: pain perception, myo-inositol, negative symptoms, schizophrenia, precision psychiatry

1. Introduction

Globally, pain presents a significant challenge, affecting approximately 20% of adults, with 10% each year diagnosed with chronic pain. Pain manifests in various forms, including acute, chronic, and intermittent, or a mix of these. Chronic pain, in particular, is a profound source of distress, disrupting daily activities and often leading to significant suffering [1].

Pain is recognized as a multifaceted phenomenon, integrating the complex interplay of neuroanatomy and neurochemistry with cognitive and emotional mechanisms [2, 3].

The International Association for the Study of Pain (IASP) defines pain as "an unpleasant sensory and emotional experience associated with, or resembling that associated with, actual or potential tissue damage" [4]. Pain is a subjective experience shaped significantly by biological, psychological, and societal influences.

The experience of pain varies greatly in its intensity, nature, and duration. Pain transcends mere symptoms, and chronic pain is acknowledged as a distinct medical condition with its own unique developmental course and clinical features [5]. People's pain perception thresholds vary significantly, making it challenging to accurately predict the level of injury that will cause pain [6].

Meta-analyses have elucidated that individuals with psychosis generally exhibit a lower pain sensitivity compared to those in the general population [7]. The recognition of reduced pain sensitivity in schizophrenia dates back to the foundational psychiatric studies by Bleuler and Kraepelin in the early twentieth century [8, 9]. Originally, Kraepelin described Dementia Praecox, noting that such patients could endure burns from cigarettes and tolerate needle punctures or wounds without typical adaptive responses. Bleuler, who coined the term "schizophrenia" for Kraepelin's Dementia Praecox, made similar findings about reduced pain responses to harmful stimuli on the body or skin of these individuals.

A significant number of case reports and series have documented that individuals with schizophrenia exhibit a lower sensitivity to pain, a phenomenon that often confounds clinicians, especially when these patients fail to report pain despite having painful physical conditions [10, 11]. Studies have consistently shown that this demographic is prone to a higher incidence of physical health issues that are typically painful, such as fractures [12], diabetes [13], cancer [14], and cardiovascular diseases [15]. This paradoxical situation underscores the complex relationship between schizophrenia and pain perception. About 40% of individuals with schizophrenia experiencing clinical pain did not communicate their pain to a healthcare provider [16].

These meta-analyses reveal a general trend toward diminished pain sensitivity in schizophrenia, yet findings are not uniform [7, 10]. Some studies suggest that individuals with schizophrenia perceive pain similarly to the general population [17, 18], while others observe an increased sensitivity to acute pain but a decreased sensitivity to prolonged, chronic pain [19]. Additionally, it has been revealed that schizophrenia patients may actually be hypersensitive to pain induction compared to healthy controls, suggesting that their apparent hypoalgesia may stem more from a reduced tendency to report pain rather than a decreased perception of pain itself [17].

Research has shown that one in three individuals with psychosis indicates experiencing pain that is clinically significant. Furthermore, the existence of pain has been identified as an indicator of a reduced quality of life related to health in those with psychosis [20].

The explanation for the altered perception of pain in schizophrenia may be related to described neuro-metabolic changes involving significant differences in levels of neuron-glia activation. Reduced pain sensations in schizophrenia may be associated with decreased levels of anterior cingulate cortex (ACC) myo-inositol (compared to controls) [21] linked to astrocyte activation, among other factors such as the lack of response to conventional antipsychotic medications [22]. Conversely, decreased levels of N-acetylaspartate (NAA), most likely reflect a neuronal process supported by myo-inositol, which reflects a characteristic neurometabolic process characterizing the mutual interactions of neuron-glia in altered pain perception. Insensitivity to pain in schizophrenia is a complex phenomenon. Impairment of cognitive function and an excess of negative symptoms can strongly influence the expression of pain by patients with schizophrenia [23]. Chronic pain in the context of schizophrenia presents a complex issue, combining neurobiological dysfunction with manifesting psychotic symptoms. Understanding this phenomenon requires considering the role of N-methyl-D-aspartate (NMDA) receptors and the intricate interactions between Src kinase and neuregulin 1 (NRG1) signaling and its ErbB4 receptors [24]. The phenomenon of excessive NRG1-ErbB4 signaling, genetically associated with the positive symptoms of this disease, may lead to the suppression of physiological enhancement of NMDA receptor function by Src, resulting in NMDAR hypofunction [25–29]. Such a state may serve as the basis for many psychopathological symptoms characteristic of schizophrenia, including cognitive impairments and hallucinations, and may also contribute to the occurrence of chronic pain by disrupting the adequate processing of pain signals. Excessive NRG1-ErbB4 signaling, through the suppression of Src activity and NMDA receptor regulation, may lead to the persistence of pain states by disrupting adaptive pain mechanisms, thus contributing to the chronic nature of pain in schizophrenia [24].

The altered perception of pain underlies many theories regarding suicide [30]. In the case of individuals attempting suicide, "interoceptive numbness" has been demonstrated, characterized by increased tolerance for aversive experiences and decreased awareness of non-aversive sensations. Hence, blunted interoception may be associated with suicidal behaviors [31]. Researchers have always tried to understand the motivations of suicide victims, however, our current scientific knowledge about the factors contributing to suicidal behaviors and the increasing number of suicides each year are insufficient [32].

Based on the International Suicide Prevention Guidelines (InterSePT) in schizophrenia, factors that may contribute to reducing suicidal tendencies include improvement of positive and negative symptoms, reduction of extrapyramidal side effects (EPS), direct antidepressant effects, improvement of cognitive function, and strict adherence to recommendations [33].

It is hypothesized that the phenomenon of altered pain perception in schizophrenia may be intricately associated with neurochemical imbalances within the brain, specifically a diminution in myo-inositol levels in the anterior cingulate cortex and decreased levels of NAA. This reduction, alongside myo-inositol's critical function in modulating glial cell volume amid neuroinflammatory events, might underpin the unique sensory processing aberrations observed in this condition. Consequently, it is further postulated that therapeutic strategies aimed at rectifying these neurobiological discrepancies, particularly through the administration of inositol, could not only ameliorate the aberrant pain perception but also confer wider benefits. These could potentially encompass the alleviation of associated affective disturbances and an enhancement in the overall functioning of individuals with schizophrenia, thereby suggesting a broader scope of inositol's therapeutic efficacy.

2. The aim of the study

The extent to which myo-inositol levels in the anterior cingulate cortex correlate with hematologic and neurochemical markers as well as with psychometric assessments, thus contributing to understanding of the neurobiological basis of psychiatric conditions primarily related to changes in pain perception in patients with schizophrenia.

3. Material and methods

This endeavor sought to determine the extent to which myo-inositol levels correlate with hematological and neurochemical markers, as well as with psychometric assessments, thereby contributing to a more integrated understanding of the neurobiological underpinnings of psychiatric conditions, mainly associated with changes in pain sensation.

3.1 Participants

Clinical assessment and recruitment of study participants were carried out at the Clinical Department of Adult, Child, and Adolescent Psychiatry at the University Hospital in Krakow, Poland. Diagnosis of schizophrenia (code F20 according to the 10th revision of the International Statistical Classification of Diseases and Related Health Problems, ICD-10), confirmed by two psychiatrists, was the inclusion criterion for participants in the research [34, 35]. The Positive and Negative Syndrome Scale (PANSS) was used for evaluation of symptomatology and severity of disease [36]. Study participants, in age ranging from 13 to 40 years, provided written consent for the research procedures. In the case of study participants under the age of 18, consent was signed by legal guardians. Study participants were inpatients. Duration of the disease ranged from 2 months to 2 years. The research was approved by Jagiellonian University Bioethics Committee: 1072.6120.252.2021 and 1072.6120.178.2022.

The study's exclusion criteria include a lot of aspects. Excluded were participants with limited legal capacity, intellectual disabilities and under court-ordered treatment. Individuals with insulin resistance, diabetes, metabolic syndrome, severe cardiovascular diseases, or a history of central nervous system disorders were not included in the study. Additionally, taking specific medications, such as clozapine treatment within the last 3 months before the study, recent use (within 3 days before the study) of non-steroidal anti-inflammatory drugs, corticosteroids, vitamin supplements, antibiotics, probiotics, antioxidants, psychoactive, narcotic substances, and changes or modifications of antipsychotic treatment within 12 weeks before the study, were also exclusion criteria. Furthermore, ineligible were also individuals with substance dependence (diagnosed according to ICD-10) and participants with alcohol or substance abuse (excluding tobacco) within 3 months before the study. Hyperactivity, psychomotor agitation, intense affective symptoms, pregnancy, breastfeeding, inability to remain in a supine position (due to spinal deformity), severe claustrophobia, the presence of pacemakers, cochlear implants, neurostimulators, drug delivery pumps or other implanted electronic devices, vascular clips, artificial heart valves, metallic orthopedic implants such as screws, artificial joints, stabilizers, and wires, were encompassed as exclusion criteria. Grounds for exclusion were also metallic foreign bodies like iron filings or other metal instrumentation which are contraindicated in magnetic resonance techniques. The criterion for exclusion was age ≤ 13 and ≥ 40 years. Excluded were also participants without a diagnosis by a psychiatrist according to ICD-10.

The control group embraced 45 healthy volunteers, aged between 13 and 40 years, and with an equal gender distribution. These participants, based on the ICD-10 criteria, did not have a diagnosis of schizophrenia or other mental disorders.

The General Health Questionnaire-28 (GHQ-28) [37, 38], used for detecting possible mental disorders and emotional distress in general population, was completed by all participants [39]. The Global Assessment of Functioning (GAF) [40] (Axis V in the

Diagnostic and Statistical Manual of Mental Disorders, Fourth Edition, DSM-IV-TR) was conducted for assessment of current social, occupational and mental functioning [41]. The Gastrointestinal Symptom Rating Scale (GSRS) was used to evaluate gastrointestinal symptoms [42, 43]. The Beck Depression Inventory (BDI-II) [44], the State and Trait Anxiety Inventory (STAI) [45], and the Experiences in Close Relationships-Revised Short (ECR-RS), were completed by all participants in order to assess attachment styles on the two dimensions of anxiety and avoidance in close relationships [46, 47]. The Traumatic Experiences Checklist (TEC) [48] was also conducted to self-assessment of potentially traumatic experiences in childhood and adulthood and to reflect the number of potentially adverse and traumatic events in life.

3.2 Treatment

Pharmacological treatment of schizophrenia patients was conducted in accordance with the guidelines of the American Psychiatric Association. Medications were received by patients in oral (p.o.) and intramuscular (i.m.) forms. Antipsychotic medications include perazine, levomepromazine, chlorpromazine, aripiprazole, risperidone, cariprazine, lurasidone, haloperidol, olanzapine, zuclopenthixol, amisulpride and quetiapine. One of the study participants was not prescribed any medications. Eight of the patients were on monotherapy, and the remainder 42 were undergoing polytherapy. Dose conversion of antipsychotics was based on the methods described by Davis and Chen (2004) [49], or Andreasen et al. (2010) [50], and conducted using chlorpromazine equivalent dose (CPZE). In the case of amisulpride the daily dose was determined using the WHOCC—ATC/DDD Index, 2023 [51]. Additionally, as recommended by Leucht et al. (2016), lurasidone was administered to seven study participants [52].

3.3 Blood collection for routine laboratory tests

From both patients and healthy volunteers, blood for comprehensive laboratory tests was collected in the morning, after overnight rest, an 8-h fasting period and in the case of chronic medications, before medication intake. These laboratory examinations included complete blood count, serum creatinine concentration, uric acid, ionogram (K^+, Na^+, Mg^{2+}), lipid profile (low-density lipoprotein, high-density lipoprotein, LDL and HDL; total cholesterol, TC and triglycerides, TG), alanine aminotransferase (ALT) activity, glucose, insulin, HOMA-IR index, inflammatory markers (high-sensitivity C-reactive protein, hsCRP), complement components C3 and C4, thyroid function tests (free triiodothyronine, FT3, free thyroxine, FT4, and thyroid-stimulating hormone, TSH), as well as antibodies against thyroid peroxidase (anti-TPO), serum ferritin level and adrenal parameter assessment (dehydroepiandrosterone sulfate, DHEA-S).

Analyses were performed with using automated analyzers, in the laboratory of the University Hospital in Krakow. The University Hospital laboratory in Krakow, in accordance with standards for medical diagnostic laboratories, undergoes daily internal and systematic external quality control.

3.4 Magnetic resonance techniques

Magnetic resonance examinations were performed in the Diagnostic Imaging Department at the University Hospital in Krakow, Poland.

The determined metabolites were: Creatine (Cr 3.02 and 3.9 ppm), Phosphocreatine (PCr 3.02 ppm and 3.93 ppm), L-Alanine (Ala 1.48 ppm), Aspartate (Asp 3.8 ppm), Glutamine (Gln 2.45 and 3.7 ppm), Glutamate (Glu 2.1 and 3.7 ppm), Glucose (Glc 3.43 and 3.8 ppm), γ-aminobutyric acid (GABA 2.3 ppm),, Phosphocholine (PCh 4.2 ppm), Glycerophosphocholine (GPC 3.6 ppm), Glutathione (GSH 3.7 ppm), N-Acetylaspartate (NAA 2.02 ppm), N-Acetylaspartylglutamate (NAAG 4.1 ppm), L-Lactate (Lac 1.33 ppm), myo-Inositol (Ins 3.6 ppm), scyllo-Inositol (Scyllo 3.35 ppm), Taurine (Tau 3.42 ppm), macromolecule (MM09 0.9 ppm, MM12 1.2 ppm, MM14 1.4 ppm, MM17 1.7 ppm, MM20 2.0 ppm) and Lipids (Lip09 0.9 ppm, Lip13a and Lip13b 1.3 ppm, Lip20 2.0 ppm). Calculated were concentrations of the sums of individual metabolites: Cr + PCr, Glu + Gln, NAA + NAAG, GPC + PCh, Lip13a + Lip13b, MM20 + Lip20, MM09 + Lip09, MM14 + Lip13a + Lip13b + MM12. The ratios of every metabolite to the sum of creatine and phosphocreatine were also calculated, e. g. NAA/(Cr + PCr). The MRS results were subjected to both qualitative and quantitative analysis.

Quality control was carried out in relation to the signal-to-noise ratio and to width of the spectral lines.

3.5 Statistical analysis

For the analysis presented, the threshold for statistical significance was set at an alpha level of 0.05. This means that results with p-values less than or equal to 0.05 were considered statistically significant, indicating a less than 5% probability that the observed effects were due to chance.

Descriptive statistics such as central tendency (mean, median), variability (standard deviation), positioning (the first and third quartiles), and extreme values (minimum and maximum), were employed to characterize the distributions of the parameters under study. These statistical measures provide a comprehensive summary of the dataset, aiding in the interpretation of the results and offering valuable insights into the underlying distribution and characteristics of the studied clinical parameters. This statistical approach ensures that the results are not only assessed for significance but also thoroughly described in terms of their distributional properties, which is essential for understanding the full context of the findings within the clinical research framework.

The investigation into the effects of inositol exposure on clinical outcomes was conducted using regression analyses that accounted for a set of critical covariates to ensure that the findings were adjusted for potential confounding variables. These covariates encompass demographic characteristics, specifically sex and age, which are fundamental factors known to influence clinical outcomes. Additionally, the analysis controlled for the variability in psychotropic medication dosages by standardizing them to chlorpromazine equivalents (further – CPZ equivalent), a common metric used to facilitate the comparison of antipsychotic drug potencies.

By including these covariates in the regression models, the analysis aimed to isolate the association between inositol exposure and the clinical outcomes from the effects of these other influential variables. This approach enhances the validity of the findings by reducing the likelihood that the observed associations are confounded by demographic differences or variations in psychotropic medication dosages. By doing so, it strengthens the inference that any significant associations uncovered between inositol exposure and the clinical outcomes are likely attributable to the effects of inositol itself, rather than extraneous factors.

3.5.1 Doubly robust generalized estimating equations (DGREE)

To mitigate the potential errors that might stem from incorrect model specifications, a doubly robust estimation approach was employed [53–56]. This method relies on two separate models: one that predicts the outcome and another that estimates the exposure. The strength of this technique lies in its ability to provide unbiased estimates of the relationship between the exposure and the outcome, provided at least one of the two models is accurately specified — it is not required for both to be perfectly correct.

The generic equations for a doubly robust estimation are (1), (2):

Outcome model (structural model):

$$Y = g^{-1}\left(\beta_0 + \beta_1 \cdot X_1 + \beta_2 \cdot X_2 + \ldots + \beta_k \cdot X_k + \varepsilon\right), \tag{1}$$

where Y – is the outcome variable (every single studied parameter), g^{-1} – is the inverse of the link function for the outcome (log as a result of the fact that some of the outcome variables were skewed), β_0 – is the intercept, β_k were the coefficients for confounders X_k and ε is the error term, k – number of confounders.

Exposure model:

$$E = h^{-1}\left(\alpha_0 + \alpha_1 \cdot Z_1 + \alpha_2 \cdot Z_2 + \ldots + \alpha_m \cdot Z_m\right), \tag{2}$$

where E – is the exposure variable (inositol concentration), h^{-1} – is the inverse of the link function for the exposure (log as well), α_0 – is the intercept, α_i were the coefficients for confounders Z_i, m – number of confounders.

The doubly robust estimation combines these two models, and it will yield unbiased estimates if either the outcome model or the exposure model is correctly specified. It does this by incorporating the predicted exposure (from the exposure model) and the observed exposure into the analysis of the outcome, thus adjusting for confounding factors and potential errors in model specification.

3.5.2 Statistical environment

Analyses were conducted using the R Statistical language (version 4.3.1, [57]) on Windows 10 Pro 64 bit (build 19,045), using the packages *drgee* (version 1.1.10, [58]), psych (version 2.3.9, [59]), dplyr (version 1.1.3, [60]) and readxl (version 1.4.3, [61]).

3.6 Characteristics of the studied cohort

In this study, we conducted a comprehensive analysis of a cohort consisting of 51 patients diagnosed with schizophrenia. The demographic breakdown of the cohort included 21 women, representing 41.2% of the sample, and 30 men, accounting for the remaining 58.8%.

The primary data metrics encompassed demographic profiles, hematological indices, neurochemical markers, and outcomes of standardized questionnaires. These variables were meticulously collated to furnish a descriptive summary. The aggregated data are methodically delineated in **Table 1**.

Parameter	*n*	*M*	*SD*	*Mdn*	*Q1*	*Q3*	*Min*	*Max*
Age, years	51	27,71	9,36	30,00	18,00	35,50	14,00	46,00
Hematological measurements and drug intake								
Chlorpromazine equivalent dose (100 mg CPZ equivalent)	51	390.61	250.15	370.00	200.00	565.00	0.00	970.00
WBC [$\times 10^3/\mu L$]	51	7.42	2.30	6.93	5.74	8.45	3.55	14.03
Neut, %	51	60.31	16.17	58.50	52.05	65.40	37.70	79.7
Lymphocyte count [$\times 10^3/\mu L$]	51	2.15	0.66	2.24	1.60	2.60	0.71	3.52
Neurochemical measurements								
Myo-inositol [$\times 10^{-6}/\mu L$], ACC ET 30,[1]	50	152.66	18.83	154.00	145.00	166.00	94.20	188.00
Myo-inositol /cr + pcr, ACC TE 30[2]	50	0.91	0.10	0.92	0.85	0.98	0.65	1.07
NAA conc. [$\times 10^{-6}$], ACC 30,[3]	50	200.14	21.47	199.00	185.00	213.25	138.00	244.00
NAA /Cr + PCr, ACC 30[4]	50	1.19	0.12	1.18	1.12	1.24	0.88	1.69
Mio-inositol, ACC 144[5]	50	967.88	283.08	978.87	793.73	1107.50	437.34	2280.00
Mio-inositol /Cr + PCr, AC 144[6]	50	0.98	0.26	0.94	0.86	1.11	0.45	2.24
NAA, ACC 144[7]	50	1443.69	219.91	1440.00	1322.50	1557.50	888.31	2050.00
NAA/Cr + PCr, ACC 144[8]	50	1.46	0.20	1.44	1.36	1.56	0.86	2.40
Myo-inositol [$\times 10^{-6}$], PCC 30[9]	50	118.23	14.71	118.00	107.25	128.75	87.30	145.00
Myo -inositol /Cr + Pcr, PCC 30[10]	50	0.85	0.09	0.85	0.80	0.90	0.65	1.09
NAA conc. [$\times 10^{-6}$], PCC 30	50	188.78	14.56	188.00	180.00	198.25	151.00	217.00
NAA /Cr + PCr, PCC 30	50	1.36	0.13	1.34	1.27	1.46	1.06	1.64
Myo-inositol, PCC 144[11]	50	680.54	170.02	663.08	564.07	775.42	372.01	1130.00
Myo-inositol/Cr + PCr, PCC 144[12]	50	0.88	0.17	0.86	0.76	0.99	0.58	1.26
NAA, PCC 144	50	1323.40	129.58	1325.00	1235.00	1415.00	1030.00	1580.00
NAA/cr + pcr, PCC 144	50	1.73	0.17	1.73	1.61	1.87	1.35	2.03

Parameter	*n*	*M*	*SD*	*Mdn*	*Q1*	*Q3*	*Min*	*Max*
PANSS questionnaire								
Positive symptoms score	50	21.24	7.66	22.00	17.25	25.75	0.00	42.00
Negative symptoms score	50	20.72	7.32	23.00	16.25	25.75	0.00	33.00
Disorganized speech score	50	16.88	5.95	17.00	13.00	21.00	0.00	31.00
Uncontrolled hostility/excitement score	50	7.26	2.67	8.00	5.00	9.00	0.00	13.00
Anxiety/depression score	50	11.70	4.17	12.00	9.00	14.00	0.00	22.00
Positive scale score	50	17.34	6.32	19.00	14.00	22.00	0.00	33.00
Negative scale score	50	20.98	7.29	22.00	15.00	26.00	0.00	34.00
General psychopathology scale score	50	39.38	12.00	39.50	35.00	47.00	0.00	63.00
Total score	50	78.20	23.93	80.00	70.00	93.00	0.00	126.00
Gastrointestinal symptoms								
Total score	46	18.83	16.49	17.50	7.25	27.75	0.00	83.00
SANS questionnaire								
Total score	50	51.28	24.53	54.00	31.00	69.50	6.00	93.00
Calgary questionnaire								
Total score	50	8.58	6.26	6.50	4.00	11.00	0.00	22.00
BDI-II questionnaire								
Total score	46	18.76	14.28	18.50	5.25	29.00	0.00	51.00
CISS questionnaire								
Task-oriented coping scale score	39	49.77	10.51	48.00	43.00	56.00	27.00	73.00

Parameter	*n*	*M*	*SD*	*Mdn*	*Q1*	*Q3*	*Min*	*Max*
Emotion-oriented coping scale score	39	47.87	12.18	45.00	37.50	57.50	26.00	75.00
Avoidance-oriented coping scale score	39	44.23	8.51	44.00	39.00	50.00	23.00	61.00
Distraction scale score	39	20.46	5.64	21.00	18.00	24.00	2.00	30.00
Social diversion scale score	39	14.97	4.36	15.00	12.00	17.50	6.00	25.00
Total score	39	141.87	19.87	143.00	128.00	155.00	100.00	181.00
ITQ questionnaire								
Reexperiencing trauma score	42	2.88	2.20	3.00	1.00	5.00	0.00	8.00
Avoidance score	42	3.74	2.52	4.00	2.00	6.00	0.00	8.00
Threat score	42	3.98	2.41	4.00	2.00	6.00	0.00	8.00
Affective dysregulation score	42	4.00	2.13	4.00	2.00	5.00	0.00	8.00
Negative self-concept score	42	3.93	2.82	4.00	2.00	6.00	0.00	8.00
Disturbance relationships score	42	3.98	2.57	4.00	2.00	6.00	0.00	8.00
PTSDFI score	42	5.93	3.90	6.00	3.00	9.00	0.00	12.00
DSOFI score	42	5.60	3.77	5.00	2.25	9.00	0.00	12.00
PTSD score	42	10.60	6.34	11.00	6.00	15.00	0.00	24.00
DSO score	42	11.71	7.05	10.50	6.50	18.75	0.00	24.00
Total score	42	33.83	18.06	31.50	21.50	48.75	0.00	71.00
CTQ questionnaire								
Emotional abuse score	42	11.38	5.01	10.00	8.00	14.00	5.00	24.00
Physical abuse score	42	6.50	2.50	5.00	5.00	7.00	5.00	16.00

Parameter	n	M	SD	Mdn	Q1	Q3	Min	Max
Sexual abuse score	42	6.64	2.68	6.00	5.00	6.00	5.00	15.00
Emotional neglect score	42	11.67	5.05	11.00	7.25	14.00	5.00	23.00
Physical neglect score	42	8.26	2.88	8.00	6.00	9.00	5.00	16.00
Denial (minimization/denial) score	42	9.12	2.47	9.00	7.00	11.00	3.00	13.00
Total score	42	66.45	16.67	64.00	53.25	76.00	43.00	105.00

[1]The myo-inositol concentration in anterior cingulate cortex (ACC) at echo time (ET) 30 ms [$\times 10^{-6}/\mu L$]).
[2]The myo-inositol to Creatine and Phosphocreatine Ratio in ACC at TE 30 ms.
[3]The concentration of N-acetylaspartate in the ACC at an ET of 30 ms.
[4]The ratio of N-acetylaspartate to the sum of creatine and phosphocreatine in the ACC at an ET of 30 ms.
[5]The concentration of myo-inositol in the ACC, potentially modulated by insulin, measured at an ET of 144 ms.
[6]The ratio of insulin levels to creatine and phosphocreatine in the ACC at an ET of 144 ms.
[7]The concentration of N-acetylaspartate in the ACC measured at an ET of 144 ms.
[8]The ratio of N-acetylaspartate to the sum of creatine and phosphocreatine in the ACC at an ET of 144 ms.
[9]The concentration of myo-inositol adjusted for insulin levels in the posterior cingulate cortex (PCC) at an echo time of 30 ms.
[10]The ratio of myo-inositol to creatine and phosphocreatine adjusted for insulin levels in the PCC at an ET of 30 ms.
[11]The concentration of myo-inositol in the PCC that adjusted by insulin, measured at an ET of 144 ms.
[12]The ratios of myo-inositol to the sum of creatine and phosphocreatine in the PCC, measured at an ET of 144 ms.
Note: n – group size, M – mean, SD – standard deviation, Mdn – median, Q1 – the first quartile, Q3 – the third quartile, Min – minimal value, Max – maximum value, PANSS – Positive and Negative Syndrome Scale, SANS – Scale for Assessment of Negative Symptoms, CALGARY – Calgary Depression Scale for Schizophrenia, BDI-II – the Beck Depression Inventory, CISS – Coping Inventory for Stressful Situations, ITQ – International Trauma Questionnaire; PTSDFI – post-traumatic stress disorder functional impairment; DSOFI – disturbances in self-organization functional impairment; PTSD – post-traumatic stress disorder; DSO – disturbances in self-organization; CTQ – Childhood Trauma Questionnaire.

Table 1.
Descriptive statistics of the studied parameters.

3.6.1 Demographic

The data reflect a mean age within the late twenties, indicative of a patient cohort in which schizophrenia typically manifests, considering the peak onset of the disorder often occurs in early adulthood. Variability in age is moderate and encompasses both the prodromal phase of late adolescence and the established phase in middle adulthood.

3.6.2 Hematological measurements and drugs intake

Dosing of antipsychotics, expressed in chlorpromazine equivalents, reveals a wide distribution, suggesting a heterogeneity in the clinical presentation and severity of the disorder within the cohort, necessitating a broad range of pharmacotherapeutic interventions. This variance also implies potential differences in treatment response or tolerability, given the considerable spread in dosages required to achieve therapeutic effects or manage side effects.

The white blood cell count is within the normal reference range for the majority, which is reassuring as it indicates no widespread hematological impact that could be attributed to the chronic use of antipsychotic medications, which are known to sometimes cause agranulocytosis. However, the range does indicate that a few patients may be experiencing leukopenia or leukocytosis.

Neutrophil percentages sit within expected values for a non-acute cohort but do exhibit variability, potentially reflective of individual responses to stress, infection, or pharmacological effects. The absence of extremely high values mitigates concern for neutrophilia which could indicate acute infection or a severe stress response.

Lymphocyte counts are consistent and fall within normal limits, suggesting stable immunological profiles within the group. The lack of significant outliers in lymphocyte counts may indicate that the cohort, on the whole, is not experiencing acute immunological challenges or significant adverse effects from medication that would manifest in lymphocyte levels.

3.6.3 Neurochemical measurements

The neurochemical profile of the cohort provides data on the metabolic environment of the ACC and PCC, two regions implicated in the pathophysiology of schizophrenia. Myo-inositol levels and NAA concentrations, alongside their ratios to creatine and phosphocreatine (Cr + PCr), offer a window into neuronal health and glial activity, both of which are pertinent to the neuropsychiatric context.

Elevated myo-inositol levels, a putative glial marker, might suggest glial proliferation or altered glial function, which is consistent with neuroinflammatory hypotheses of schizophrenia. The mean myo-inositol levels in the ACC and PCC fall within a range that does not immediately indicate pronounced glial pathology, yet variability in these levels may correlate with individual differences in disease manifestation or progression.

The NAA concentration serves as an indirect marker of neuronal integrity and function, with aberrations often reflecting neuronal loss or dysfunction. The mean NAA levels in both ACC and PCC are within normal ranges but again reveal individual variability. The standard deviations and range of values intimate that subgroups within the cohort may exhibit neurochemical signatures of neuronal compromise.

DOI: http://dx.doi.org/10.5772/intechopen.1005244

Ratios of myo-inositol and NAA to Cr + PCr are critical in standardizing these metabolite concentrations against a relatively stable reference, which mitigates inter-individual and instrumental variability. The reported mean ratios are suggestive of preserved metabolic homeostasis in the context of schizophrenia, though the breadth of the data indicates a spectrum of neurochemical states within the cohort.

The extended echo time (TE) of 144 ms compared to the standard TE of 30 ms provides an enhanced specificity in the metabolite resonance and suggests a more robust signal for myo-inositol and NAA. The discrepancies in metabolite concentrations and ratios at different echo times may reflect the complex interplay of relaxation times and signal-to-noise ratios inherent to magnetic resonance spectroscopy.

3.6.4 PANSS questionnaire

Positive symptoms, characterized by the presence of psychopathology such as hallucinations, delusions, and disorganized thought processes, exhibited a mean score that suggests a moderate level of severity across the cohort. The range and standard deviation indicate substantial heterogeneity in the presentation of positive symptoms, with some individuals experiencing minimal symptomatology while others may be grappling with severe manifestations.

Negative symptoms, which reflect deficits such as blunted affect, social withdrawal, and anhedonia, also show a moderate mean score with variability comparable to that of positive symptoms. The breadth of negative symptom scores underscores the diverse impact of schizophrenia on emotional responsiveness and social functioning, which are crucial determinants of long-term outcomes and functional capacity.

Disorganized speech is a cardinal feature of schizophrenia, indicative of formal thought disorder. The scores here suggest a modest mean level of disorganization, which could impact communication and cognitive coherence. The range of scores points to the presence of subgroups within the cohort with varying degrees of communicative and cognitive disruption.

Uncontrolled hostility and excitement are less prevalent than other symptom domains, as reflected by the lower mean score.

Anxiety and depression, which can be secondary to the core symptomatology or intrinsic to the schizophrenia spectrum, present with a lower mean score relative to other symptom domains but are non-negligible.

The positive and negative scale scores, which are composite measures, corroborate the individual symptom domain scores, with the negative scale scores slightly exceeding the positive scale scores on average. This suggests that the negative symptoms may be more prominent or persistent in the cohort studied, which aligns with clinical understanding that negative symptoms are often more resistant to current pharmacotherapies and predictive of poorer functional outcomes.

General psychopathology scores, which encompass a wider range of symptoms such as guilt feelings, tension, and active social avoidance, are the highest among the domains. This reflects the broad impact of schizophrenia beyond the core symptom clusters of positive and negative symptoms, highlighting the complex interplay of affective, cognitive, and behavioral components in this disorder.

The total PANSS score, encompassing the spectrum of symptomatology, demonstrates considerable variability, indicative of the heterogeneity inherent in schizophrenia. The mean total score suggests a moderate to severe overall symptom burden, with implications for global functioning and prognosis.

3.6.5 Gastrointestinal symptoms

The gastrointestinal (GI) symptomatology in the cohort, as reflected by the descriptive statistics, suggests a varied presentation with a mean score that may be indicative of mild to moderate distress. The wide range in scores, extending to a maximum of 83, denotes that while some patients experience minimal GI complaints, others may suffer from severe symptoms.

3.6.6 SANS questionnaire

Turning to the Scale for the Assessment of Negative Symptoms (SANS), the mean total score suggests a moderate level of negative symptom burden. This scale measures affective flattening, alogia, avolition, anhedonia, and attentional impairment, which are core features of schizophrenia and have substantial implications for social and occupational functioning. The relatively high standard deviation indicates a diverse expression of negative symptoms within the cohort.

3.6.7 Calgary questionnaire

The Calgary Depression Scale for Schizophrenia (CDSS) is specifically designed to assess depressive symptoms in the context of schizophrenia, distinguishing them from negative and extrapyramidal symptoms. The mean score here is indicative of mild depressive symptoms, although the range of scores suggests that some patients may experience more pronounced depressive features.

3.6.8 BDI-II questionnaire

The Beck Depression Inventory-II (BDI-II) is a self-report inventory that measures the severity of depression. The mean score in the cohort suggests mild to moderate depression, while the range of scores implies that the severity of depressive symptoms is highly variable among patients.

3.6.9 CISS questionnaire

The cohort's responses to the Coping Inventory for Stressful Situations (CISS) questionnaire offer a comprehensive overview of coping strategies employed in the face of stress. The data elucidate the predilection toward task-oriented, emotion-oriented, and avoidance-oriented coping mechanisms, including subcategories such as distraction and social diversion.

Task-oriented coping emerges as a moderately utilized strategy with the mean score leaning toward the upper half of the available range. This suggests a general tendency within the cohort to adopt an active and problem-focused approach when managing stress. Given the relatively moderate standard deviation, the cohort exhibits a semblance of uniformity in this coping style, though individual variations are present.

Emotion-oriented coping, with a mean score closely aligned with that of task-oriented coping, indicates a comparable reliance on internal processes characterized by emotional expression, rumination, and self-blame in response to stress. The broader range and higher standard deviation suggest a greater diversity in the use of emotion-oriented strategies, which may reflect variance in emotional self-awareness and regulation skills.

Avoidance-oriented coping, which includes distraction and social diversion, is engaged to a lesser extent than task-oriented and emotion-oriented strategies. The mean scores for these scales indicate a tendency within the cohort to sometimes defer confrontation with stressors, either by engaging in alternative activities (distraction) or seeking solace in social interactions (social diversion). The standard deviations in these scales are lower, implying a more homogenous use of avoidance strategies among the individuals.

The total score, representing the cumulative coping effort across all domains, falls within the upper mid-range of the scale. This cumulative score suggests that the cohort actively engages with stress, utilizing a repertoire of coping strategies. The range of total scores, however, indicates that while some individuals exhibit a robust and versatile coping profile, others may have a less adaptive approach, possibly indicating vulnerability to stress-related psychopathology or the need for interventions to enhance coping efficacy.

3.6.10 ITQ questionnaire

The clinical data derived from the International Trauma Questionnaire (ITQ) reflect a cohort's trauma-related psychopathology with a particular emphasis on Post-Traumatic Stress Disorder (PTSD) and complex PTSD (C-PTSD), as operationalized by scores on reexperiencing, avoidance, threat, affective dysregulation, negative self-concept, and disturbance in relationships.

Reexperiencing trauma scores indicate a lower mean relative to other ITQ subscales, suggesting that while the involuntary and distressing reliving of traumatic events is present, it is not the most dominant symptom across the cohort.

The avoidance scores are slightly higher, implying that the behavioral or cognitive efforts to evade trauma-related stimuli are a more pronounced response among the individuals assessed.

Threat perception, a cardinal symptom of PTSD reflecting heightened arousal and reactivity, is slightly more severe on average than reexperiencing or avoidance symptoms.

Affective dysregulation, emblematic of C-PTSD, presents with the highest mean score among the ITQ subscales, which are at the upper limit of the lower half of the scale, indicating emotional responses that are not adequately modulated.

Negative self-concept encapsulates feelings of worthlessness and a persistent negative belief about oneself, which is marked by a mean score that is indicative of a moderate level of severity.

Disturbances in relationships, quantified by similar mean scores to negative self-concept, reflect the impairment in forming and maintaining close relationships, often due to pervasive distrust and a preoccupation with the possibility of betrayal.

The PTSDFI and DSOFI scores highlight the differentiation between PTSD and its dissociative subtype, a form of the disorder where symptoms of depersonalization and derealization are prominent. The means of these scores suggest a moderate expression of these symptoms within the cohort, with a range indicating variability in the severity of dissociative experiences and the functional impairment they entail.

The PTSD score, which may encompass both DSM-5 PTSD symptom clusters and C-PTSD features, shows that on average, individuals experience moderate levels of PTSD symptoms. The range, however, suggests that some individuals may exhibit minimal symptoms while others have severe PTSD symptomatology.

The DSO score, representing the dissociative subtype of PTSD, has a slightly higher mean than the PTSD score, suggesting that dissociative symptoms may be particularly salient in studied cohort. This is clinically significant as the dissociative subtype often requires specialized treatment approaches.

The total score, which amalgamates the symptomatology across the PTSD and C-PTSD spectrum, indicates a moderate to severe level of trauma-related psychopathology in the cohort. The wide range of total scores reflects the heterogeneity in the severity of trauma-related symptoms among individuals.

3.6.11 CTQ questionnaire

The Child Trauma Questionnaire (CTQ) scores from the presented data offer a quantifiable measure of childhood maltreatment across different domains, including emotional abuse, physical abuse, sexual abuse, emotional neglect, physical neglect, and a minimization/denial dimension.

Emotional abuse scores indicate a mean slightly above the median, with a non-negligible standard deviation, suggesting variability in the cohort's experiences of emotional abuse during childhood. The range of scores indicates that while some individuals report low levels of emotional abuse, others have experienced higher levels, which could correlate with a greater risk for emotional dysregulation and disorders such as depression and anxiety.

Physical abuse scores are notably lower than emotional abuse scores, with a tighter range and lower standard deviation, indicating more homogeneity in experiences of physical abuse within the cohort.

Sexual abuse scores are similar to physical abuse, with a mean close to the median, suggesting that instances of sexual abuse within this cohort are relatively consistent, though the range indicates that experiences do vary among individuals.

Emotional neglect scores have a mean that is slightly above the median, with a range indicating a spread of experiences within the cohort.

Physical neglect scores, representing the failure to provide basic physical needs, show lower mean and median values relative to emotional neglect, yet with a range that reveals some individuals experienced higher levels of neglect.

The denial score, which reflects minimization or denial of maltreatment, exhibits a mean close to the median and a relatively low standard deviation, suggesting a commonality in the cohort's tendency to minimize or deny the impact of childhood trauma.

The total CTQ score, which aggregates the different forms of maltreatment, reflects a moderate mean value with a broad range of scores.

4. Results

See **Table 2**.

4.1 Hematological measurements

In the examination of inositol's modulation within the ACC at a 30 ms ET on hematological parameters in schizophrenic patients, the statistical analysis reveals that none of the observed changes in white blood cell (WBC) count, neutrophil percentage (Neut %), or lymphocyte count reach statistical significance.

This could indicate that inositol's therapeutic reach, if present, might be confined to the central nervous system without pronounced peripheral hematological effects, or there may be a lack of sensitivity in the current measurements to detect subtle changes.

Outcome variable	N_{obs}	β	*SE*	*z*	$Pr(>\vert z\vert)$
Hematological measurements					
WBC [$\times 10^3/\mu L$]	50	1.21×10^{-3}	2.45×10^{-3}	−0.50	0.620
Neut %	50	0.19×10^{-3}	1.53×10^{-3}	0.12	0.903
Lymphocyte count [$\times 10^3/\mu L$]	50	-2.23×10^{-3}	2.30×10^{-3}	−0.97	0.330
Neurochemical measurements					
Myo-inositol /Cr + PCr, ACC TE 30	50	3.94×10^{-3}	$0.57 \times 10^{-3-}$	6.87	**< 0.001**
NAA conc. ACC 30, [$\times 10^{-6}$]	50	1.26×10^{-3}	$0.48 \times 10^{-3-}$	2.62	**0.009**
NAA /Cr + PCr ACC 30	50	-1.72×10^{-3}	$0.64 \times 10^{-3-}$	−2.71	**0.007**
Myo-inositol, ACC 144	50	7.23×10^{-3}	1.60×10^{-3}	4.52	**< 0.001**
Mio-inositol /Cr + PCr, AC 144	50	4.23×10^{-3}	1.85×10^{-3}	2.29	**0.022**
NAA, ACC 144	50	1.43×10^{-3}	0.83×10^{-3}	1.72	0.085
NAA/Cr + PCr, ACC 144	50	-1.41×10^{-3}	0.84×10^{-3}	−1.67	0.095
Myo-inositol [$\times 10^{-6}$], PCC 30	50	2.70×10^{-3}	0.77×10^{-3}	3.52	**< 0.001**
Myo-inositol /Cr + PCr, PCC 30	50	2.47×10^{-3}	0.61×10^{-3}	4.03	**< 0.001**
NAA conc. [$\times 10^{-6}$], PCC 30	50	0.78×10^{-3}	0.35×10^{-3}	2.20	**0.028**
NAA /Cr + PCr, PCC 30	50	0.51×10^{-3}	0.78×10^{-3}	0.65	0.513
Myo-inositol, PCC 144	50	0.46×10^{-3}	2.08×10^{-3}	0.22	0.824
Myo-inositol/Cr + PCr, PCC 144	50	7.65×10^{-6}	1.69×10^{-3}	0.01	0.996
NAA, PCC 144	50	1.23×10^{-3}	0.40×10^{-3}	3.09	0.002
NAA/Cr + PCr, PCC 144	50	0.63×10^{-3}	0.69×10^{-3}	0.92	0.356
Gastrointestinal symptoms					
Total score	45	-5.80×10^{-3}	5.02×10^{-3}	−1.16	0.248
PANNS questionnaire					
positive symptoms score	49	0.79×10^{-3}	3.12×10^{-3}	0.25	0.801
negative symptoms score	49	-0.94×10^{-3}	2.43×10^{-3}	−0.39	0.700
disorganized speech score	49	-0.75×10^{-3}	3.47×10^{-3}	0.22	0.830
uncontrolled hostility/excitement score	49	0.71×10^{-3}	3.56×10^{-3}	0.20	0.842
anxiety/depression score	49	-1.36×10^{-3}	3.22×10^{-3}	−0.42	0.672
positive scale score	49	1.76×10^{-3}	2.93×10^{-3}	0.60	0.547
negative scale score	49	-1.28×10^{-3}	2.62×10^{-3}	−0.49	0.625
general psychopathology scale score	49	-0.24×10^{-3}	3.10×10^{-3}	−0.08	0.938
total score	49	-0.67×10^{-6}	2.77×10^{-3}	−0.02	0.981
SANS questionnaire					
Total score	49	-1.87×10^{-3}	4.08×10^{-3}	−0.46	0.646

Outcome variable	N_{obs}	β	SE	z	Pr(>|z|)
Calgary questionnaire					
Total score	49	-2.94×10^{-3}	7.31×10^{-3}	−0.40	0.687
BDI-II questionnaire					
Total score	45	-11.37×10^{-3}	6.05×10^{-3}	−1.88	0.060
CISS questionnaire					
Task-oriented coping scale score	39	2.47×10^{-3}	1.96×10^{-3}	1.26	0.208
Emotion-oriented coping scale score	39	-2.52×10^{-3}	1.87×10^{-3}	−1.35	0.179
Avoidance-oriented coping scale score	39	0.51×10^{-3}	1.22×10^{-3}	0.42	0.677
Distraction scale score	39	-2.82×10^{-3}	2.15×10^{-3}	−1.31	0.191
Social diversion scale score	39	3.05×10^{-3}	1.89×10^{-3}	1.61	0.108
Total score	39	0.24×10^{-3}	0.96×10^{-3}	0.25	0.805
ITQ questionnaire					
Reexperiencing trauma score	41	-12.66×10^{-3}	7.62×10^{-3}	−1.66	0.097
Avoidance score	41	-11.16×10^{-3}	4.93×10^{-3}	−2.26	**0.024**
Threat score	41	-3.01×10^{-3}	4.63×10^{-3}	−0.65	0.516
Affective dysregulation score	41	-6.24×10^{-3}	4.11×10^{-3}	−1.52	0.129
Negative self-concept score	41	-12.25×10^{-3}	6.55×10^{-3}	−1.87	0.061
Disturbance relationships score	41	-9.67×10^{-3}	4.59×10^{-3}	−2.11	**0.035**
PTSDFI score	41	-6.29×10^{-3}	4.72×10^{-3}	−1.33	0.182
DSOFI score	41	-7.23×10^{-3}	4.52×10^{-3}	−1.60	0.109
PTSD score	41	-8.33×10^{-3}	4.28×10^{-3}	−1.95	0.051
DSO score	41	-11.17×10^{-3}	4.53×10^{-3}	−2.46	**0.014**
Total score	41	-8.62×10^{-3}	3.40×10^{-3}	−2.54	**0.011**
CTQ questionnaire					
Emotional abuse score	41	-6.79×10^{-3}	2.77×10^{-3}	−2.45	**0.014**
Physical abuse score	41	-3.57×10^{-3}	2.90×10^{-3}	−1.23	0.219
Sexual abuse score	41	-4.59×10^{-3}	3.37×10^{-3}	−1.36	0.173
Emotional neglect score	41	-4.25×10^{-3}	2.93×10^{-3}	−1.45	0.147
Physical neglect score	41	-2.06×10^{-3}	2.00×10^{-3}	−1.03	0.305
Denial (minimization/denial) score	41	1.56×10^{-3}	1.89×10^{-3}	0.83	0.409
Total score	41	-2.43×10^{-3}	1.79×10^{-3}	−1.36	0.174

Note: Nobs – the number of observations included in the regression model; β –the regression coefficient; SE – the standard error; z – statistic from Wald's z-test, Pr(>|z|) – the p-value, PANSS – Positive and Negative Syndrome Scale, SANS – Scale for Assessment of Negative Symptoms, CALGARY – Calgary Depression Scale for Schizophrenia, BDI-II – the Beck Depression Inventory, CISS – Coping Inventory for Stressful Situations, ITQ – International Trauma Questionnaire; PTSDFI – post-traumatic stress disorder functional impairment; DSOFI – disturbances in self-organization functional impairment; PTSD – post-traumatic stress disorder; DSO – disturbances in self-organization; CTQ – Childhood Trauma Questionnaire.

Table 2.
Modulatory impact of brain inositol [Myo-inositol [$\times 10^{-6}/\mu L$], ACC ET 30] on studied clinical outcome measures among a cohort of schizophrenic patients, adjusted for sex, age, and psychotropic medication dosage standardized to 100 mg chlorpromazine equivalents.

4.2 Neurochemical measurements

The robust and statistically significant positive association between inositol exposure and myo-inositol levels in both the ACC and PCC at ET 30 ms, as evidenced by z-scores exceeding the critical threshold and $p < 0.001$, suggests a potentiation effect of inositol on its own concentration in these regions. This is consistent with the hypothesis that inositol supplementation could augment its cerebral bioavailability, which has been postulated to modulate synaptic plasticity and cellular osmolarity, potentially providing a neuroprotective milieu.

The myo-inositol/creatinine plus phosphocreatinine (Cr + PCr) ratio also demonstrates a significant increase in the PCC at ET 30 ms and in the ACC at both ET 30 ms and ET 144 ms. These findings further reinforce the notion that inositol exposure has a consistent impact on its relative concentration, perhaps indicating a compensatory or regulatory mechanism in cerebral metabolic processes that could be dysregulated in schizophrenia.

NAA, a surrogate marker for neuronal integrity and function, shows a significant increase in concentration in the PCC at ET 30 and 144 ms, as well as in the ACC at ET 30 ms, with corresponding p-values of 0.028, 0.002, and 0.009, respectively. These data suggest that inositol may have a beneficial effect on neuronal health or may indicate an upregulation of mitochondrial activity, which could be of substantial interest in the context of the neurodegenerative aspects of schizophrenia.

However, when assessing the ratios of NAA/Cr + PCr, results yield a more complex interpretation. In the ACC at ET 30 ms, there is a significant decrease in this ratio, as evidenced by $p = 0.007$. This could suggest that while NAA levels increase, the rise is not in proportion with creatinine and phosphocreatinine levels, which may indicate altered energy metabolism or a shift in the neurochemical balance that warrants further investigation.

At ET 144 ms, both the NAA concentrations and ratios in the ACC, while showing positive beta coefficients, do not achieve statistical significance, suggesting that the effect of inositol may be time-dependent, or that the homeostatic mechanisms may equilibrate beyond the initial response period.

Clinically, these findings suggest that inositol has the potential to modulate neurochemical profiles in schizophrenia, particularly by increasing the availability of myo-inositol and possibly supporting neuronal integrity as indicated by changes in NAA levels. These neurochemical shifts could hypothetically translate into clinical improvements, given the association of myo-inositol with signaling pathways and NAA with neuronal health. However, the translation of these biochemical changes to clinical practice requires cautious interpretation and further validation through clinical trials assessing symptomatology and cognitive functions.

Additionally, these findings must be contextualized within the broader scope of schizophrenic pathophysiology, noting that the etiology of schizophrenia is multifactorial and the modulation of a single neurochemical parameter may not yield substantial therapeutic benefits in isolation. Further research should elucidate the implications of these neurochemical changes for the neurocognitive deficits and psychopathology inherent in schizophrenia.

4.3 Gastrointestinal symptoms, SANS, Calgary, and BDI-II questionnaires

While inositol appears to have a minimal impact on gastrointestinal, negative, and depressive symptoms in the studied schizophrenia cohort, it is essential to recognize the limitations of the current analysis. These include the relatively small sample size and the potential for idiosyncratic responses to inositol within the heterogeneous cohort of individuals with schizophrenia. Furthermore, the assessment tools used, although validated, may not capture subtle changes in symptomatology that could be clinically meaningful for patients.

4.4 PANSS questionnaire

The analysis suggests that inositol exposure does not lead to a notable amelioration in the positive symptoms of schizophrenia, which includes hallucinations and delusions, as evidenced by a positive beta coefficient that failed to reach statistical significance (p = 0.801). Similarly, the negative symptoms, which encompass affective flattening, alogia, and avolition, also did not show significant improvement (p = 0.700). The scores for disorganized speech – a core symptom of thought disorder in schizophrenia—likewise remained unchanged in a statistically meaningful way (p = 0.830).

The subcomponent of uncontrolled hostility/excitement, indicative of the potential for agitation and aggression, also displayed insubstantial change post-inositol exposure (p = 0.842). Furthermore, the anxiety/depression score of the PANSS, which is critical given the high prevalence of comorbid anxiety and depression in studied cohort, did not demonstrate significant variation with inositol (p = 0.672).

When dissected into the positive and negative scale scores, again, no significant effects were observed. The positive scale score reflects the cumulative severity of the positive symptoms, and the data indicate no substantial response to inositol (p = 0.547). Correspondingly, the negative scale score, reflective of the aggregate severity of negative symptoms, similarly did not display statistically significant change (p = 0.625).

The general psychopathology scale score, which encompasses a broader range of symptoms including somatic concern, anxiety, guilt feelings, and active social avoidance, showed negligible change (p = 0.938), underscoring the absence of a substantial impact of inositol on these psychopathological features.

Lastly, the total PANSS score, which is a holistic measure of the overall symptom severity in schizophrenia, indicated no significant modulation by inositol exposure, as the negligible beta coefficient and very high p-value (p = 0.981) attest.

In drawing conclusions from this data, it is important to consider that while inositol's neuromodulatory roles have been explored in various psychiatric conditions, this particular set of results does not support its efficacy in modifying the symptomatology of schizophrenia when assessed at a specific time point post-exposure. These findings should not negate the possible neurochemical benefits of inositol observed in other studies, but rather highlight the complexity of schizophrenia's pathophysiology, where multiple interacting neurobiological pathways contribute to the manifestation of symptoms, and the therapeutic response can be highly individualized.

Furthermore, in considering the translation of these findings to clinical practice, one must weigh the absence of significant outcomes against the backdrop of extant treatment modalities for schizophrenia, which often involve antipsychotic medications with considerable side effect profiles.

4.5 CISS questionnaire

The numerical trends in the data suggest a nuanced modulation of coping strategies, albeit without reaching statistical significance across the different scales of coping measured. The task-oriented coping scale score shows a positive beta coefficient, suggesting a potential increase in task-focused coping strategies with inositol exposure, but the $p = 0.208$ indicates that this increase is not statistically significant.

Conversely, the emotion-oriented coping scale score indicates a negative beta coefficient, implying a possible decrease in emotion-focused coping strategies with inositol intervention. However, the statistical analysis yields a $p = 0.179$, which does not confer statistical significance to this finding.

The avoidance-oriented coping scale score, which encompasses strategies to divert attention from stressors, presents a very slight positive beta coefficient, yet this effect is statistically unsubstantial with a $p = 0.677$. This is similarly echoed in the distraction scale score, where there is an insinuated reduction in this coping style post-inositol exposure, but again without statistical support ($p = 0.191$).

The social diversion scale score, indicative of seeking social contact as a means of coping, shows a positive beta coefficient and the lowest p-value among the scales at 0.108. While this could suggest a tendency toward increased utilization of social diversion coping strategies with inositol exposure, the lack of statistical significance precludes definitive conclusions.

The total score for the CISS, which amalgamates the coping strategies into an overall assessment of coping effectiveness, shows an insignificant beta coefficient and a high p-value of 0.805. This further corroborates the lack of significant impact of inositol on coping mechanisms in studied cohort.

From a clinical and analytical standpoint, these findings suggest that inositol, within the parameters of this study, does not exert a significant modulatory effect on coping strategies as measured by the CISS in individuals with schizophrenia. The implications for clinical practice remain limited given the lack of statistical significance, yet the trends observed may inform future hypotheses and research directions.

4.6 ITQ questionnaire

The avoidance score, reflecting efforts to circumvent trauma-related thoughts or reminders, shows a statistically significant reduction in the case of highest inositol concentrations ($p = 0.024$), which may imply a potential utility for inositol in mitigating avoidance symptoms in this cohort.

The disturbance in relationships score, indicative of impairments in forming and maintaining close relationships as a result of trauma, also presents a statistically significant decrease ($p = 0.035$), suggesting that inositol may confer benefits in enhancing social functioning and interpersonal relations among those afflicted with schizophrenia.

The DSO score, a cumulative measure of pervasive changes in affect regulation, self-concept, and relational difficulties, demonstrates a statistically significant decrement ($p = 0.014$), potentially pointing toward a broader ameliorative effect of inositol on the complex sequelae of trauma and stress disorders beyond the primary PTSD symptoms.

The total score, encapsulating the overall impact of trauma-related sequelae, shows a statistically significant reduction ($p = 0.011$), reinforcing the notion that inositol might play a role in alleviating the overarching burden of trauma-related symptoms in studied patient cohort.

While the reexperiencing trauma score, affective dysregulation score, negative self-concept score, and PTSD score all exhibit negative β coefficients, suggesting a downward trend in symptomatology with inositol exposure, the lack of statistical significance precludes definitive assertions regarding their clinical relevance.

Notably, the threat score, which addresses hypervigilance and exaggerated startle response, and the PTSDFI and DSOFI scores, representing indices of PTSD and DSO respectively, do not indicate significant changes with inositol treatment. This underscores the multifaceted and heterogeneous nature of trauma-related disorders and the possibility that inositol's efficacy may vary across different symptom clusters.

From a psychiatric perspective, these findings highlight a potential therapeutic niche for inositol in addressing specific facets of trauma-related psychopathology in schizophrenia, particularly avoidance behaviors and disturbances in relationships, which can profoundly affect the quality of life and functional outcomes. The data also suggest that inositol might contribute to improvements in the broader constellation of difficulties subsumed under DSO, warranting further research into its neuromodulatory effects within this domain.

4.7 CTQ questionnaire

Analyzing the data, the emotional abuse score exhibits a significant decrement with inositol exposure, as evidenced by a $p = 0.014$. This finding is clinically pertinent, as emotional abuse in childhood has been robustly linked to the exacerbation of psychotic symptoms and can contribute to poorer prognostic outcomes in schizophrenia. The significant reduction in the emotional abuse score with inositol treatment may indicate a therapeutic potential for mitigating the long-standing impact of such trauma, potentially leading to an attenuation of trauma-related symptomatology in studied cohort.

While the other categories of abuse and neglect—physical abuse, sexual abuse, emotional neglect, and physical neglect—also demonstrate negative β coefficients, suggesting a trend toward symptom reduction with inositol, these results do not meet the threshold for statistical significance. Hence, while there is an indication of a potentially beneficial effect, these data do not provide robust support for the clinical efficacy of inositol in these domains of historical trauma within the schizophrenia cohort.

The denial score interestingly shows a positive β coefficient, although without statistical significance, indicating no substantial evidence for inositol's impact on patients' tendency to minimize or deny their traumatic experiences. This could imply that inositol does not influence the cognitive or psychological processes underpinning the acknowledgment or reporting of historical trauma as measured by the CTQ.

The total score, which aggregates the sum of the subscales, similarly does not reach statistical significance, suggesting that the overall effect of inositol on the combined dimensions of childhood trauma is not compelling within the confines of this dataset.

From a clinical psychiatry perspective, these findings suggest that inositol may possess specific modulatory properties on emotional abuse-related sequelae in schizophrenia, which can be significant considering the pervasive effects of emotional maltreatment on mental health. However, the absence of significant findings in other trauma-related domains signals the need for cautious interpretation and the necessity for further inquiry.

5. Discussion

5.1 Part I

The heterogeneity of the clinical picture and severity of the disorder within the examined group of individuals with schizophrenia, and consequently insensitivity to pain, can be explained by the wide variability in the doses of antipsychotic drugs used, expressed in chlorpromazine equivalents. This, on the one hand, suggests a wide range of pharmacotherapeutic interventions in the studied cohort, and on the other hand, confirms the theory that the lesser experience of pain in schizophrenia may be due to the use of chronic neuroleptic pharmacotherapy [62]. The obtained range of results also implies potential differences in response to treatment or increased tolerance, considering the significant variability in doses required to achieve therapeutic effects or manage side effects. A systematic review conducted in 2004 indicated that up to 90% of atypical neuroleptics exhibited analgesic effects [63]. Our findings provide evidence suggesting that analgesia depends on both the dose and type of antipsychotic drug, although the use of neuroleptics remains problematic in improving depressive symptoms or cognitive functions and reducing suicide attempts associated with them in schizophrenia [64–66].

Positive symptoms, characterized by the presence of psychopathology such as hallucinations, delusions, and disorganized thought processes, among the examined individuals, showed a mean score suggesting a moderate level of severity in the entire cohort. However, the range and standard deviation indicate significant heterogeneity in the presentation of positive symptoms. The wide range of scores for negative symptoms emphasizes the diverse impact of schizophrenia on emotional response and social functioning, which are key determinants of long-term outcomes and functional abilities.

The results on the negative scale among the examined cohort slightly exceeded those on the positive scale, suggesting that negative symptoms may be more prominent or enduring in the studied cohort. This is consistent with the clinical understanding of the association of negative symptoms with altered pain perception, resistance to current pharmacotherapies, and poorer functional outcomes. Additionally, we cannot exclude the influence of a broader range of symptoms, such as guilt feelings, tension, and active avoidance of social contacts, which were highest among these domains in the studied group. This reflects the broad impact of the complex interaction of affective, cognitive, and behavioral elements in pain perception in schizophrenia.

5.2 Part II

Through conducting proton magnetic resonance spectroscopy (1H-MRS) in a group of individuals with schizophrenia, we evaluated the metabolic activity of the anterior cingulate cortex (ACC) and posterior cingulate cortex (PCC) involving myo-inositol. Myo-inositol is an inert osmolyte abundantly present in glial cells. One of its important functions is the regulation of cell volume during morphological changes, such as those occurring during glial activation in neuroinflammatory processes and neuropathic pain [67]. Evaluating the correlation of this indicator with other measured parameters of clinical and neurometabolic assessment and based on available literature, elevated levels of myo-inositol may suggest glial proliferation or altered glial function, consistent with neuroinflammatory hypotheses of schizophrenia. Elevated levels of myo-inositol have been observed in viral infections such as HIV infection [68, 69], progressive multiple sclerosis [70], or in diffusion imaging models confirming glial activation [71, 72]. Higher levels of myo-inositol have been observed with aging [73–75]. Transcriptomic data indicate that aging is associated with increased markers of astrocytes and microglia [76], particularly with increased markers of reactive astrocytes in the prefrontal cortex [77]. Presumably, these glial changes may constitute a common mechanism responsible for similar neurometabolic profiles observed in aging and in the process of altered pain perception in schizophrenia. In our study, the average levels of myo-inositol in the ACC and PCC fall within a range that does not immediately indicate clear glial pathology; however, the variability of these levels may correlate with individual differences in symptoms or disease progression. The prolonged echo time (TE) of 144 ms compared to the standard TE of 30 ms provides increased specificity of metabolite resonance and suggests a stronger signal for myo-inositol and N-acetylaspartate (NAA).

There are individual studies indicating that changes in the concentration of myo-inositol in the orbitofrontal cortex may be associated with specific mood/affective states such as extreme pain perception. Additional support for altered pain perception may come from the reduced level of N-acetylaspartate in the dorsolateral prefrontal cortex, confirming the hypothesis that N-acetylaspartate depletion in the prefrontal cortex is a chemical marker of chronic pain, indicating neuronal degeneration which may be related to possible glutamate's excitotoxicity [78–81]. Inositol has neuromodulatory potential, particularly by increasing its availability and supporting neuronal integrity [82], as indicated by a wide range of changes in N-acetylaspartate levels. The observed neurochemical changes may hypothetically translate into clinical improvement and reduced pain perception in schizophrenia, considering the association of myo-inositol with signaling pathways and NAA with neuronal health. Translating these brain biochemistry changes into clinical practice requires careful interpretation and further validation through clinical studies assessing symptomatology and evaluating neuronal-glial mechanisms underlying pain modulation by cognitive and emotional states as pillars of cognitive-behavioral therapy. Key metabolites considered useful in assessing altered pain perception in schizophrenia are myo-inositol and NAA, which have previously been linked to increased pain symptoms in complex regional pain syndrome. Interestingly, there is also evidence that chronic pain itself alters brain circuits, including those related to endogenous pain control, suggesting that pain control becomes increasingly difficult as pain becomes chronic. In this case, the hypothesis of the existence of a negative feedback loop between impaired pain-modulating circuits and pain processing is justified, leading not only to exacerbation of chronic pain among individuals with schizophrenia but also to accompanying cognitive and emotional deficits associated with pain, which in the studied group indicated an average slightly above the median, with insignificant standard deviation, suggesting variability in cohort experiences related to emotional violence. Affective dysregulation, characteristic of C-PTSD, was characterized by the highest average score among the ITQ subscales, confirming the significant influence of emotional reactions that are not adequately modulated in the studied group of patients. The justification for the obtained results is that both the ACC region and the insula have long been considered components of the emotional brain [83, 84] responsible for encoding the emotional and motivational aspects of pain. Patients with alterations in these areas exhibit altered emotional responses to pain [85–88] and imaging and stimulation studies demonstrate a relationship between emotional and motivational aspects of pain perception and neuronal activation in the ACC and insula [89–92]. Another explanation for altered pain perception in schizophrenia may be reduced gray matter content in patients with chronic pain associated with possible glutamate excitotoxicity [93]. In schizophrenia at a very early stage of the disease, even before antipsychotic treatment, increased presynaptic dopamine release with a characteristic small increase in glutamate concentration was observed in PET studies [94]. Conversely, in healthy individuals, positron emission tomography studies have shown that reduced density of D2 receptors in the striatum was associated with an increased pain threshold [95]. These studies suggest that changes in neurotransmitter systems may mean that patients with chronic pain have reduced receptor availability or increased endogenous release of these neurotransmitters [96].

Understanding the pathophysiology of altered pain perception in schizophrenia and developing effective therapeutic interventions seems crucial for curbing the wave of adverse consequences of schizophrenia, including suicide attempts. Changes in the neurometabolic integrity of brain areas involved in both pain control and cognitive and/or emotional functioning may explain why patients suffering from schizophrenia with chronic pain develop cognitive deficits, as well as anxiety disorders or depression. Ongoing research suggests that emotional and cognitive changes may begin long after the onset of pain. For example, patients with psychotic symptoms may exhibit anxiety-like behaviors and attention deficits for several years after injury and onset of hypersensitivity, temporally coinciding with anatomical changes in the frontal cortex [97, 98]. The concept of pain control dependent on the level of myo-inositol in the prefrontal cortex in individuals with schizophrenia is confirmed in this study, where the result of emotional violence shows a significant decrease with exposure to inositol. This finding has significant clinical potential, as childhood emotional violence is strongly associated with exacerbation of psychotic symptoms and may contribute to worse prognostic outcomes in schizophrenia. Adversities in early life and mechanisms of altered pain perception may further explain the relationship between suicide risk and abnormalities in brain circuits and neurochemistry in schizophrenia [99].

A significant reduction in the index of emotional violence after treatment with inositol may indicate therapeutic potential in alleviating the long-term consequences of childhood trauma, potentially leading to a reduction in trauma-related symptomatology in the studied cohort. The presented study provides evidence that pain can be harmful to the brain and that chronic pain itself may decrease an individual's ability to control pain endogenously and lead to numerous comorbidities that accompany schizophrenia.

5.3 Part III

Analyzing the results regarding emotional violence, it is evident that they show an average slightly above the median, with an insignificant standard deviation, suggesting variability in the experiences of the studied cohort related to childhood emotional violence. The range of results indicates that while some individuals reported low levels of emotional violence, others experienced higher levels, which may correlate with a greater risk of emotional dysregulation and future disorders such as depression and anxiety states. Results for physical neglect, representing unmet basic physical needs, showed lower mean and median values compared to emotional neglect. The literature on the subject suggests that while physical and sexual abuse in childhood are known risk factors for chronic pain in adulthood, the relationship between childhood emotional violence and chronic pain remains insufficiently explored [100].

In most studies describing hypoalgesia in schizophrenia, the subjective response of the patient to painful stimuli had strong emotional underpinnings. Insensitivity to pain in this case may reflect deficits in the patient's expression of emotions. In other words, indifference to pain in patients with schizophrenia may not signify actual hypoalgesia. The aforementioned interoception is essentially supported by the insular cortex, with primary visceral sensation being associated with the mid and posterior insula regions, and integration of interoceptive information with cognitive functions, emotions, and other higher-order processes occurring in more anterior areas of the cerebral cortex [101, 102]. The medial prefrontal cortex, including the anterior cingulate cortex, prefrontal cortex, and infralimbic cortex, which are associated with shaping pain sensations in the central nervous system, is involved in these mechanisms [103]. The coexistence of psychological pain has been found to be an important moderator of the lasting benefits of treating patients with schizophrenia prone to suicide [104]. The analgesic action of schizophrenia treatment may explain the anti-suicidal effects of ketamine [104]. Research has revealed new possibilities for the use of this drug. It has been used in the treatment of acute, chronic, and cancer pain. The most interesting reports come from studies on the antidepressant and anti-suicidal properties of ketamine, offering hope for the development of an effective drug for major depressive disorders [105], although retrospective studies suggest that these effects may be short-lived [106].

In studies assessing the impact of childhood emotional violence on pain perception disturbances in populations with diagnosed mental health disorders, attention was drawn to the fact that among individuals receiving injectable drugs for chronic pain, experiences of childhood emotional violence were common, partly influenced by a history of diagnosed mental health disorders [107]. Similarly, it is known that individuals with mental health disorders have a high incidence of childhood trauma; however, little is known about how childhood emotional violence may be associated with chronic pain in this population [108]. Available data suggest that physicians should consider childhood trauma when treating psychiatric disorders in individuals experiencing chronic pain. Awareness of trauma-informed care may lead to more effective treatment in cases perceived as treatment-resistant [109], including suicide attempts. Childhood emotions, as demonstrated by this study, can be significant predictors of poor health outcomes in psychiatric patients, remaining unnoticed even with normal psychiatric assessment results. Considering the detrimental impact of high levels of pain disturbances, examining the potential influence of childhood emotions on altered pain perception in patients with schizophrenia appears crucial in designing interventions to improve the quality of life for this patient group. This approach may also facilitate identifying potential factors affecting the final clinical assessment outcomes for patients with schizophrenia and provide a better understanding of possible early interventions before pain interferes with daily activities. To the best of our knowledge, this is the first study to address the impact of childhood emotional exposure on the occurrence of chronic pain among individuals with schizophrenia. Further efforts are needed to determine pain perception intervention indicators to develop standards for therapeutic interventions among individuals with schizophrenia.

Emotional violence in childhood shapes interpersonal relationships, leading to weakened abilities to initiate and maintain connections. This factor has been identified as an important component of the experience of altered pain perception [110]. Addressing the issue of disruptions related to altered pain perception through effective psychosocial treatment and improving emotional awareness may result in a measurable indicator of pain control and the reduction of adverse effects on the quality of life and functioning of individuals with the condition [111, 112]. Increased access to effective prevention programs is therefore an urgent need, especially among marginalized populations, including schizophrenia, about which little is yet known regarding the assessment of pain expression by the patient. Interestingly, affective dysregulation, characteristic of C-PTSD, showed the highest mean score among the ITQ subscales, which fell within the upper limit of the lower half of the scale, clearly indicating emotionally reactive responses that were not adequately controlled. Conversely, the DSO score, representing the dissociative subtype of PTSD, exhibited a higher mean score than PTSD, suggesting that dissociative symptoms were particularly prominent in the studied cohort. This has clinical significance as the dissociative subtype often requires specialized treatment methods.

In investigating the relationship between inositol and its impact on emotional reactions in the studied cohort, attention is drawn to the significant decrease in emotional violence scores with exposure to inositol. This discovery has significant clinical implications, as childhood emotional violence has been strongly linked to exacerbating psychotic symptoms and may contribute to poorer prognostic outcomes in schizophrenia. The substantial reduction in the emotional violence index following inositol treatment may indicate its therapeutic potential in alleviating the long-term effects of such trauma, potentially leading to a reduction in trauma-related symptomatology in the studied cohort.

From a psychiatric perspective, these findings illuminate the potential role of inositol as a therapeutic agent in addressing specific aspects of psychopathology associated with a history of trauma in schizophrenia. This appears particularly pertinent in the context of avoidance behaviors and disturbances in relationships, which directly affect patients' quality of life and functionality. Furthermore, these findings indicate that inositol may provide benefits in tackling the broadly defined challenges often linked to continuous, repeated, and diverse traumatic exposures, such as affective dysregulation, negative self-concept, and disturbances in relationships, underscoring the necessity for further investigation into its neuromodulatory effects.

Inositol, an endogenous biologically active compound in the human body, plays a pivotal role in neurocommunication, serving as a crucial component in the signal transduction processes within neuronal cells. It possesses the capacity to modulate various neurochemical pathways, which could be exceptionally advantageous in the context of schizophrenia and related trauma-induced disorders. It has been demonstrated that inositol exerts its therapeutic effect in depression and associated anxiety disorders, partly by reducing the function of the serotonin-2A receptor (5HT2A-R) and specifically by diminishing the receptor's signaling capacity through Gq proteins. Additionally, inositol inhibits the function of the muscarinic acetylcholine receptor (mAChR), which may also contribute to its therapeutic effect in depression [113]. Through its influence on the neurotransmitter system, such as serotonin, inositol may aid in mitigating certain psychopathological symptoms, including anxiety, depression, and social-emotional processing issues related to trauma.

Moreover, owing to its potential neuroprotective [114] and anti-inflammatory actions [115], inositol may support the protection and regeneration of neural tissue, crucial in the face of chronic stress and trauma exposure, frequently observed in individuals with schizophrenia. This could, in turn, lead to enhancements in socio-emotional functioning, as well as patients' quality of life. The role of inositol in promoting neuroplasticity and its anti-inflammatory properties could be a critical mechanism in mitigating the neurological impacts of trauma. Neuroplastic changes are crucial for recovery from traumatic experiences, and inositol's contribution to synaptic formation and repair could facilitate the re-establishment of healthy neural networks disrupted by trauma. Trauma and stress induce inflammatory states within the brain, contributing to neuronal damage and deterioration of brain function [116]. Inositol, owing to its anti-inflammatory properties, may aid in reducing neuroinflammation, thereby protecting neural cells from damage and supporting their regeneration. Future research might explore how inositol influences neuroplastic pathways in the traumatized brain, potentially offering insights into its therapeutic effects in schizophrenia.

In summary, these insights herald new avenues for research and therapy focused on neuromodulation with inositol as a potential strategy to address specific trauma-related challenges in schizophrenia. Nonetheless, additional research is necessary to validate these initial findings and to elucidate the mechanisms of action of inositol, alongside establishing the best practices for its application in psychiatric therapy.

5.4 Limitations of the study

We failed to consider other important variables related to pain expression by patients, such as pain intensity, catastrophizing, and pain quality, as data that could provide significant measurable information allowing for the assessment of pain threshold cutoffs for which further diagnostic and therapeutic guidelines can be defined in the group of individuals with schizophrenia showing clear emotional neglect.

Emotional abuse in childhood may imply changes in pain perception among individuals diagnosed with schizophrenia. Childhood emotional abuse remained independently associated with neuroglial disturbances related to myo-inositol levels in the anterior cingulate cortex in adults with schizophrenia. Individuals with chronic pain should be assessed for childhood psychological trauma and the presence of mental disorders, and appropriate therapeutic measures should be provided to reduce distorted pain perception. Lastly, these findings underscore the importance of socio-behavioral interventions, including coping skills training and interpersonal skills enhancement, to mitigate disruptions in pain perception and improve the quality of life for patients with schizophrenia experiencing concurrent chronic pain and reporting a history of emotional abuse.

A limitation of this study was its reliance on retrospective self-reports of childhood trauma history, rather than employing a prospective approach, which could have provided greater accuracy. This retrospective methodology may introduce recall bias and affect the validity of the trauma histories reported, potentially influencing the study's findings and interpretations.

6. Conclusion

The complex nature of pain and its impact on the daily lives of millions of people entails the need for a thorough analysis of the processes and chemical compounds contributing to its development. Disturbed pain perception in patients with schizophrenia poses an additional diagnostic challenge for this disease. Reduced levels of myo-inositol in the anterior cingulate cortex may be the cause of reduced pain perception in patients with schizophrenia. One of the most important functions of myo-inositol, an osmolyte present in glial cells, is the regulation of the volume of glial cells during morphological changes occurring in the course of neuroinflammatory processes and neuropathic pain. The glial changes associated with increased levels of myo-inositol may be the cause of altered pain perception in schizophrenia. However, it is important to remember that schizophrenia is a complex disorder with a wide range of affective, cognitive, and behavioral symptoms, all of which may affect pain perception in patients. Understanding the basis of impaired pain perception in patients with schizophrenia may enable the introduction of appropriate therapy. Proper therapeutic intervention should reduce the emotional violence index, thus reducing the number of future disorders such as depression and anxiety, hopefully reducing the number of suicides in patients with schizophrenia. The use of inositol in therapy may result in a significant reduction in emotional violence which could be a future approach in the treatment of pain in schizophrenia.

Future research should delve into the intricate relationship between myo-inositol levels and the modulation of pain perception in individuals diagnosed with schizophrenia. It is crucial to conduct prospective, longitudinal studies to map out the changes in myo-inositol concentrations within the brain over time and to understand how these fluctuations correlate with the development and alteration of pain perception in this population. Investigating the neuroinflammatory and neuropathic mechanisms underlying pain perception in schizophrenia is paramount, with an emphasis on exploring how glial cell activity and the regulatory role of myo-inositol contribute to these processes. Additionally, a thorough analysis of the diverse symptomatology of schizophrenia, encompassing affective, cognitive, and behavioral dimensions, and their cumulative effect on pain perception is imperative. Such comprehensive research efforts are essential for uncovering the neurobiological and psychosocial dynamics influencing pain perception in schizophrenia, paving the way for more effective treatments and interventions.

Author's contribution

Wirginia Krzyściak (WK) contributed to conceptualization, software, validation, data analysis, investigation, data curation, writing—original draft, writing—review and editing, visualization, supervision, project administration, funding acquisition; **Paulina Karcz (PK)** contributed to methodology and software; **Amira Bryll (AB)** and **Robert Chrzan (RC)** contributed to methodology; **Aleksander Turek (AT)** contributed to methodology and curated data; **Paulina Mazur (PM)** contributed to writing—original draft; **Natalia Śmierciak (NŚ)** contributed to methodology; **Marta Szwajca (MS)** contributed to methodology, writing—original draft, writing—review and editing; **Tadeusz Popiela (TP)** contributed to supervision, methodology, software; **Katarzyna Furman (KF)** contributed to methodology; **Maciej Pilecki (MP)** contributed to supervision and methodology.

Conflict of interest

The authors declare no conflict of interest.

Author details

Wirginia Krzyściak[1*], Marta Szwajca[2], Paulina Karcz[3], Aleksander Turek[2], Natalia Śmierciak[2], Amira Bryll[4], Paulina Mazur[1], Robert Chrzan[4], Katarzyna Furman[2], Maciej Pilecki[2] and Tadeusz Popiela[4]

1 Faculty of Pharmacy, Department of Medical Diagnostics, Jagiellonian University Medical College, Krakow, Poland

2 Faculty of Medicine, Department of Child and Adolescent Psychiatry and Psychotherapy, Jagiellonian University Medical College, Krakow, Poland

3 Faculty of Health Sciences, Department of Electroradiology, Jagiellonian University Medical College, Krakow, Poland

4 Faculty of Medicine, Department of Radiology, Jagiellonian University Medical College, Krakow, Poland

*Address all correspondence to: wirginiakrzysciak@cm-uj.krakow.pl and wirginia.krzysciak@uj.edu.pl

References

[1] Goldberg DS, McGee SJ. Pain as a global public health priority. BMC Public Health. 2011;**11**(1):1-5

[2] Garland EL. Pain processing in the human nervous system: A selective review of nociceptive and Biobehavioral pathways. Primary Care. 2012;**39**(3):561

[3] Bushnell MC, Čeko M, Low LA. Cognitive and emotional control of pain and its disruption in chronic pain. Nature Reviews. Neuroscience. 2013;**14**(7):502-511. DOI: 10.1038/nrn3516

[4] Raja SN, Carr DB, Cohen M, Finnerup NB, Flor H, Gibson S, et al. The revised International Association for the Study of Pain definition of pain: Concepts, challenges, and compromises. Pain. 2020;**161**(9):1976-1982

[5] Treede RD, Rief W, Barke A, Aziz Q, Bennett MI, Benoliel R, et al. Chronic pain as a symptom or a disease: The IASP classification of chronic pain for the international classification of diseases (ICD-11). Pain. 2019;**160**(1):19-27

[6] Farrar JT. Cut-points for the measurement of pain: The choice depends on what you want to study. Pain. 2010;**149**(2):163-164

[7] Potvin S, Marchand S. Hypoalgesia in schizophrenia is independent of antipsychotic drugs: A systematic quantitative review of experimental studies. Pain. 2008;**138**(1):70-78

[8] Bleuler E, Dover P. Textbook of Psychiatry (Trans. Brill HA, 1951). New York: Dover Publications; 1911

[9] Kraepelin E. Dementia praecox and paraphrenia. In: Textbook of Psychiatry. 8th ed. Livingston, Edinburgh: Robert E. Kreiger Publishing Co.; 1919

[10] Stubbs B, Thompson T, Acaster S, Vancampfort D, Gaughran F, Correll CU. Decreased pain sensitivity among people with schizophrenia: A meta-analysis of experimental pain induction studies. Pain. 2015;**156**(11):2121-2131

[11] O'Connell F, Osiyemi N, Saliba Z, Mortimer N, Pourmand A. Reduced pain perception in patients with schizophrenia; a missed case of hand fracture. The American Journal of Emergency Medicine. 2021;**49**:440.e1-440.e3. DOI: 10.1016/j.ajem.2021.04.080

[12] Howard L, Kirkwood G, Leese M. Risk of hip fracture in patients with a history of schizophrenia. The British Journal of Psychiatry. 2007;**190**(FEB.):129-134

[13] Peet M. Diet, diabetes and schizophrenia: Review and hypothesis. The British Journal of Psychiatry. Supplement. 2004;**47**:102-105

[14] Nordentoft M, Plana-Ripoll O, Laursen TM. Cancer and schizophrenia. Current Opinion in Psychiatry. 2021;**34**(3):260-265

[15] Hennekens CH, Hennekens AR, Hollar D, Casey DE. Schizophrenia and increased risks of cardiovascular disease. American Heart Journal. 2005;**150**(6):1115-1121

[16] Kuritzky A, Mazeh D, Levi A. Headache in schizophrenic patients: A controlled study. Cephalalgia. 1999;**19**(8):725-727

[17] Stubbs B, Mitchell AJ, De Hert M, Correll CU, Soundy A, Stroobants M,

et al. The prevalence and moderators of clinical pain in people with schizophrenia: A systematic review and large scale meta-analysis. Schizophrenia Research. 2014;**160**(1-3):1-8

[18] Nagamine T. Pain threshold paradox in schizophrenia: A narrative review based on the lastest neuroscience. Psychiatria Danubina. 2023;**35**(2):174-179. DOI: 10.24869/psyd.2023.174

[19] Lévesque M, Potvin S, Marchand S, Stip E, Grignon S, Pierre L, et al. Pain perception in schizophrenia: Evidence of a specific pain response profile. Pain Medicine. 2012;**13**(12):1571-1579

[20] Stubbs B, Gardner-Sood P, Smith S, Ismail K, Greenwood K, Patel A, et al. Pain is independently associated with reduced health related quality of life in people with psychosis. Psychiatry Research. 2015;**230**(2):585-591

[21] Das TK, Dey A, Sabesan P, Javadzadeh A, Théberge J, Radua J, et al. Putative astroglial dysfunction in schizophrenia: A meta-analysis of 1H-MRS studies of medial prefrontal Myo-inositol. Frontiers in Psychiatry. 2018;**9**:1-10

[22] Labonté C, Zhand N, Park A, Harvey PD. Complete blood count inflammatory markers in treatment-resistant schizophrenia: Evidence of association between treatment responsiveness and levels of inflammation. Psychiatry Research. 2022;**308**:114382

[23] Urban-Kowalczyk M, Pigońska J, Śmigielski J. Pain perception in schizophrenia: Influence of neuropeptides, cognitive disorders, and negative symptoms. Neuropsychiatric Disease and Treatment. 2015;**11**:2023-2030. DOI: 10.2147/NDT.S87666

[24] Salter MW, Pitcher GM. Dysregulated Src upregulation of NMDA receptor activity: A common link in chronic pain and schizophrenia. The FEBS Journal. 2012;**279**(1):2

[25] Balu DT, Coyle JT. Neuroplasticity signaling pathways linked to the pathophysiology of schizophrenia. Neuroscience and Biobehavioral Reviews. 2011;**35**(3):848-870

[26] Hahn CG, Wang HY, Cho DS, Talbot K, Gur RE, Berrettini WH, et al. Altered neuregulin 1-erbB4 signaling contributes to NMDA receptor hypofunction in schizophrenia. Nature Medicine. 2006;**12**(7):824-828

[27] Banerjee A, MacDonald ML, Borgmann-Winter KE, Hahn CG. Neuregulin 1 - erbB4 pathway in schizophrenia: From genes to an interactome. Brain Research Bulletin. 2010;**83**(3-4):132

[28] Huang YZ, Won S, Ali DW, Wang Q, Tanowitz M, Du QS, et al. Regulation of neuregulin signaling by PSD-95 interacting with ErbB4 at CNS synapses. Neuron. 2000;**26**(2):443-455

[29] Pitcher GM, Beggs S, Woo RS, Mei L, Salter MW. ErbB4 is a suppressor of long-term potentiation in the adult hippocampus. Neuroreport. 2008;**19**(2):139-143

[30] Risch N, Dupuis-Maurin K, Dubois J, Courtet P, Olié E. Sensitivity to ostracism is blunted in suicide attempters only when they report suicidal ideation. Journal of Affective Disorders. 2023;**337**:169-174. DOI: 10.1016/j.jad.2023.05.045

[31] DeVille DC, Kuplicki R, Stewart JL, Paulus MP, Khalsa SS, Aupperle RL, et al. Diminished responses to bodily threat and blunted interoception in suicide attempters. eLife. 2020;**9**:1-28. DOI: 10.7554/eLife.51593

[32] Hedegaard H, Curtin SC, Warner M. Suicide rates in the United States continue to increase key findings data from the National Vital Statistics System. Mortality. 2018;**309**:1-8

[33] Meltzer HY. Treatment of suicidality in schizophrenia. Annals of the New York Academy of Sciences. 2001;**932**:44-60. DOI: 10.1111/j.1749-6632.2001.tb05797.x

[34] World Health Organization. Comprehensive mental health action plan 2013-2030. 2021

[35] American Psychiatric Association. Diagnostic and Statistical Manual of Mental Disorders: DSM-5. Washington, DC: American Psychiatric Association; 2013

[36] Kay SR, Fiszbein A, Opler LA. The positive and negative syndrome scale (PANSS) for schizophrenia. Schizophrenia Bulletin. 1987;**13**(2):261-276

[37] Goldberg D. Use of the general health questionnaire in clinical work. British Medical Journal (Clinical Research Ed.). 1986;**293**(6556):1188-1189

[38] Goldberg DP, Hillier VF. A scaled version of the general health questionnaire. Psychological Medicine. 1979;**9**(1):139-145

[39] Sterling M. General health questionnaire - 28 (GHQ-28). Journal of Physiotherapy. 2011;**57**(4):259

[40] Aas IM. Global assessment of functioning (GAF): Properties and frontier of current knowledge. Annals of General Psychiatry. 2010;**9**(20):1-11

[41] American Psychiatric Association. Diagnostic and Statistical Manual of Mental Disorders. 4th ed. Washington, DC: American Psychiatric Association; 1994

[42] Svedlund J, Sjödin I, Dotevall G. GSRS–A clinical rating scale for gastrointestinal symptoms in patients with irritable bowel syndrome and peptic ulcer disease. Digestive Diseases and Sciences. 1988;**33**(2):129-134

[43] Kulich KR, Madisch A, Pacini F, Piqué JM, Regula J, Van Rensburg CJ, et al. Reliability and validity of the gastrointestinal symptom rating scale (GSRS) and quality of life in reflux and dyspepsia (QOLRAD) questionnaire in dyspepsia: A six-country study. Health and Quality of Life Outcomes. 2008;**6**(12):1-12

[44] Beck A, Steer R, Brown G. Manual for the BDI-II. San Antonio: TX: Psychological Corporation; 1996

[45] Spielberger C, Gorsuch R, Lushene R, Vagg PR, Jacobs GA. Manual for the State-Trait Anxiety Inventory (Form Y1-Y2). 1st ed. Palo Alto, CA, USA: Consulting Psychologists Press; 1983

[46] Fraley RC, Waller NG, Brennan KA. An item response theory analysis of self-report measures of adult attachment. Journal of Personality and Social Psychology. 2000;**78**(2):350-364

[47] Lubiewska K, Głogowska K, Mickiewicz K, Wojtynkiewicz E, Izdebski P, Wiśniewski C. Skala experience in close relationships-revised: struktura, rzetelność oraz skrócona wersja skali w polskiej próbie. Psychologia Rozwojowa. 2016;**1**:49-63

[48] Nijenhuis E, Van der Hart O, Kruger K. The psychometric characteristics of the traumatic experiences checklist (TEC): First findings among psychiatric outpatients. Clinical Psychology & Psychotherapy. 2002;**9**(3):200-210

[49] Davis JM, Chen N. Dose response and dose equivalence of antipsychotics.

Journal of Clinical Psychopharmacology. 2004;**24**:192-208

[50] Andreasen NC, Pressler M, Nopoulos P, Miller D, Ho BC. Antipsychotic dose equivalents and dose-years: A standardized method for comparing exposure to different drugs. Biological Psychiatry. 2010;**67**(3):255-262

[51] WHOCC. ATC/DDD index. 2023. Available from: https://www.whocc.no/atc_ddd_index/

[52] Leucht S, Samara M, Heres S, Davis JM. Dose equivalents for antipsychotic drugs: The DDD method. Schizophrenia Bulletin. 2016;**42**:90-94

[53] Robins JM, Mark SD, Newey WK. Estimating exposure effects by modelling the expectation of exposure conditional on confounders. Biometrics. 1992;**48**(2):479

[54] Robins JM, Rotnitzky A. Comment on "inference for semiparametric models: Some questions and an answer" by P. Bickel and J. Kwon. Statistica Sinica. 2001;**11**:920-936

[55] Bang H, Robins JM. Doubly robust estimation in missing data and causal inference models. Biometrics. 2005;**61**(4):962-973

[56] Tchetgen Tchetgen EJ, Robins JM, Rotnitzky A. On doubly robust estimation in a semiparametric odds ratio model. Biometrika. 2010;**97**(1):171

[57] R Core Team. R: A Language and Environment for Statistical Computing. R Foundation for Statistical Computing. Vienna, Austria: R-project; 2023

[58] Zetterqvist J, Sjölander A. Doubly robust estimation with the R Package degree, Version 1.1.10. Epidemiologic Methods. 2015;**4**(1):69-86

[59] Revelle W. Procedures for Psychological, Psychometric, and Personality Research [R Package Psych Version 2.3.9]. Evanston, Illinois: Northwestern University, R project; 2023

[60] Wickham H, François R, Henry L, Müller K, Vaughan D. Dplyr: A Grammar of Data Manipulation. R Package Version 1.1.3. 2023

[61] Wickham H, Bryan J. Readxl: Read Excel Files. R Package Version 1.4.3. 2023.

[62] Zitman FG, Linssen ACG, Edelbroek PM, Van Kempen GMJ. Does addition of low-dose flupentixol enhance the analgetic effects of low-dose amitriptyline in somatoform pain disorder? Pain. 1991;**47**(1):25-30

[63] Fishbain DA, Cutler RB, Lewis J, Cole B, Rosomoff RS, Rosomoff HL. Do the second-generation "atypical neuroleptics" have analgesic properties? A structured evidence-based review. Pain Medicine. 2004;**5**(4):359-365. DOI: 10.1111/j.1526-4637.2004.04054.x

[64] Gupta S, Black DW, Arndt S, Hubbard WC, Andreasen NC. Factors associated with suicide attempts among patients with schizophrenia. Psychiatric Services. 1998;**49**(10):1353-1355

[65] Meltzer HY, Alphs L, Green AI, Altamura AC, Anand R, Bertoldi A, et al. Clozapine treatment for suicidality in schizophrenia: International suicide prevention trial (InterSePT). Archives of General Psychiatry. 2003;**60**(1):82-91. DOI: 10.1001/archpsyc.60.1.82

[66] Schreiber S, Getslev V, Backer MM, Weizman R, Pick CG. The atypical neuroleptics clozapine and olanzapine differ regarding their antinociceptive mechanisms and potency. Pharmacology, Biochemistry, and Behavior. 1999;**64**(1):75-80

[67] Chang L, Munsaka SM, Kraft-Terry S, Ernst T. Magnetic resonance spectroscopy to assess neuroinflammation and neuropathic pain. Journal of Neuroimmune Pharmacology. 2013;**8**(3):576-593

[68] Chelala L, O'Connor EE, Barker PB, Zeffiro TA. Meta-analysis of brain metabolite differences in HIV infection. Neuroimage Clin. 2020;**28**:1-14

[69] Taylor MJ, Schweinsburg BC, Alhassoon OM, Gongvatana A, Brown GG, Young-Casey C, et al. Effects of human immunodeficiency virus and methaphetamine on cerebral metabolites measured with magnetic resonance spectroscopy. Journal of Neurovirology. 2007;**13**(2):150-159

[70] Swanberg KM, Landheer K, Pitt D, Juchem C. Quantifying the metabolic signature of multiple sclerosis by in vivo proton magnetic resonance spectroscopy: Current challenges and future outlook in the translation from proton signal to diagnostic biomarker. Frontiers in Neurology. 2019;**10**:1-34

[71] Ligneul C, Palombo M, Hernández-Garzón E, Carrillo-De Sauvage MA, Flament J, Hantraye P, et al. Diffusion-weighted magnetic resonance spectroscopy enables cell-specific monitoring of astrocyte reactivity in vivo. NeuroImage. 2019;**191**:457-469

[72] Ebert T, Heinz DE, Almeida-Corrêa S, Cruz R, Dethloff F, Stark T, et al. Myo-inositol levels in the dorsal hippocampus serve as glial prognostic marker of mild cognitive impairment in mice. Frontiers in Aging Neuroscience. 2021;**13**:1-17

[73] Cleeland C, Pipingas A, Scholey A, White D. Neurochemical changes in the aging brain: A systematic review. Neuroscience and Biobehavioral Reviews. 2019;**98**:306-319

[74] Lind A, Boraxbekk CJ, Petersen ET, Paulson OB, Siebner HR, Marsman A. Regional Myo-inositol, Creatine, and choline levels are higher at older age and scale negatively with visuospatial working memory: A cross-sectional proton MR spectroscopy study at 7 tesla on Normal cognitive ageing. The Journal of Neuroscience. 2020;**40**(42):8149-8159

[75] Gong T, Hui SCN, Zöllner HJ, Britton M, Song Y, Chen Y, et al. Neurometabolic timecourse of healthy aging. NeuroImage. 2022;**264**:119740

[76] González-Velasco O, Papy-García D, Le Douaron G, Sánchez-Santos JM, De Las RJ. Transcriptomic landscape, gene signatures and regulatory profile of aging in the human brain. Biochim Biophys Acta Gene Regul Mech. 2020;**1863**(6):194491-194491

[77] Payán-Gómez C, Rodríguez D, Amador-Muñoz D, Ramírez-Clavijo S. Integrative analysis of global gene expression identifies opposite patterns of reactive Astrogliosis in aged human prefrontal cortex. Brain Sciences. 2018;**8**(12):227-247

[78] Grachev ID, Thomas PS, Ramachandran TS. Decreased levels of N-acetylaspartate in dorsolateral prefrontal cortex in a case of intractable severe sympathetically mediated chronic pain (complex regional pain syndrome, type I). Brain and Cognition. 2002;**49**(1):102-113

[79] Harris RE, Sundgren PC, Pang Y, Hsu M, Petrou M, Kim SH, et al. Dynamic levels of glutamate within the insula are associated with improvements in multiple pain domains in fibromyalgia. Arthritis and Rheumatism. 2008;**58**(3):903-907

[80] Grachev ID, Fredrickson BE, Apkarian AV. Abnormal brain chemistry

in chronic back pain: An in vivo proton magnetic resonance spectroscopy study. Pain. 2000;**89**(1):7-18. DOI: 10.1006/brcg.2001.1489

[81] Harris RE, Sundgren PC, Craig AD, Kirshenbaum E, Sen A, Napadow V, et al. Elevated insular glutamate in fibromyalgia is associated with experimental pain. Arthritis and Rheumatism. 2009;**60**(10):3146-3152

[82] Jung YH, Kim H, Jeon SY, Kwon JM, Kim YC, Lee WJ, et al. Neurometabolite changes in patients with complex regional pain syndrome using magnetic resonance spectroscopy: A pilot study. Neuroreport. 2019;**30**(2):108-112. DOI: 10.1097/WNR.0000000000001168

[83] Penfield W, Boldrey E. Somatic motor and sensory representation in the cerebral cortex of man as studied by electrical stimulation. Brain. 1937;**60**(4):389-443

[84] MacLean PD. Psychosomatic disease and the visceral brain; recent developments bearing on the Papez theory of emotion. Psychosomatic Medicine. 1949;**11**(6):338-353

[85] Foltz EL, White LE. The role of rostral cingulumotomy in "pain" relief. International Journal of Neurology. 1968;**6**(3-4):353-373

[86] Foltz EL, White LE. Pain "relief" by frontal cingulumotomy. Journal of Neurosurgery. 1962;**19**:89-100

[87] Corkin S, Hebben N. Subjective estimates of chronic pain before and after psychosurgery or treatment in a pain unit. Pain. 1981;**11**:S150

[88] Berthier M, Starkstein S, Leiguarda R. Asymbolia for pain: A sensory-limbic disconnection syndrome. Annals of Neurology. 1988;**24**(1):41-49

[89] Rainville P, Duncan GH, Price DD, Carrier B, Bushnell MC. Pain affect encoded in human anterior cingulate but not somatosensory cortex. Science. 1997;**277**(5328):968-971

[90] Tölle TR, Kaufmann T, Siessmeier T, Lautenbacher S, Berthele A, Munz F, et al. Region-specific encoding of sensory and affective components of pain in the human brain: a positron emission tomography correlation analysis. Annals of Neurology. 1999;**45**(1):40-47

[91] Zubieta JK, Smith YR, Bueller JA, Xu Y, Kilbourn MR, Jewett DM, et al. Regional mu opioid receptor regulation of sensory and affective dimensions of pain. Science. 2001;**293**(5528):311-315

[92] Ostrowsky K, Magnin M, Ryvlin P, Isnard J, Guenot M, Mauguière F. Representation of pain and somatic sensation in the human insula: A study of responses to direct electrical cortical stimulation. Cerebral Cortex. 2002;**12**(4):376-385

[93] Strittmatter M, Ostertag D, Hoffmann KH, Paulus C, Fischer C, Meyer S. Monoaminergic transmitters in the cerebrospinal fluid of patients with acute, chronic, and intermittent pain. Interface between pain and depression? Der Nervenarzt. 2005;**76**(4):443-452. DOI: 10.1007/s00115-004-1746-z

[94] Kruse AO, Bustillo JR. Glutamatergic dysfunction in schizophrenia. Translational Psychiatry. 2022;**12**(1):1-13. DOI: 10.1038/s41398-022-02253-w

[95] Hagelberg N, Jääskeläinen SK, Martikainen IK, Mansikka H, Forssell H, Scheinin H, et al. Striatal dopamine D2 receptors in modulation of pain in humans: A review. European Journal of Pharmacology. 2004;**500**(1-3):187-192. DOI: 10.1016/j.ejphar.2004.07.024

[96] Narita M, Kuzumaki N, Narita M, Kaneko C, Hareyama N, Miyatake M, et al. Chronic pain-induced emotional dysfunction is associated with astrogliosis due to cortical delta-opioid receptor dysfunction. Journal of Neurochemistry. 2006;**97**(5):1369-1378

[97] Seminowicz DA, Laferriere AL, Millecamps M, Yu JSC, Coderre TJ, Bushnell MC. MRI structural brain changes associated with sensory and emotional function in a rat model of long-term neuropathic pain. NeuroImage. 2009;**47**(3):1007-1014

[98] Low LA, Millecamps M, Seminowicz DA, Naso L, Thompson SJ, Stone LS, et al. Nerve injury causes long-term attentional deficits in rats. Neuroscience Letters. 2012;**529**(2):103-107

[99] van Heeringen K, Mann JJ. The neurobiology of suicide. Lancet Psychiatry. 2014;**1**(1):63-72. DOI: 10.1016/S2215-0366(14)70220-2

[100] Lampe A, Doering S, Rumpold G, Sölder E, Krismer M, Kantner-Rumplmair W, et al. Chronic pain syndromes and their relation to childhood abuse and stressful life events. Journal of Psychosomatic Research. 2003;**54**(4):361-367

[101] Barrett LF, Simmons WK. Interoceptive predictions in the brain. Nature Reviews Neuroscience. 2015;**16**(7):419-429. DOI: 10.1038/nrn3950

[102] Hassanpour MS, Simmons WK, Feinstein JS, Luo Q, Lapidus RC, Bodurka J, et al. The insular cortex dynamically maps changes in cardiorespiratory Interoception. Neuropsychopharmacology. 2017;**43**:426-434. DOI: 10.1038/npp.2017.154

[103] Chen J, Li Z, Lv YF, Li CL, Wang Y, Wang RR, et al. Empathy for pain: A novel bio-psychosocial-behavioral laboratory animal model. Sheng Li Xue Bao. 2015;**67**(6):561-570

[104] Abbar M, Demattei C, El-Hage W, Llorca PM, Samalin L, Demaricourt P, et al. Ketamine for the acute treatment of severe suicidal ideation: Double blind, randomised placebo controlled trial. BMJ. 2022;**376**:1-9. DOI: 10.1136/bmj-2021-067194

[105] Nowacka A, Borczyk M. Ketamine applications beyond anesthesia - A literature review. European Journal of Pharmacology. 2019;**860**:1-14. DOI: 10.1016/j.ejphar.2019.172547

[106] Siegel AN, Di Vincenzo JD, Brietzke E, Gill H, Rodrigues NB, Lui LMW, et al. Antisuicidal and antidepressant effects of ketamine and esketamine in patients with baseline suicidality: A systematic review. Journal of Psychiatric Research. 2021;**137**:426-436. DOI: 10.1016/j.jpsychires.2021.03.009

[107] Prangnell A, Shoveller J, Voon P, Shulha H, Grant C, Milloy MJ, et al. The impact of childhood emotional abuse on pain interference among people with chronic pain who inject drugs in Vancouver, Canada. Pain Medicine. 2020;**21**(4):704-713. DOI: 10.1093/pm/pnz233

[108] Prangnell A, Voon P, Shulha H, Nosova E, Shoveller J, Milloy MJ, et al. The relationship between childhood emotional abuse and chronic pain among people who inject drugs in Vancouver, Canada. Child Abuse & Neglect. 2019;**93**:119-127. DOI: 10.1016/j.chiabu.2019.05.006

[109] Ee JS, Culp PA, Bevis ZJ, Dogbey GY, Agnello RN, Chang MH. Chronic pain

and childhood adversity experiences among U.S. military personnel. Military Medicine. 2023;**188**(6):561-566. DOI: 10.1093/milmed/usad244

[110] Guillory J, Chang P, Henderson CR, Shengelia R, Lama S, Warmington M, et al. Piloting a text message-based social support intervention for patients with chronic pain: Establishing feasibility and preliminary efficacy. The Clinical Journal of Pain. 2015;**31**(6):548-556

[111] Burger AJ, Lumley MA, Carty JN, Latsch DV, Thakur ER, Hyde-Nolan ME, et al. The effects of a novel psychological attribution and emotional awareness and expression therapy for chronic musculoskeletal pain: A preliminary, uncontrolled trial. Journal of Psychosomatic Research. 2016;**81**:1-8

[112] Hanley MA, Raichle K, Jensen M, Cardenas DD. Pain catastrophizing and beliefs predict changes in pain interference and psychological functioning in persons with spinal cord injury. The Journal of Pain. 2008;**9**(9):863-871

[113] Brink CB, Viljoen SL, De Kock SE, Stein DJ, Harvey BH. Effects of myo-inositol versus fluoxetine and imipramine pretreatments on serotonin 5HT2A and muscarinic acetylcholine receptors in human neuroblastoma cells. Metabolic Brain Disease. 2004;**19**(1-2):51-70

[114] Villalba H, Shah K, Albekairi TH, Sifat AE, Vaidya B, Abbruscato TJ. Potential role of myo-inositol to improve ischemic stroke outcome in diabetic mouse. Brain Research. 2018;**1699**:166-176. DOI: 10.1016/j.brainres.2018.08.028

[115] Claxson A, Morris C, Blake D, Sirén M, Halliwell B, Gustafsson T, et al. The anti-inflammatory effects of D-myo-inositol-1.2.6-trisphosphate (PP56) on animal models of inflammation. Agents and Actions. 1990;**29**(1-2):68-70. DOI: 10.1007/BF01964724

[116] Hori H, Kim Y. Inflammation and post-traumatic stress disorder. Psychiatry and Clinical Neurosciences. 2019;**73**(4):143-153. DOI: 10.1111/pcn.12820

Chapter 4

Existing and Newer Therapies in the Management and Diagnosis of Schizophrenia

Shreshth Khanna

Abstract

Schizophrenia is a serious mental health disorder that affects a person's overall well-being. It is a functional psychosis in which severe personality changes and thought disorders occur with no evidence of organic cerebral damage. The disease manifestation primarily includes the presence of two types of symptoms "positive" and "negative." Positive symptoms include delusions, illusions, auditory hallucinations, thought disorders with irrational conclusions, poor sentence formation, and stereotypic or aggressive behavior, whereas negative symptoms include withdrawn behavior, poor socialization, emotional dampening, absence of enthusiasm, and cognitive deficits. Usually, the onset is at the age of 15–30 years. Starting treatment as early as possible is an important step in the recovery process. Cognitive symptoms include problems in attention, concentration, and memory. Antipsychotic medications can help to alleviate the frequency and intensity of psychotic symptoms. These medications are usually taken in tablet or liquid form on a daily basis. Some antipsychotic medications are given as injections at intervals of 2–4 weeks. Psychosocial treatments help people find solutions to everyday challenges and manage symptoms while attending school, working, and forming relationships. Educational programs can help family and friends learn about symptoms of schizophrenia, treatment options, and strategies for helping loved ones with the illness.

Keywords: schizophrenia, psychosis, antipsychotic medicines, hallucinations, disorganized thoughts, cognitive behavioral therapy

1. Introduction

Schizophrenia is a mental disorder characterized by disruptions in thought processes, perceptions emotional responsiveness, and social interactions. Schizophrenia is a severe and disabling disorder. It is one of the leading causes of years lost to disability worldwide.

The term schizophrenia finds its roots from "schizo" (split) and "phrene" (mind) to define the disorganized thinking of people with schizophrenia.

Characteristic presentation of the patients with schizophrenia includes symptoms such as hallucinations, delusions, and disorders in thought perception and execution, reduced emotional expression, reduced enthusiasm to focus and achieve goals, tumultuous relationships, motor, and cognitive impairment [1].

Antipsychotic medications remain the mainstay treatment modality of schizophrenia. Evidence-based psychosocial interventions in conjunction with pharmacotherapy can help patients achieve better compliance and recovery.

Negative and positive symptoms of schizophrenia include abulia, anhedonia, social withdrawal, alogia, and affective flattening. Positive schizotypy comprises ideas of reference, delusions, illusions, and hallucinations [2].

2. Causes

The exact cause/s of schizophrenia are still unknown. Some of the postulated causes include:

Traumatic brain injury.

Childhood traumatic events.

Imbalance of the neurotransmitters, birth defects.

3. Pathogenesis of schizophrenia

3.1 Genetic predisposition

The genetic studies have provided some insights that inheritance can account for at least some proportion of schizophrenic disorders. Identical twins possess up to 60% chance of disease development. The risk in first-degree relatives is about 10% [3]. Reports of linkages of schizophrenia to loci on chromosomes 1, 2, 5, 6, 8, 10, 13, 15, and 22 have been identified [4]. Despite the evidence for genetic linkages, the results are inconclusive.

3.2 Dopamine hypothesis of schizophrenia

The dopamine hypothesis was based on the discovery that haloperidol bound to dopamine sites with higher affinity compared to the other neurotransmitters. These sites were named antipsychotic/dopamine receptor sites (D2 receptors). Subsequently, it was also established that a minimum of 65% receptor occupancy of the D2 receptors was needed for appropriate antipsychotic benefit [5].

Evidence that suggests excessive dopaminergic activity underlies the disorder:

Positron emission tomography (PET) scan shows increased dopamine (DA) receptor density in both schizophrenic patients. Post-mortem studies in the patients with schizophrenia reveal the presence of increased DA receptor densities [6].

Drugs that increase the DA activity such as levo-dopa (DA precursor) or amphetamine (DA releaser) either aggravate or precipitate symptoms of schizophrenia.

The levels of homo-vanillic acid (HVA), a metabolite of DA, in the cerebrospinal fluid (CSF), plasma, and urine increase during the early phases of therapy.

The "dopamine hypothesis" thus came into being and has been used since then to describe the underlying pathophysiology of schizophrenia.

However, in the wake of recent literature dysregulation of the serotonergic, glutamatergic, GABA-ergic, opioid, cholinergic, and probably other systems are incriminated [7].

3.3 Serotonin hypothesis of schizophrenia

According to this hypothesis, an increased excitatory neuromodulation in the serotonergic pathway in the dorsolateral frontal lobe and the anterior cingulate cortex forms an important pathophysiological basis of the disease. The concept of excessive serotonergic stimulation can also be validated by nuclear magnetic resonance (NMR) spectroscopy [8].

Additionally, the implication of serotonin as a neurotransmitter in schizophrenia stems from several observations including post-mortem human studies in patients of schizophrenia demonstrating decreased cortical 5-HT_{2A} receptor density, the psychotogenic effects of lysergic acid diethylamide (LSD) mimicking the symptoms of schizophrenia, and the ability of atypical antipsychotic drugs to bind to the serotonin receptors to bring about the antipsychotic response [8].

3.4 Glutamate hypothesis of schizophrenia

The glutamate hypothesis of schizophrenia was initially proposed based on the observation that the N-methyl-D-aspartate (NMDA) receptor antagonists like phencyclidine and ketamine induced positive and negative symptoms in healthy individuals that resembled symptoms of schizophrenia and exacerbated the symptoms in schizophrenia patients. The N-methyl-D-aspartate (NMDA) receptor is a glutamatergic receptor that may be involved in brain overactivity that is usually seen with the withdrawal of sedatives such as alcohol, resulting in agitation and seizures. Reduced glutamate receptor densities have been reported in post-mortem brains of schizophrenics [9].

Glutamate exerts excitatory and DA exerts inhibitory role over GABAergic striatal neurons which project to thalamus and serve as a sensory gate. An increase in glutamate or decrease in DA facilitates GABAergic activity at this gate. In contrast, decreased glutamate and increased DA activity will disable the gate to allow uninhibited sensory inputs to reach the cortex [10].

Additionally, studies using NMR spectroscopy neuroimaging have linked GABA and glutamate NMDA receptors to abnormal brain connectivity in individuals with schizophrenia [11].

Abnormal NMDA glutamate receptor activity is implicated in sensory and cognitive deficits, thought disorders, negative and positive symptoms of schizophrenia, and executive dysfunction [12].

4. Clinical presentation

Schizophrenia is a heterogeneous group of disorders characterized by perturbations of language, thinking, and social activity. The disorder mostly begins in the adolescent age group and has an insidious onset and a poor outcome. Social withdrawal, perceptual distortions, recurrent delusions, and hallucinations are the common presentations in the patients suffering from schizophrenia.

The manifestations of the disease include two types of symptoms: "positive" and "negative."

Patients may present with positive symptoms such as conceptual distortions, delusions, illusions, auditory hallucinations, thought disorders, garbled sentences and stereotypical aggressive behavior, delusions and hallucinations, and/or negative symptoms such as loss of functions, anhedonia, decreased emotional expression, impaired concentration, introvert behavior, poor socialization, emotional blunting, lack of motivation, and cognitive deficits.

According to the DSM-5 criteria to diagnose schizophrenia, two (or more) of the following, each of which should be present for a significant portion of time during 1-month period (or less if successfully treated).

At least one of these must be delusions, hallucinations, or disorganized speech:

Delusions
Hallucinations
Disorganized speech (e.g., frequent derailment or incoherence)

Grossly disorganized or catatonic behavior.

Negative symptoms (i.e., diminished emotional expression or avolition).

Continuous signs of the disturbance persist for at least 6 months. This 6-month period must include at least 1 month of symptoms (or less if successfully treated) that meet the above criteria (i.e., active phase symptoms) and may include periods of prodromal or residual symptoms [13].

During these prodromal or residual periods, the signs of the disturbance may be manifested only by negative symptoms or by two or more symptoms listed above present in an attenuated form.

For a significant portion of time since the onset of the disturbance, level of functioning in one or more major areas, such as work, interpersonal relations, or self-care is markedly below the level achieved prior to the onset (or when the onset is in childhood or adolescence, there is a failure to achieve the expected level of interpersonal, academic, or occupational functioning) [13].

5. Lab investigations/neuroimaging

The neuroimaging studies have highlighted a considerable cortical tissue loss of up to 5% of the brain volume and enlargement of cerebral ventricles in the patients of schizophrenia. The affected tissue structures include the hippocampus, superior temporal, and the prefrontal cortex which are also present with reduced gray matter volumes [14].

Hyperactivity in the hippocampal and the dorsal lateral prefrontal cortex regions has been observed in various MRI studies, leading to a postulation that a loss of inhibitory functions of the neurons may be responsible to an extent for the symptoms in schizophrenia.

A plentitude of structural and functional imaging modalities is currently being contemplated to discern the patterns of brain connectivity particularly to outline the factors that cause a transition to full-blown psychosis [15].

6. Differential diagnosis

It is impertinent to diagnose and delineate schizophrenia from a wide range of mental disorders, including but not limited to:

- Substance-induced psychotic disorder
- Mood disorders with psychotic features

DOI: http://dx.doi.org/10.5772/intechopen.1005073

- Sleep-related disorders
- Delusional disorder
- Paranoid personality disorder
- Schizotypal personality disorder
- Pervasive developmental disorder
- Psychosis secondary to organic cause

7. Management of schizophrenia

7.1 Non-pharmacological

A range of effective care options for people with schizophrenia exists including cognitive behavioral therapy, medication, psychoeducation, and psychosocial therapy.

Facilitated and assisted living, societal support systems, and employment environments are quintessential care options for patients living with schizophrenia.

A recovery-oriented treatment practice, that is, giving people the agency in treatment decisions, is crucial for people with schizophrenia and their guardians.

7.2 Pharmacological

Antipsychotic medications remain the cornerstone in the management of schizophrenia. They are thought to control psychotic symptoms by affecting the level of neurotransmitter dopamine in the brain.

The treatment goal is to manage signs and symptoms at the lowest possible dose. Different drugs, different doses, or combinations can be implemented over time to achieve the desired result. Other symptoms accompanying psychosis could be addressed with medications such as anti-depressants or anti-anxiety drugs. It can take several weeks to notice an improvement in symptoms.

The Texas Medication Algorithm Project (TMAP) entails a six-stage pharmacotherapeutic algorithm in the treatment of schizophrenia.

Stage 1 involves treatment initiation with a second-generation antipsychotic (SGA) as a first-line therapy. In case of little to no therapeutic response, proceed to stage 2.

Stage 2 includes monotherapy with either another SGA or a first-generation antipsychotic (FGA). In case of absence of any therapeutic response, proceed to stage 3.

Stage 3 consists of clozapine monotherapy with a constant monitoring of the white blood cell (WBC) count. In case of agranulocytosis, clozapine therapy should be suspended. In case of absence of therapeutic response in stage 3, proceed to stage 4.

↓

Stage 4 entails a combination of clozapine therapy with an FGA or an SGA or electroconvulsive therapy (ECT). In case of resistance to treatment, proceed to stage 5.

↓

Stage 5 calls for monotherapy with an FGA or an SGA that has not been tried. Finally, in case of stage 5 treatment is still unsuccessful, proceed to stage 6.

↓

Stage 6 consists of combination therapy with an SGA, an FGA, ECT, and/or a mood stabilizer.

Combination therapy is recommended only in the later stages of the treatment algorithm [16].

Due to an increased predisposition to cause drug interactions, treatment nonadherence, and medication errors, routinely prescribing two or more antipsychotics is not endorsed.

8. Choice of antipsychotic medication

The choice between typical (FGA) and atypical antipsychotic (SGA) is of paramount importance.

As per the American Psychiatric Association, second-generation or the atypical antipsychotics (SGAs) except for clozapine are the agents of first choice in the treatment of schizophrenia. SGAs are usually preferred over first-generation antipsychotics (FGAs) because of their disposition for lesser extrapyramidal symptoms [17].

The clinical potencies of typical antipsychotic drugs are proportional to their respective affinities for the dopaminergic D2 receptor. The available antipsychotic agents are effective in only up to 70% of patients presenting with a first episode and full remission of symptoms may take up to 6–8 weeks. Appropriate clinical and drug history of the patient should be taken to help delineate and commence treatment with a new antipsychotic agent.

Lack of response to an antipsychotic drug for at least 6–8 weeks with good compliance should mandate a change in the antipsychotic.

Clozapine needs to be considered after failure of sequential trials of two antipsychotics (one of which is an SGA) or if the patient has an aggressive behavior, suicidal tendencies, not responding to their prescribed antipsychotic medication, and those experiencing unbearable side effects with two different classes of antipsychotic medications.

First-generation or typical antipsychotics are better suited to treating positive symptoms of schizophrenia, whereas the newer agents appear to be more effective in handling the positive and the negative as well as improving the cognitive symptoms.

Long-acting injectable preparations (risperidone, paliperidone, olanzapine, and aripiprazole) are considered when there is noncompliance with the therapy.

9. Treatment-resistance

Up to 30% of patients with schizophrenia show only little symptomatic improvement or unacceptable side effects after multiple trials of FGAs therapy. Clozapine is the most effective oral antipsychotic in terms of managing treatment-resistant schizophrenia.

10. First-generation antipsychotics

The first-generation antipsychotics have numerous and serious neurological side effects, that may or may not be irreversible. First-generation antipsychotics include:

- Chlorpromazine
- Fluphenazine
- Haloperidol
- Pimozide
- Sulpiride
- Perphenazine

11. Second-generation antipsychotics

These groups of newer generation medications are chosen as they possess a lower risk of serious side effects compared to the first-generation antipsychotic agents. Second-generation antipsychotics include:

- Aripiprazole
- Asenapine
- Brexpiprazole
- Cariprazine
- Clozapine
- Iloperidone
- Lurasidone
- Olanzapine

- Paliperidone
- Quetiapine
- Risperidone
- Ziprasidone

12. Long-acting injectable antipsychotics

In patients where non-adherence due to pill burden or side effects to oral medications is an impedance, some long-acting injectable antipsychotics can be given as intramuscular or subcutaneous injections. Depending on the medication they are usually given once every 2–4 weeks.

Common medications that are available as an injection include:

- Aripiprazole
- Fluphenazine decanoate
- Haloperidol decanoate
- Paliperidone
- Risperidone

13. Antipsychotic treatment

13.1 Dose

The dose of the antipsychotic needs to be tailored for every patient. A fine balance between relapse prevention and reducing the side effects should be maintained. Patients not experiencing positive symptoms during therapy may be candidates for reduction in doses, while monitoring for potential relapse. According to literature the dose of the medication needs to be tapered gradually by about 20% every 6 months till a stable effective dose is reached [18].

13.2 Duration of treatment

The duration of treatment depends on a number of factors and should be personalized. The suggested guidelines are as follows:

- First-episode patients ought to receive 1–2 years of maintenance treatment.
- Patients with several episodes or exacerbations are to receive maintenance treatment for 5 years or longer after the last episode.
- Patients with a history of suicide attempts or showcasing aggressive behavior should receive treatment for longer time periods.

Rapid initiation of drug treatment is of utmost importance, specifically within the first 5 years after an acute episode, as this is the duration where most neurological changes in the brain take place [19].

13.3 Augmentation and combination therapy

In case of inadequate or subtherapeutic response to clozapine therapy in the patients both the augmentation (i.e., ECT and or a mood stabilizer) and combination therapy (with another antipsychotic) may be considered.

However, exposure to multiple antipsychotics at the same time may increase the risk of serious side effects [20].

The practicing physicians should contemplate the following factors before administering the augmentation therapy: [21].

- The augmentation therapy should be considered in patients with a prior inadequate or subtherapeutic response to therapy.
- Augmentation agents are effective in treating symptoms of schizophrenia when given in conjunction with other treatment modalities.
- In case of lack of clinical response to the augmentation strategy, the therapy should be withheld and other options should be contemplated.

Mood stabilizers, anxiolytics, anti-depressants, and anti-convulsant are commonly used as drugs in the augmentation therapy [22].

Treatment during the acute phase of schizophrenia is followed by a maintenance phase of treatment which aims at increasing socialization and improving self-care and mood.

Maintenance treatment is essential to help prevent relapse of symptoms. In most schizophrenia patients, it is difficult to implement effective rehabilitation programs without using antipsychotic agents [19].

14. Mechanism of drug action

The exact mechanism by which the antipsychotic drugs produce their effects remains obscure. Depending on their receptor affinities, they are mainly categorized as follows:

1. Typical or older antipsychotic agents, which produce their therapeutic effects primarily via high dopamine (D_2) antagonism and low serotonin (5-HT_{2A}) antagonism;
2. The therapeutic efficiency of atypical neuroleptics, revolves around the antagonism of the N-methyl-D-aspartate (NMDA) and α1 and α2 adrenergic activity, thereby modifying the balance between 5-HT2 and D2 receptor activity. These agents demonstrate moderate to high D_2 and 5-HT2A receptor antagonism [23].

To contain the positive symptoms of schizophrenia, at least 60–65% of D_2 receptors must be occupied by the antipsychotic agents, whereas ≥77% of D_2 receptor blockade has been associated with the extrapyramidal symptoms [23].

The improvement in the negative paradigms of schizophrenia and the cognitive benefits with the use of atypical antipsychotics has been attributed primarily to the 5-HT_{2A} antagonism in combination with the D_2 antagonism, resulting in the release of dopamine into the prefrontal cortex [17].

15. Side effects of the antipsychotic drugs

15.1 Endocrine system

Hyperprolactinemia has been seen to occur in up to 80% of patients treated with antipsychotic agents like risperidone or paliperidone, which may lead to sexual dysfunction, decreased libido, menstrual irregularities, or gynecomastia. Some of the newer atypical antipsychotic agents like aripiprazole or ziprasidone may serve as possible replacement treatment options in the patients with increased prolactin levels [24].

Weight gain is another significant side effect in patients receiving antipsychotic drugs and may eventually lead to non-adherence.

Antipsychotic drugs also can increase the risk of type-II diabetes. Olanzapine has the greatest risk of diabetes, followed by risperidone and quetiapine [24].

15.2 Cardiovascular system

Orthostatic or postural hypotension and tachycardia are attributed to the $\alpha 1$ adrenoceptor blockade and vagal inhibition, respectively. These have been seen to occur in up to 75% of patients treated with an antipsychotic agent. Patients with diabetes, pre-existing cardiovascular disease, or elderly age appear to be at a greater risk, and counseling regarding the same should be practiced [17].

ECG changes, especially QTc prolongation, can occur with the use of antipsychotic agents such as thioridazine, clozapine, iloperidone, and ziprasidone. QTc prolongation should be constantly monitored throughout the therapy, and treatment must be discontinued if this interval consistently exceeds 500 msec. The choice of an antipsychotic agent should be based on the patient profile taking into consideration patients' pre-existing cardiac or cerebrovascular disease or the use of drugs like diuretics or the drugs that have a tendency to prolong the QTc interval [17].

15.3 Lipid changes

Hypertriglyceridemia, hypercholesterolemia, and dyslipidemia are a possible squeal in the patients of schizophrenia treated with SGAs or typical antipsychotics like phenothiazines. Newer antipsychotics that are safer in this regard include drugs such as risperidone, ziprasidone, and aripiprazole. Olanzapine has been shown to have negative effects on cholesterol levels and lipids [21].

15.4 Central nervous system

15.4.1 Dystonia

This disorder often results in non-adherence and can be life-threatening. Dystonic reactions typically accompany treatment with FGAs. Dystonia may be minimized by using SGAs or by initiating FGAs at lower doses [17].

15.4.2 Akathisia

Akathisia is an inability to remain still and has been seen in up to 40% of patients treated with high-potency older antipsychotic agents such as haloperidol and fluphenazine. Novel antipsychotics such as quetiapine and clozapine appear to have the lowest risk for this side effect. The use of propranolol and diphenhydramine may be helpful in providing relief in this regard [25].

15.4.3 Pseudoparkinsonism

The incidence of this disorder has ranged from 15% to 36% in patients treated with FGAs. There is an increased risk of drug induced Parkinsonism with higher doses of risperidone. Although the incidence of the same taking into consideration, the use of novel antipsychotics in the treatment of schizophrenia-increased risk is relatively low. Treatment of drug-induced Parkinsonism is with the use of anti-cholinergic agents such as trihexyphenidyl and procyclidine [17].

15.4.4 Tardive dyskinesia

Characterized by involuntary oro-buccal-lingual dyskinesias. The prevalence of the disorder is up to 25% among patients receiving FGA therapy. The risk of tardive dyskinesia is significantly lower with the use of newer generation antipsychotic agents. The management of tardive dyskinesias involves increasing the cholinergic activity along with "neurolept-holidays" [17].

15.4.5 Sedation

Chlorpromazine, thioridazine, mesoridazine, clozapine, olanzapine, and quetiapine have the highest sedation potential. The potential of these agents could be exploited in patients of schizophrenia accompanied by irritation and insomnia. Studies have shown that SGAs offer superior cognitive benefits compared with FGAs [17].

15.4.6 Seizures

All antipsychotic agents carry an increased predisposition to cause seizures. The antipsychotic agents that are the most infamous for causing seizures are clozapine and chlorpromazine. Antipsychotic agents including risperidone, molindone, thioridazine, haloperidol, pimozide, trifluoperazine, and fluphenazine are associated with the lower risk in this regard.

15.4.7 Poikilothermia

One of the severe side effects of antipsychotic therapy is poikilothermia. Patients may be at increased risk of heat stroke because of the inability to dissipate excess body heat, especially during exercise or physical exertion. These side effects most commonly occur during treatment with the older antipsychotics such as chlorpromazine, but they have also been associated with the SGAs such as clozapine [17].

15.4.8 Neuroleptic malignant syndrome (NMS)

It is a life-threatening side effect of antipsychotic drug therapy in extremely sensitive to the extrapyramidal side effects of neuroleptics. The incidence of NMS is up to 1.0% in the patients treated with the older antipsychotics such as fluphenazine and haloperidol. The novel antipsychotic agents appear to be relatively safer in this regard. The treatment of NMS involves the use of drugs such as dantrolene, diazepam, and bromocriptine [17].

15.4.9 Miscellaneous adverse effects

Schizophrenia medications can cause a variety of other adverse effects, including the following:

- Chlorpromazine is commonly associated with opaque deposits in the lens.
- Quetiapine is associated with an increased risk of cataracts. Whereas, thioridazine at doses ≥800 mg daily is at risk of retinitis pigmentosa.
- Clozapine has been associated with urinary hesitancy and retention.
- FGAs and risperidone have a greater tendency to cause sexual dysfunction.
- Treatment with antipsychotics can cause transient leukopenia.
- Clozapine, chlorpromazine, and olanzapine are associated with a risk of hematological complications such as neutropenia or agranulocytosis.
- Both FGAs and SGAS can cause photosensitivity reactions.

The varying safety profiles of antipsychotic medications may be due to their effects on various neuroreceptor systems.

16. Progress evaluation

The progress of recovery during the treatment of schizophrenia is both objective and subjective.

Objectively, the recovery can be quantified by the relief of symptoms and the return of the patient to work. The use of various scales including the Brief Psychiatric Rating Scale (BPRS) and the Positive and Negative Syndrome Scale (PANSS) serve as valuable pointers in the improvement of schizophrenia.

Subjective parameters of recovery are measured by the patient themselves in terms of his or her life satisfaction, feeling of hope, and knowledge about his or her mental illness [26].

Despite continuous recent therapeutic advances into the treatment, there is a significant number of years lost to disability and a substantial reduction in life expectancy in the patients suffering from schizophrenia by about 10–25 years [26].

17. Antipsychotic drugs

17.1 Typical antipsychotic drugs (older generation antipsychotic drugs)

17.1.1 Butyrophenone

Butyrophenones are synthetic compounds employed as antipsychotic medications. Besides treating psychotic conditions, certain members have demonstrated effectiveness in controlling nausea and vomiting. A few examples within this class include haloperidol, droperidol, melperone, domperidone, and benperidol.

17.1.2 Haloperidol

Haloperidol, a widely used first-generation typical antipsychotic, is used to address the positive symptoms of schizophrenia. It blocks the dopaminergic D2 receptors in the brain. It reaches its peak effectiveness at 72% receptor blockade. However, besides blocking the D2 receptors, haloperidol also blocks the noradrenergic, cholinergic, and histaminergic receptors, which amount to several adverse drug reactions.

17.1.2.1 Pharmacokinetics

Absorption: Haloperidol is a highly lipophilic drug, and its oral bioavailability is 70%. The time to reach peak plasma concentration is 6 hours after oral administration. It is approximately 93% plasma protein bound. It undergoes extensive metabolism in the liver via sulfoxidation and CYP3A4, 2D6, and 1A2 enzymes [27].

Approximately 30% of haloperidol is primarily excreted in the urine.

Schizophrenia: The recommended dosing involves oral administration of 5–20 mg, taken 2–3 times a day. The maximum recommended oral dosage should not exceed 100 mg/d.

17.1.2.2 Extrapyramidal adverse effects

Acute dystonia, akathisia, neuroleptic malignant syndrome (NMS), Parkinsonism, and tardive dyskinesia (TD) are commonly observed in haloperidol therapy.

Other less common adverse effects include orthostatic hypotension, lens opacities, anxiety, cerebral edema, depression, dizziness, confusion, anorexia, constipation, dyspepsia, ileus, QT prolongation, and torsades de pointes [28].

17.1.3 Pimozide

Pimozide is commonly used as an antipsychotic agent. It works by affecting the balance of certain neurotransmitters in the brain, helping to alleviate symptoms of delusions and hallucinations.

17.1.3.1 Pharmacokinetics

Pimozide is well-absorbed orally and reaches peak concentrations within a few hours. It is widely distributed throughout the body, including the central nervous system (CNS). It is metabolized through the CYP450 enzyme system. Its long half-life leads to a sustained duration of action. The drug and its metabolites are excreted in the feces, with a smaller portion excreted in the urine.

17.1.3.2 Dosage

The dosage of pimozide is usually started from 1 to 2 mg/day.

17.1.3.3 Adverse reactions

Changes in prolactin levels, menstrual irregularities, and blood dyscrasias. Neuroleptic malignant syndrome, QTc prolongation, sedation, drowsiness, affecting alertness and concentration dry mouth, constipation, urinary retention, blurred vision, and weight gain.

Extrapyramidal symptoms including tremors, rigidity, bradykinesia, tardive dyskinesia are seen with the use of pimozide.

17.1.4 Phenothiazines

17.1.4.1 Chlorpromazine

Chlorpromazine belongs to the first-generation antipsychotic (FGA) or typical antipsychotics. It exerts its antipsychotic effect by blocking post-synaptic D2 receptors in the mesolimbic pathway. However, its extrapyramidal side effects are attributed to the blockade of D2 receptors in the nigrostriatal pathway. The antiemetic effect of chlorpromazine is attributed to the combined blockade of histaminergic H1, dopaminergic D2, and muscarinic M_1 receptors in the vomiting center.

17.1.4.2 Pharmacokinetics

Chlorpromazine is metabolized primarily by the CYP1A2 and 2D6 enzymes. Elimination takes place through urine, bile, and feces, with a half-life ranging from 10 to 40 hours for its active metabolite.

The medication is available as tablets and can also be administered as intramuscular and intravenous injections.

17.1.4.3 Dosage

The dose is initially started from 25 to 75 mg/day orally twice a day to a range of 100–1000 mg/day.

The parenteral route of the drug is initially started at 25 mg, followed by 25–50 mg after 1–4 hours. The usual dose can be up to 800 mg/day.

17.1.4.4 Adverse drug reactions (ADRs)

It causes non-neurologic side effects such as dryness of mouth, blurring of vision, dizziness, postural hypotension, urinary retention, and constipation by blocking the muscarinic receptors. Elderly age patients are particularly at an increased risk of angle-closure glaucoma. Due to the blockade of the histamine H1 receptors, there is an increased potential for sedation.

It also causes hyperprolactinemia, gynecomastia, galactorrhea, erectile dysfunctions irregular menstruation, oligomenorrhea, amenorrhea, and galactorrhea.

Corneal depositions, QT interval prolongation, cholestatic jaundice, and drug induced hepatotoxicity, which may significantly increase the alanine aminotransferase level (ALT). Regular monitoring of the liver enzymes should be done during chlorpromazine therapy, and in case of the early detection of liver injury, the drug should be stopped.

Chlorpromazine can also cause EPS such as acute dystonia, akathisia, Parkinsonism, and tardive dyskinesia (TD) [29].

17.1.5 Thioridazine

It is a typical antipsychotics used to effectively treat the positive symptoms of schizophrenia, such as hallucinations, delusions, and disorganization by blocking D2 receptors in the mesolimbic pathway. Thioridazine is a substrate of the hepatic enzyme CYP450 2D6 and is also an inhibitor of the same enzyme.

17.1.5.1 Dosage

Thioridazine is initiated from 50 to 100 mg three times per day to a maximum of 800 mg/day.

17.1.5.2 ADRs

17.1.5.2.1 Extrapyramidal side effects

It is associated with a risk of developing EPS including dystonia, Parkinsonism, and tardive dyskinesia. The neuroleptic malignant syndrome (NMS) is another serious side effect.

Thioridazine is associated with prolonged QTc intervals, such as torsades de pointes. Hence, initiating this medicine at a lower dose is advised, and a prior ECG should be done.

Pigmentary retinopathy is specific to thioridazine. Nonspecific symptoms include dry mouth, dry eyes, sedation, orthostatic hypotension, weight gain, dizziness, erectile dysfunction, pruritus, photosensitivity, and constipation. Rare ADRs include irreversible retinal pigmentation, poikilothermia, and agranulocytosis [29].

17.1.6 Fluphenazine

Fluphenazine is a high-potency antipsychotic agent which brings about its therapeutic effect largely through antagonism of post-synaptic D-2 dopaminergic receptors in mesolimbic, nigrostriatal, and the tuberoinfundibular pathways. The blockage of post-synaptic dopaminergic D-2 receptors in the mesolimbic pathway addresses the positive symptoms of schizophrenia.

Owing to the antagonistic actions on the α1 adrenergic receptors, fluphenazine is known to cause various cardiac side effects. Fluphenazine has strong antagonistic effects at both muscarinic M-1 and histaminergic H-1 receptors.

17.1.6.1 Dosage

Fluphenazine is typically initiated from 2.5 to 10 mg/day divided every 6 to 8 hours.

Fluphenazine has a relatively half-life of about 15 hours. The injection formulations are dosed from 12.5 to 25 mg I.M. or S.C. every 28 days. The maximum dose of fluphenazine is 40 mg/day.

17.1.6.2 Pharmacokinetics

It is extensively metabolized and undergoes "first pass" metabolism in the hepatocytes and is excreted both via the urinary and fecal route. It is ≥90% plasma protein bound. With oral fluphenazine, peak plasma/serum levels are attained within a few hours. Fluphenazine crosses the blood-brain barrier and the blood-placental barrier easily and cannot be removed by dialysis.

17.1.6.3 ADR

Due to the dopamine receptor antagonism as well as its anticholinergic antihistaminic and alpha receptor blocking actions, fluphenazine has a wide range of adverse effect profile. Fluphenazine is commonly associated with sedation, dryness of mouth and eyes, blurring of vision, urinary retention and constipation, orthostatic hypotension, reflex tachycardia, and dizziness. Extrapyramidal side effects including akathisia, pseudo-parkinsonism and tardive dyskinesia are also observed [30].

Endocrinal side effects such as galactorrhea, gynecomastia, sexual dysfunction, amenorrhea in females, and on off-cycle bleeding can occur. Various serious side effects including neuroleptic malignant syndrome, liver function abnormalities, jaundice, seizures, and agranulocytosis have been observed. It carries a black-box warning for increased risk of cerebrovascular events and death especially in the elderly patients. QT interval prolongation and T-wave abnormalities have been also been associated with its use [30].

17.1.7 Thioxanthenes

17.1.7.1 Flupentixol

It is a typical antipsychotic drug of the thioxanthene class.

Although commonly prescribed as an oral tablet formulation, it is mainly used is as a long-acting injectable formulation that can be given once or twice a month to individuals with schizophrenia having poor compliance and adherence with the oral medications and/or a history of frequent relapses.

17.1.7.2 Pharmacokinetics

It is absorbed 40% after oral administration. It is widely distributed throughout the body including the CNS. It is 99% plasma protein bound. It is extensively metabolized. The metabolites are excreted in the feces and urine. The dihydrochloride metabolite has a half-life of 35 hours.

The dose range of flupenthixol varies from 10 to 200 mg/2 to 4 weeks.

17.1.7.3 Adverse drug reactions

Hypokinesia, muscle rigidity, Parkinsonism, tremors, akathisia, dystonia, dry mouth, dizziness, blurring of vision, agranulocytosis, and osteoporosis on long-term use [31].

17.1.8 Sulpiride

Sulpiride is an antipsychotic medication that belongs to the benzamide class. Sulpiride exerts its therapeutic effects by blocking dopamine D2 and D3 receptors.

17.1.8.1 Pharmacokinetics

Following oral administration, it has a bioavailability of 30%. It is approximately 40% plasma protein bound particularly to albumin. It is has a plasma half-life around 8 hours. It has an aVD of about 2.72 ± 0.66 L/kg.

17.1.8.2 Dosage

The usual dosage is started from 4 mg twice a day.

Side effects include extrapyramidal symptoms, sedation, weight gain, dyslipidemia, and hyperprolactinemia [32].

17.2 Atypical neuroleptics

17.2.1 Clozapine

It is a second-generation or atypical antipsychotic. It acts as an atypical antipsychotic to dopamine and serotonin receptors. It binds to the 5-HT1A and D4 receptor more than the D2 receptor, contributing to decrease adverse events and extrapyramidal symptoms. Unlike other antipsychotics, clozapine does not cause a rise in prolactin level.

17.2.1.1 Pharmacokinetics

The peak concentrations are attained in 2.5 hours. It exhibits approximately 97% plasma protein binding. The uptake of clozapine in the liver is by solute carrier family (SLC) transporter protein. Clozapine is metabolized by CYP3A4. It has a half-life up to 12 hours. Approximately 50% of clozapine is excreted in the urine and 30% in the feces.

Treatment is started from 12.5 mg once or twice daily and increased by 25–50 mg daily to target 150–600 mg daily in divided doses by day 14.

17.2.1.2 Adverse effects

Agranulocytosis mandating weekly WBC count especially for first 3 months of therapy, myocarditis, metabolic syndrome, hyperglycemia, hypertriglyceridemia, seizures, excessive salivation, pulmonary embolism, and neuroleptic malignant syndrome [33].

17.2.2 Olanzapine

Olanzapine is a second-generation (atypical) antipsychotic medication. It works as D2 receptor antagonist at the post-synaptic receptors leading to a decrease in positive symptoms in patients, including hallucinations, delusions, disorganized speech, thoughts, and behavior. Olanzapine is similar neurochemically to clozapine but has a significant risk of inducing weight gain.

Olanzapine works similarly on serotonin 5HT2A receptors in the frontal cortex as an antagonist and decreases negative symptoms, including anhedonia, flat affect, alogia, avolition, and poor attention.

17.2.2.1 Pharmacokinetics

Absorption: Steady-state plasma concentration in about 1 week. The time to peak concentration is 6 hours for oral formulation. The volume of distribution is approximately 1000 L, and it is 93% plasma protein bound.

Olanzapine is extensively metabolized by glucuronidation and the cytochrome P450 system primarily CYP1A2 and 2D6. The half-life of olanzapine is approximately 30 hours. Olanzapine is excreted primarily via the renal route (57%) and feces (30%).

The usual dosage is started from 2.5, 5, 7.5, 10, 15, and 20 mg dosages to targeted 10–30 mg/day.

17.2.2.2 Adverse drug reaction

Impaired glucose tolerance, metabolic syndrome, increased akathisias, and extrapyramidal symptoms [34].

17.2.3 Risperidone

It exhibits their therapeutic effects through some D2 and 5HT2A blockade. Their binding affinity to the D2 receptors is low accounting for the lesser likelihood of causing EPS. The relative potency is more toward the 5-HT2 receptor sites than the D2 receptor sites. Risperidone also exerts considerable α2 antagonism.

Paliperidone is a recently approved agent that is a metabolite of risperidone and shares many of its properties.

They are agonist at the 5HT1A receptor, besides it also has additional serotonin and norepinephrine reuptake inhibiting effects. The blockade of the D2 receptors specifically in the mesolimbic pathway is thought to be the reason for the improvement in the positive symptoms of schizophrenia.

The dosage is started from 1 mg daily, to a maximum dose of 16 mg daily.

17.2.3.1 ADR

Acute dystonia, akathisia, tardive dyskinesia, weight changes, metabolic changes, and sedation are significant concerns with risperidone [35].

17.2.4 Quetiapine

Quetiapine has many complex mechanisms, but it mediates its pharmacological effect via its 5HT2 antagonistic action. Quetiapine has a strong affinity for the 5-HT2 and on the dopaminergic D1 and D2 receptors, where they act as an antagonist to bring about the therapeutic response. Additionally, it has anxiolytic and antidepressant properties owing to the blockade of the norepinephrine transporter (NET) and partial agonistic activity at the 5 HT1A receptor, respectively. Quetiapine is distinct in having a weak D2 effect but potent α1 and histamine blockade.

The usual dose is 300–800 mg/day. The half-life for quetiapine is about 7 hours.

17.2.4.1 Adverse drug reactions

It is associated with an increased risk of death in dementia-related psychosis in elderly patients. Neuroleptic malignant syndrome, increased suicidal ideations, somnolence, orthostatic hypotension, and dizziness are the most common side effects of quetiapine [36].

17.2.5 Ziprasidone

Ziprasidone is another atypical antipsychotic agent that has a substantial binding affinity for the 5HT2A receptors compared to the D2, α1, and H1 receptors.

Antagonism at the dopamine (D2) receptor in the mesolimbic pathway may be responsible in diminishing the positive symptoms, whereas the antagonism at the 5HT2A receptor sites in the mesocortical pathway may be responsible for the reduction of negative symptoms of psychosis. Ziprasidone causes minimal weight gain and is unlikely to increase prolactin but may increase QT prolongation.

17.2.5.1 Pharmacokinetics

Ziprasidone has a half-life of 7–10 hours. It attains its steady-state plasma concentration within 1–3 days of initiation of dosing. The average systemic clearance of ziprasidone is 7.5 ml/min/kg. Elimination of ziprasidone is primarily via the hepatic route.

17.2.5.2 Dosage

Ziprasidone is started at 20 mg twice per day with meals, to a maximum of 120–200 mg/day. As several days are needed to attain steady-state plasma concentrations, dose adjustments should occur gradually after a few days.

17.2.5.3 ADR

Patients treated with antipsychotic drugs may develop tardive dyskinesia [37].

17.2.6 Aripiprazole

Aripiprazole, an atypical antipsychotic, has shown effectiveness in reducing irritability, hyperactivity. Acting as a partial agonist at D2 and 5HT-1a receptors and an antagonist at the 5HT-2a receptor. Aripiprazole stabilizes dopamine and serotonin in specific brain regions, effectively managing positive, negative, and cognitive symptoms in schizophrenia.

17.2.6.1 Pharmacokinetics

Aripiprazole has an oral availability is 87%. The mean elimination half-life is about 75 hours. Aripiprazole acts as a substrate of both the cytochrome P-450 3A4 and 2D6 isoenzymes, predisposing to various drug-drug interactions.

Dosage aripiprazole should be started at a dose of 10 or 15 mg/day, preferably administered along with the meals. The maximum dose should not exceed 30 mg/day.

17.2.6.2 ADR

The most frequent adverse effects are headache, anxiety, insomnia, nausea, vomiting, lightheadedness, weight gain, or prolactin increase as a result of its partial agonist properties [38].

17.2.7 Zotepine

Zotepine is an antipsychotic medication used in the treatment of various psychiatric disorders, primarily schizophrenia.

17.2.7.1 Pharmacokinetics

Zotepine is typically administered orally, and its absorption may be influenced by factors such as the formulation of the drug and the individual's gastrointestinal function. After absorption, it is distributed throughout the body, including the central nervous system, where it exerts its therapeutic effects. It undergoes metabolism in the liver, through the cytochrome P450 system. Zotepine and its metabolites occurs through renal excretion and possibly through hepatic routes.

17.2.7.2 Dosage

25 mg tid increased at 4-day interval to a maximum of 100 mg tid.

17.2.7.3 Adverse reactions

Common side effects of zotepine may include sedation, weight gain, orthostatic hypotension, and anticholinergic effects such as dry mouth. Metabolic effects, including changes in blood glucose and lipid levels, are also seen with its use [39].

17.2.8 Sertindole

Sertindole is an atypical antipsychotic medication. It works by blocking the dopaminergic and serotonin receptors which helps to normalize the imbalance of these neurotransmitters associated with psychotic disorders.

17.2.8.1 Pharmacokinetics

Sertindole is typically administered orally, and its absorption may be influenced by factors such as the formulation of the drug and individual variations in gastrointestinal function. After absorption, sertindole is likely to be distributed throughout the body, including the central nervous system, where it exerts its therapeutic effects. Sertindole undergoes extensive hepatic metabolism, primarily through the cytochrome P450 enzyme system. The elimination of sertindole and its metabolites primarily occurs through renal excretion and possibly through hepatic routes.

17.2.8.2 Dosage

Initially started with 4 mg/day to a maximum of 24 mg/day.

17.2.8.3 Adverse reactions

Common side effects may include sedation, weight gain, increased appetite, orthostatic hypotension, and QT interval prolongation [40].

17.2.9 Asenapine

It is an atypical antipsychotic medication that is used for the treatment of schizophrenia and bipolar disorder.

17.2.9.1 Pharmacokinetics

Absorption: It is formulated for sublingual administration. The sublingual route allows for rapid absorption and onset of action. It is extensively plasma protein bound. It undergoes hepatic metabolism, through the cytochrome P450 (CYP) enzyme system. The elimination half-life of asenapine is relatively short, and it is eliminated through both hepatic and renal routes.

Drug Interactions: Asenapine may interact with other medications that are strong inhibitors or inducers of CYP1A2 and CYP2D6 influencing their plasma concentrations.

Dosage: Asenapine is typically administered sublingually in doses of 5–10 mg twice daily.

Adverse reactions: Common side effects may include sedation, somnolence, weight gain, metabolic effects, orthostatic hypotension, and increased blood glucose levels. It is also associated with a risk of extrapyramidal side effects [41].

17.2.10 Lurasidone

Lurasidone is an atypical antipsychotic. The mechanism of action of lurasidone involves both the dopaminergic and serotonergic receptors. It acts as an atypical antipsychotic owing to the antagonism at the D2, 5-HT2A receptors, whereas antagonism at the 5-HT7 and partial agonism at the 5-HT1A receptors contribute to the antidepressant properties of lurasidone.

17.2.10.1 Dosage

Lurasidone is available in various strengths, that is, 20, 40, 60, 80, and 120 mg tablets. It is poorly soluble after oral ingestion. It should be administered with a slightly high calories diet, regardless of the fat content, which helps in increasing its oral bioavailability. Upon administration the time to peak plasma concentration takes about 3 hours, and a steady-state concentration is achieved in 7 days. Lurasidone is primarily metabolized by CYP3A4 isoenzyme.

Usually started from 40 mg/day to a maximum dose of 160 mg/day in adults and 80 mg/day in adolescents. In the case of renal and hepatic impairment, the maximum dose is 80 mg/day.

17.2.10.2 Adverse effects

Lurasidone is a relatively safety advantage with a reduced risk of metabolic side effects such as hypercholesterolemia, hyperlipidemia, hyperglycemia, and weight gain when compared with the other atypical antipsychotic agents.

The most common adverse effects experienced are nausea, akathisia, somnolence, weight gain, sedation, and drug-induced Parkinsonism [42].

18. Newer approaches

18.1 Ulotaront

Ulotaront (SEP-363856) is a trace-amine-associated receptor 1 (TAAR1) agonist having a 5-HT1A receptor agonist activity. It is in phase III clinical development, with FDA breakthrough therapy designation, for the treatment of schizophrenia. Population-based pharmacokinetic analysis showed that ulotaront was rapidly absorbed and quickly cleared from plasma after oral administration to subjects with schizophrenia. The plasma protein binding of ulotaront is relatively low. It has been shown to inhibit CYP2D6, and it induces CYP2B6 [43].

18.2 Ralmitaront

Ralmitaront (RO6889450) is a TAAR1 partial agonist presently undergoing phase II clinical trials.

Further results are awaited.

18.3 KarXT (xanomeline-trospium)

Xanomeline is a dual M_1 and M_4 muscarinic receptor agonist having negligible D_2 dopamine receptor blockage, which is unlike the presently available therapies for schizophrenia. Xanomeline-trospium (KarXT) combines xanomeline with the peripherally restricted muscarinic receptor antagonist trospium chloride with the goal of improving xanomeline-related adverse events associated with peripheral muscarinic receptors. In the phase III EMERGENT-2 trials, it has been shown to decrease positive and negative symptoms of schizophrenia [44].

18.4 Emraclidine (CVL-231)

Emraclidine is a novel, brain-penetrant, highly selective M_4 receptor positive allosteric modulator in development for the treatment of schizophrenia. It is presently in phase II clinical trials. M_4 receptor subtypes are selectively expressed in the striatum and activation of these receptors has been shown to indirectly regulate dopamine levels without blocking D2/D3 receptors, which may lead to unwanted motor side effects seen in current antipsychotics [45].

18.5 Pimavanserin

It is a selective serotonin receptor-modulating agent with a preferable inverse agonist/antagonist activity at serotonergic 5-HT_{2A} receptors. Steady-state C_{max} and $AUC_{0–24}$ values are approximately 3- to 5-fold greater after once-a-day oral administration (50–150 mg) for 14 days, which is consistent with pimavanserin's long plasma half-life (57 hours). The oral bioavailability of pimavanserin is 99.7% [46].

18.6 Luvadaxistat (TAK-831)

Luvadaxistat (also known as TAK-831 and NBI-1065844) is a potent investigational, first-in-class oral selective inhibitor with high binding affinity to DAAO inhibitor and supposedly increases the NMDA activity. It is developed for the management of negative symptoms and cognitive impairment associated with schizophrenia (CIAS) [47].

18.7 Cannabidiol

Cannabidiol (CBD) is a phytocannabinoid that is an important constituent of *Cannabis sativa* and has been postulated to be of pharmacological benefits in schizophrenia. Delta-9-tetrohydrocannabinol (THC) is the main psychoactive ingredient in cannabis having anxiogenic, psychotomimetic, and amnestic effects. CBD has been seen to possess anxiolytic, antipsychotic, and anticonvulsant properties. Several trials are underway to establish its therapeutic potential [48].

18.8 Brexpiprazole

Brexpiprazole has been approved by the FDA for treatment of schizophrenia in adults. Its indication was expanded to the treatment of agitation and dementia associated with Alzheimer's disease. It has a high affinity for the D2 and the 5-HT2A receptors and is a potent partial agonist at the 5-HT1A and 5-HT2C receptors. Brexpiprazole has been found to be efficacious for long-term management of schizophrenia as it shows a relatively favorable adverse effect profile besides reducing both positive and negative symptoms and has low tendencies to cause EPS [49].

18.9 Samidorphan and olanzapine

Samidorphan, a μ-opioid receptor antagonist, and olanzapine combination marketed as Lybalvi, is used in the treatment of adults with schizophrenia and bipolar disorder 1. The combination is available as an oral tablet composed of multiple strengths of olanzapine (5–20 mg) and a fixed dose of 10 mg of samidorphan. In studies enrolling healthy adults and adults with schizophrenia, the combination of olanzapine with samidorphan, a μ-opioid receptor antagonist, mitigated weight gain associated with olanzapine monotherapy [50].

18.10 Sarcosine

N-methyl-glycine (sarcosine) is a potent inhibitor of glycine transporter-1. Sarcosine generally has negligible side effects and is very well tolerated by people with schizophrenia. Larger and longer studies with adequate sample sizes are mandated to better estimate the long term effectiveness and safety and to establish the therapeutic potential of sarcosine as an augmentation therapy to present antipsychotic therapy [51].

18.11 Bitopertine

It is an alternative formulation for schizophrenia that focuses primarily on the disturbances of brain glutamatergic neurotransmission, particularly at the NMDA receptors (NMDAR). Long-term trials are needed to establish its therapeutic benefits [52].

18.12 Repetitive transcranial magnetic stimulation (rTMS)

rTMS is widely used in the treatment of various psychiatric disorders. Stimulation of patients' temporoparietal areas may treat schizophrenic patients' hallucinatory symptoms, and stimulation of patients' frontal areas may improve patients' negative symptoms and cognition. Because of the slow disease progression, patients often have to take the medication for a long time, so the side effects of the medication cannot be ignored. The side effects of long term anti-schizophrenia medication can cause a plethora of side effects including insulin antagonism, adrenaline antagonism affecting glucose and lipid metabolism, cardiac arrhythmias, and other various adverse reactions. Although several trials are underway, large-scale studies are needed to establish their therapeutic benefits [53].

19. Conclusion

Schizophrenia is a serious mental disorder that affects the patients and their relatives. The management of schizophrenia involves an interplay of both the pharmacological and non-pharmacological interventions. A total of ≥30% of patients remain resistant to the existing treatment. Newer drugs targeting various targets are in different phases of drug development. The quest for an optimally designed drug with desirable safety and efficacy is still on.

Author details

Shreshth Khanna
Hamdard Institute of Medical Sciences and Research, Jamia Hamdard, New Delhi, India

*Address all correspondence to: shreshthkhanna@gmail.com

References

[1] Schizophrenia National Institute of Mental Health. 2023. Available from: https://www.nimh.nih.gov/health/statistics/schizophrenia#:~:text=Symptoms%20of%20schizophrenia%20include%20psychotic,motor%20impairment%2C%20and%20cognitive%20impairment [Accessed: February 20, 2024]

[2] Correll CU, Schooler NR. Negative symptoms in schizophrenia: A review and clinical guide for recognition, assessment, and treatment. Neuropsychiatric Disease and Treatment. 2020;**16**:519-534. DOI: 10.2147/NDT.S225643

[3] Lo LE et al. Risk of schizophrenia in relatives of individuals affected by schizophrenia: A meta-analysis. Psychiatry Research. Available from: https://www.sciencedirect.com/science/article/abs/pii/S0165178119318608. 2020 [Accessed: February 20, 2024]

[4] Bassett AS, Chow EW, Weksberg R. Chromosomal abnormalities and schizophrenia. American Journal of Medical Genetics. 2000;**97**(1):45-51. DOI: 10.1002/(sici)1096-8628(200021)97:1<45::aid-ajmg6>3.0.co;2-9

[5] Madras BK. History of the discovery of the antipsychotic dopamine D2 receptor: A basis for the dopamine hypothesis of schizophrenia. Journal of the History of the Neurosciences. 2013;**22**:62-78

[6] Weinstein JJ, van de Giessen E, Rosengard RJ, Xu X, Ojeil N, Brucato G, et al. PET imaging of dopamine-D2 receptor internalization in schizophrenia. Molecular Psychiatry. 2018;**23**(6):1506-1511. DOI: 10.1038/mp.2017.107. Epub 2017 May 16. Erratum in: Mol Psychiatry. 2017 Jul 25

[7] Deng C, Dean B. Mapping the pathophysiology of schizophrenia: Interactions between multiple cellular pathways. Frontiers in Cellular Neuroscience. 2013;7:238

[8] Eggers AE. A serotonin hypothesis of schizophrenia. Medical Hypotheses. 2013;**80**(6):791-794. DOI: 10.1016/j.mehy.2013.03.013. Epub 2013 Apr 1

[9] Correll CU, Kane JM. Schizophrenia: Mechanism of action of current and novel treatments. The Journal of Clinical Psychiatry. 2014;**75**:347-348

[10] van den Pol AN, Gao XB, Patrylo PR, Ghosh PK, Obrietan K. Glutamate inhibits GABA excitatory activity in developing neurons. The Journal of Neuroscience. 1998;**18**(24):10749-10761. DOI: 10.1523/JNEUROSCI.18-24-10749.1998

[11] McGlashan TH, Hoffman RE. Schizophrenia as a disorder of developmentally reduced synaptic connectivity. Archives of General Psychiatry. 2000;**57**:637-648

[12] Coyle JT, Tsai G, Goff D. Converging evidence of NMDA receptor hypofunction in the pathophysiology of schizophrenia. Annals of the New York Academy of Sciences. 2003;**1003**:318-327

[13] American Psychiatric Association. Diagnostic and Statistical Manual of Mental Disorders. 5th ed. Arlington, VA: American Psychiatric Association; 2013

[14] Shenton ME, Dickey CC, Frumin M, et al. A review of MRI

findings in schizophrenia. Schizophrenia Research. 2001;**49**:1-52

[15] Kerns JG, Lauriello J. Can structural neuroimaging be used to define phenotypes and course of schizophrenia? The Psychiatric Clinics of North America. 2012;**35**:633-644

[16] American Psychiatric Association Choosing Wisely. Five Things Physicians and Patients Should Question. 2013. Available from: http://www.choosingwisely.org/wp-content/uploads/2013/09/102913_F64_46-APA-5things-List_Draft-5.pdf [Accessed: February 21, 2024]

[17] Crismon L, Argo TR, Buckley PF. Schizophrenia. In: DiPiro JT, Talbert RL, Yee GC, et al., editors. Pharmacotherapy: A Pathophysiologic Approach. 9th ed. New York, New York: McGraw-Hill; 2014. pp. 1019-1046

[18] Grover S, Chakrabarti S, Kulhara P, Avasthi A. Clinical practice guidelines for management of schizophrenia. Indian Journal of Psychiatry. 2017;**59**(Suppl 1):S19-S33. DOI: 10.4103/0019-5545.196972

[19] Lehman AF, Lieberman JA, Dixon LB, et al. Practice guidelines; work group on schizophrenia. Practice guideline for the treatment of patients with schizophrenia, second edition. The American Journal of Psychiatry. 2004;**161**(suppl 2):1-56

[20] Lieberman JA, Stroup TS, McEvoy JP, et al. Effectiveness of anti-psychotic drugs in patients with chronic schizophrenia. The New England Journal of Medicine. 2005;**353**(12):1209-1223

[21] Nasrallah HA. Metabolic findings from the CATIE trial and their relation to tolerability. CNS Spectrums. 2006;**11**(suppl. 7):32-39

[22] Leucht S, Barnes TR, Kissling W, et al. Relapse prevention in schizophrenia with new-generation antipsychotics: A systematic review and exploratory meta-analysis of randomized controlled trials. The American Journal of Psychiatry. 2003;**160**(7):1209-1222

[23] Kapur S, Mamo D. Half a century of antipsychotics and still a central role for dopamine D2 receptors. Progress in Neuro-Psychopharmacology & Biological Psychiatry. 2003;**27**(7):1081-1090

[24] Monteleone P, Martiadis V, Maj M. Management of schizophrenia with obesity, metabolic and endocrinological disorders. The Psychiatric Clinics of North America. 2009;**32**(4):775-794

[25] Haddad PM, Dursun SM. Neurological complications of psychiatric drugs: Clinical features and management. Human Psychopharmacology. 2008;**23**(suppl. 1):15-26

[26] Laursen TM, Munk-Olsen T, Vestergaard M. Life expectancy and cardiovascular mortality in persons with schizophrenia. Current Opinion in Psychiatry. 2012;**25**(2):83-88

[27] Hiemke C, Bergemann N. Consensus guidelines for therapeutic drug monitoring in neuropsychopharmacology: Update 2017. Pharmacopsychiatry. 2018;**51**(1-02):9-62

[28] Beach SR, Celano CM. QT prolongation, torsades de pointes, and psychotropic medications: A 5-year update. Psychosomatics. 2018;**59**(2):105-122

[29] Morris E, Green D, Graudins A. Neuroleptic malignant syndrome developing after acute overdose with olanzapine and chlorpromazine. Journal of Medical Toxicology. 2009;**5**(1):27-31

[30] Brodeur S, Vanasse A, Courteau J, Stip E, Lesage A, Fleury MJ, et al. Comparative effectiveness and safety of antipsychotic drugs in patients with schizophrenia initiating or reinitiating treatment: A Real-World Observational Study. Acta Psychiatrica Scandinavica. 2022;**145**(5):456-468

[31] Mahapatra J, Quraishi SN, David A, Sampson S, Adams CE. Flupenthixol decanoate (depot) for schizophrenia or other similar psychotic disorders. Cochrane Database of Systematic Reviews. 2014;**2014**(6):CD001470. DOI: 10.1002/14651858.CD001470.pub2

[32] Davis C. Sulpiride, Sulpiride—An Overview. ScienceDirect Topics. Available from: https://www.sciencedirect.com/topics/chemistry/sulpiride; 2007 [Accessed: February 20, 2024]

[33] De Berardis D, Rapini G, Olivieri L. Safety of antipsychotics for the treatment of schizophrenia: A focus on the adverse effects of clozapine. Therapeutic Advances in Drug Safety. 2018;**9**(5):237-256

[34] Thomas K, Saadabadi A. Olanzapine. In: StatPearls. Treasure Island (FL): StatPearls Publishing; 2024. Available from: https://www.ncbi.nlm.nih.gov/books/NBK532903/ [Updated 2023 Aug 28]

[35] McNeil SE, Gibbons JR, Cogburn M. Risperidone. In: StatPearls. Treasure Island (FL): StatPearls Publishing; 2024. Available from: https://www.ncbi.nlm.nih.gov/books/NBK459313/ [Updated 2023 Jan 16]

[36] Maan JS, Ershadi M, Khan I, et al. Quetiapine. In: StatPearls. Treasure Island (FL): StatPearls Publishing; 2024. Available from: https://www.ncbi.nlm.nih.gov/books/NBK459145/ [Updated 2023 Aug 28]

[37] Bouchette D, Fariba KA, Marwaha R. Ziprasidone. In: StatPearls. Treasure Island (FL): StatPearls Publishing; 2024. Available from: https://www.ncbi.nlm.nih.gov/books/NBK448157 [Updated 2022 May 8]

[38] Gettu N, Saadabadi A. Aripiprazole. In: StatPearls. Treasure Island (FL): StatPearls Publishing; 2024. Available from: https://www.ncbi.nlm.nih.gov/books/NBK547739 [Updated 2023 May 16]

[39] DeSilva P, Fenton M, Rathbone J. Zotepine for schizophrenia. Cochrane Database of Systematic Reviews. 2006;**2006**(4):CD001948. DOI: 10.1002/14651858.CD001948.pub2

[40] Juruena MF, de Sena EP, de Oliveira IR. Sertindole in the management of schizophrenia. Journal of Central Nervous System Disease. 2011;**3**:75-85. DOI: 10.4137/JCNSD.S5729

[41] Balaraman R, Gandhi H. Asenapine, a new sublingual atypical antipsychotic. Journal of Pharmacology and Pharmacotherapeutics. 2010;**1**(1):60-61. DOI: 10.4103/0976-500X.64538

[42] Azhar Y, Shaban K. Lurasidone. In: StatPearls. Treasure Island (FL): StatPearls Publishing; 2024. Available from: https://www.ncbi.nlm.nih.gov/books/NBK541057 [Updated 2023 Jun 12]

[43] Heffernan MLR, Herman LW, Brown S, Jones PG, Shao L, Hewitt MC, et al. Ulotaront: A TAAR1 agonist for the treatment of schizophrenia. ACS Medicinal Chemistry Letters. 2021;**13**(1):92-98. DOI: 10.1021/acsmedchemlett.1c00527

[44] Kaul I, Sawchak S, Correll CU. Efficacy and safety of the muscarinic receptor agonist KarXT (xanomeline-trospium) in schizophrenia

(EMERGENT-2) in the USA: Results from a randomised, double-blind, placebo-controlled, flexible-dose phase 3 trial. Lancet. 2024;**403**(10422):160-170. DOI: 10.1016/S0140-6736(23)02190-6. Epub 2023 Dec 14

[45] Krystal JH. The Lancet. Emraclidine, a novel positive allosteric modulator of cholinergic M4 receptors, for the treatment of schizophrenia: A two-part, randomized, double-blind, placebo-controlled, phase 1b trial. 2023;**401**(10383):1131-1240. Available from: https://www.thelancet.com/journals/lancet/article/PIIS0140-6736(01)06225-0/abstract [Accessed: February 21, 2024]

[46] Cusick E, Gupta V. Pimavanserin. In: StatPearls. Treasure Island (FL): StatPearls Publishing; 2024. Available from: https://www.ncbi.nlm.nih.gov/books/NBK557712 [Updated 2023 May 1]

[47] Fradley R, Goetghebeur P, Miller D. Luvadaxistat: A novel potent and selective D-amino acid oxidase inhibitor improves cognitive and social deficits in rodent models for schizophrenia. Neurochemical Research. 2023;**48**(10):3027-3041. DOI: 10.1007/s11064-023-03956-2. Epub 2023 Jun 8. Erratum in: Neurochemical Research 2023 Jul 13

[48] Ahmed S, Roth RM, Stanciu CN, Brunette MF. The impact of THC and CBD in schizophrenia: A systematic review. Frontiers in Psychiatry. 2021;**12**:694394. DOI: 10.3389/fpsyt.2021.694394

[49] FDA (US Food and Drug Administration). FDA Approves New Drug to Treat Schizophrenia and as an Add on to an Antidepressant to Treat Major Depressive Disorder. 2015. Available from: https://www.fda.gov/newsevents/newsroom/pressannouncements/ucm454647.htm [Accessed: March 8, 2024]

[50] Keown A. Alkermes Announces FDA Approval of LYBALVITM for the Treatment of Schizophrenia and Bipolar I Disorder. Dublin, Ireland: BioSpace; 2021. Available from: https://www.biospace.com/article/releases/alkermes-announces-fda-approval-of-lybalvi-for-the-treatment-of-schizophrenia-and-bipolar-i-disorder [Accessed: September 7, 2021]

[51] Fond G, Mallet J, Urbach M, Benros ME, Berk M, Billeci M, et al. Adjunctive agents to antipsychotics in schizophrenia: A systematic umbrella review and recommendations for amino acids, hormonal therapies and anti-inflammatory drugs. BMJ Mental Health. 2023;**26**(1):e300771. DOI: 10.1136/bmjment-2023-300771

[52] Kantrowitz JT, Javitt DC. N-methyl-d-aspartate (NMDA) receptor dysfunction or dysregulation: The final common pathway on the road to schizophrenia? Brain Research Bulletin. 2010;**83**(3-4):108-121

[53] Kumar N et al. A randomized, double blind, sham-controlled trial of repetitive transcranial magnetic stimulation (rTMS) in the treatment of negative symptoms in schizophrenia. Brain Stimulation. Available from: https://www.sciencedirect.com/science/article/pii/S1935861X20300383#:~:text=Research%20has%20implicated%20hypofrontality%20in,shown%20to%20reverse%20this%20hypofrontality. 2020 [Accessed: February 21, 2024]

Chapter 5

Artificial Intelligence and Schizophrenia: Crossing the Limits of the Human Brain

António Melo, Joana Romão and Tiago Duarte

Abstract

This chapter delves into the transformative role of Artificial Intelligence (AI) in the diagnosis, treatment, and management of schizophrenia. It explores how AI's advanced analytical capabilities can address the complexities of this psychiatric condition. The discussion begins with an overview of AI's growing significance in healthcare, highlighting its potential in enhancing diagnostic precision and personalizing treatment strategies. Then, specific AI applications in schizophrenia care are examined, including early detection in at-risk individuals, AI-driven diagnostic tools, and the role of AI in guiding treatment choices. Furthermore, it discusses the challenges in translating AI's theoretical potential into practical clinical applications, particularly in accurately distinguishing between various psychiatric conditions. The ethical, legal, and privacy concerns arising from AI's integration into healthcare are also revised, emphasizing the need for balanced strategies and policies. This comprehensive examination of AI in schizophrenia care not only underscores its potential to revolutionize patient care but also highlights the crucial need for ongoing research and development to overcome current limitations and ethical challenges.

Keywords: artificial intelligence, machine learning, schizophrenia, early detection, predictive analytics, personalized treatment

1. Introduction

1.1 Artificial intelligence (AI) and its growing role in healthcare

In recent years, AI has emerged as a transformative force in various sectors, with healthcare being one of the most promising and rapidly evolving areas [1]. The infusion of AI into healthcare promises to enhance efficiency, accuracy, and outcomes across a spectrum of processes, ranging from patient diagnosis to treatment and long-term disease management. This technological revolution is particularly significant in the context of complex and multifaceted disorders like schizophrenia, where traditional approaches often encounter limitations in terms of early detection, personalized treatment, and continuous monitoring [2].

Artificial Intelligence (AI), with its unparalleled ability to analyze large datasets, recognize patterns, and learn from outcomes, presents an opportunity to address some of the most enduring challenges in schizophrenia care [1]. By leveraging technologies, such as machine learning, natural language processing, and predictive analytics, AI can assist in unveiling subtle nuances of the disease that often go unnoticed in conventional methods [2].

1.2 World Health Organization (WHO)'s 2023 report about the current state of AI in healthcare

As we progress through 2024, AI continues to play a transformative role in the healthcare sector. This overview released by the WHO [3] discusses the current state and future prospects of AI applications in healthcare. This list is by no means exhaustive, but instead aims to provide the reader with recent updates on this constantly evolving field.

- Enhanced diagnostics and personalized medicine: As previously mentioned, through the rapid processing of large amounts of data, AI-driven diagnostic tools are significantly advancing in terms of accuracy, particularly in early disease detection. Moreover, AI is pivotal in personalized medicine, tailoring treatments based on individual patient data, genetics, and lifestyle factors. These advancements are optimizing patient outcomes by providing more precise and effective treatment plans.

- Predictive analytics for disease prevention: AI's predictive analytics not only aid in early diagnosis, but can also forecast potential health issues before they occur, based on patterns in individual health data. This proactive approach allows healthcare providers to intervene early, potentially preventing or mitigating the onset or progression of diseases.

- Improving patient care and experience: AI-powered chatbots and virtual assistants are enhancing patient engagement by providing round-the-clock support. Wearables integrated with AI monitor health metrics in real time, enabling continuous care and timely interventions [4]. These technologies are not only improving patient care but are also making healthcare more accessible and efficient.

- Revolutionizing medical imaging: AI algorithms are refining the analysis of medical imaging, aiding in the early detection of conditions like cancer, which leads to improved treatment efficacy and survival rates.

- Drug discovery and development: AI is accelerating the drug discovery process by analyzing large datasets to predict molecular interactions and identify potential compounds for treating various diseases. This acceleration could lead to faster introductions of new treatments to the market.

- Streamlining administrative tasks: AI-driven automation is alleviating administrative burdens in healthcare. This includes handling routine tasks, such as billing, scheduling, and data entry, allowing healthcare professionals to focus more on patient care.

Artificial Intelligence (AI) in healthcare is witnessing continuous growth and innovation, with its applications ranging from diagnostic accuracy to operational efficiency. The integration of AI promises a healthcare future that is more efficient, accessible, and patient-centric.

1.3 How can AI enhance diagnosis, treatment, and management of schizophrenia?

The diagnosis of schizophrenia, traditionally reliant on clinical assessments and patient self-reporting, has been fraught with challenges. AI-driven diagnostic tools promise to bring a level of precision and objectivity to this process, harnessing algorithms that can analyze and interpret complex patterns in speech, behavior, and even brain imaging, leading to more accurate and timely diagnoses [5].

In treatment, AI's role is multifaceted, spanning from facilitating drug discovery and development to personalizing therapeutic intervention. AI systems can analyze genetic, environmental, and clinical data to predict individual responses to specific treatments, paving the way for personalized medicine in schizophrenia care. This not only enhances the efficacy of treatments but also minimizes adverse effects, leading to improved patient outcomes and quality of life [6].

Moreover, the management of schizophrenia, a long-term endeavor, may also be significantly bolstered by AI. AI-powered mobile apps and wearable devices offer new avenues for continuous monitoring of symptoms and treatment adherence, enabling timely interventions and better management of the disease. These predictive analytics can play a crucial role in identifying potential relapses or deterioration, facilitating proactive care strategies [4].

1.4 Purpose and scope of the chapter

This chapter aims to delve deeply into the burgeoning field of AI-driven innovations in schizophrenia care [1]. It seeks to elucidate how AI technologies can reshape the landscape of diagnosis, treatment, and management of schizophrenia [2]. The discussion will encompass a range of AI applications, highlighting both their current impacts and future potential.

In delving into these areas, this chapter is intended to initiate a preliminary reflection on the integration of AI into healthcare, especially within the delicate realm of mental health [3]. Acknowledging the rapid pace of technological advancement, it recognizes the possibility that its insights may become outdated over time. Nonetheless, it seeks to contribute to the discourse on the potential of AI in schizophrenia care. By outlining the current state-of-the-art AI applications and their implications, this chapter aspires to provide valuable perspectives to clinicians, researchers, and stakeholders in the mental health field. It highlights the initial yet significant steps AI is taking toward transforming schizophrenia care, emphasizing its emergent role in this critical area [4].

2. Fundamentals of AI in healthcare

2.1 Basic principles of AI and machine learning

Artificial Intelligence (AI) in healthcare involves simulating human intelligence processes through technology. Machine Learning (ML), a key subset of AI, focuses on training algorithms on data to make predictions or decisions. This training can take various forms, such as supervised, unsupervised, or semi-supervised, depending on the availability and nature of the data. In healthcare, AI and ML are applied to analyze complex data, aiding in improved decision-making and patient care outcomes. A study published in PNAS Nexus highlights the critical importance of multidisciplinary collaboration in advancing health through AI/ML, emphasizing the application of these methods across a wide range of research areas in healthcare [7].

Artificial Intelligence (AI) is therefore a revolutionary field that intersects technology and human intellect, aiming to create systems capable of performing tasks that typically require human intelligence. This field spans various aspects, such as learning, reasoning, problem-solving, perception, and language understanding. Its applications are diverse, ranging from simple tasks like sorting data to complex operations like driving autonomous vehicles or assisting in medical diagnoses.

Artificial Intelligence (AI) is not a singular technology but a collection of methodologies and tools. Its development has been a journey through various phases, from the initial focus on symbolic AI, where the emphasis was on imitating the logical reasoning of humans, to the current emphasis on machine learning and neural networks.

2.2 Understanding machine learning (ML)

Machine Learning (ML) is a pivotal aspect of AI, where algorithms are designed to learn from data. As these algorithms are exposed to more data over time, they improve their ability to make predictions or decisions, a process that mimics human learning. ML can be categorized into different types based on the nature of the learning process [8]:

- Supervised Learning: In this type, algorithms learn from labeled data, which are data that have been classified or annotated in some way. The algorithm uses these data to learn and make predictions. For instance, in healthcare, an algorithm could be trained with images labeled either as showing a disease or not, enabling it to identify that disease in new images.

- Unsupervised Learning: Unlike supervised learning, unsupervised learning involves algorithms learning from unlabeled data. Here, the focus is on finding patterns or structures within the data. For example, in e-commerce, an unsupervised learning algorithm might analyze customer purchasing data to identify distinct groups of customers based on buying patterns.

- Semi-Supervised Learning: This type of learning combines elements of both supervised and unsupervised learning. It's used when you have a large amount of data, but only some of it is labeled. The algorithm learns from the labeled data and applies this learning to the unlabeled data.

- Reinforcement Learning: In reinforcement learning, algorithms learn to make a sequence of decisions by trial and error, receiving feedback in the form of rewards or penalties. This type of learning is common in robotics and gaming, where the algorithm learns to make a series of decisions to achieve a goal.

The effectiveness of ML depends significantly on the quality and quantity of the data used for training. Large datasets can lead to more accurate and robust models.

However, it's crucial to consider the ethical implications of data use, especially in sensitive areas like healthcare.

Machine Learning (ML) has wide-ranging applications, from diagnosing diseases to recommending products, detecting fraud, and powering chatbots and self-driving cars. Its ability to automate complex tasks that are either too time-consuming or impossible for humans to perform manually makes it a powerful tool in various industries.

In summary, ML is a dynamic and transformative aspect of AI, continually evolving and finding new applications across different sectors. For professionals, particularly in healthcare and psychiatry, understanding these fundamentals of ML can provide valuable insights into the potential applications and implications of AI in their fields.

2.3 Understanding deep learning

Deep Learning [9], a sophisticated subset of ML, is centered around neural networks with numerous layers, commonly known as deep neural networks (DNNs). These networks are adept at recognizing intricate patterns in data, which is invaluable for tasks like image and speech recognition.

The core concept of deep learning is to imitate the functioning of the human brain with artificial neural networks (ANNs). Each "neuron" in these networks is a mathematical function that processes input data and passes its output to the next layer. The "deep" in deep learning refers to the number of layers through which the data are transformed. More layers allow the network to learn complex patterns at multiple levels of abstraction, making it powerful for a wide range of applications.

Deep learning networks are trained using large amounts of data and computational power. During training, these networks adjust their internal parameters (weights) to minimize the difference between their predictions and the actual outcomes (known as loss). This process is iterative and continues until the network optimally performs the task it's designed for.

These networks come in various forms, each suited for different types of tasks:

- Convolutional Neural Networks (CNNs): Predominantly used in image recognition and processing, CNNs are adept at recognizing visual patterns directly from pixel images with minimal preprocessing. They can identify faces, objects, and traffic signs, making them essential for computer vision applications.

- Recurrent Neural Networks (RNNs): Suited for sequential data like speech and text, RNNs can use their internal state (memory) to process sequences of inputs. This makes them ideal for tasks like speech recognition, language modeling, and translation.

- Autoencoders: Used for unsupervised learning, autoencoders are designed to compress the input into a lower-dimensional code and then reconstruct the output from this representation. This feature is particularly useful for anomaly detection and denoising.

- Generative Adversarial Networks (GANs): Comprising two networks, a generator and a discriminator, GANs are used for generating new data that resemble the training data. They are widely used in image generation, photo editing, and creating realistic art from sketches.

The effectiveness of deep learning has been demonstrated in various fields, from autonomous vehicles to medical diagnosis, where it has been instrumental in developing systems that surpass human-level performance in certain tasks. However, deep learning models require substantial data and computational resources, and there are ongoing challenges related to understanding and interpreting the decisions made by these models.

2.4 Understanding natural language processing (NLP)

Natural Language Processing (NLP) [10] is a vital domain AI that focuses on the interaction between computers and human language. It involves the development of algorithms and systems that can read, understand, interpret, and respond to human language in a way that is both meaningful and useful. This complex field combines elements of computer science, linguistics, and machine learning to enable computers to process and analyze large amounts of natural language data.

The applications of NLP are diverse and impactful:

- Chatbots and Virtual Assistants: NLP is the technology behind chatbots and virtual assistants like Siri, Alexa, and Google Assistant. These tools can understand and respond to voice or text inputs, assist with information retrieval, perform actions, and even mimic human-like conversations.

- Translation Services: NLP enables the translation of text or speech from one language to another. Tools like Google Translate utilize NLP algorithms to interpret the text in one language and accurately translate it to another, taking into account grammar, context, and idioms.

- Sentiment Analysis: NLP is used to analyze opinions, feelings, and attitudes in written language. This is particularly useful in social media monitoring, market research, and customer service, where it's essential to gauge public opinion or customer sentiment.

- Information Extraction: NLP can be used to extract key pieces of information from large texts, such as extracting names, dates, and places from news articles or identifying key terms in legal documents.

- Speech Recognition: NLP algorithms are fundamental in transcribing spoken language into text, used in voice-controlled devices and for creating subtitles or transcripts of audio recordings.

- Content Generation: Advanced NLP models, like Generative Pre-trained Transformer 3 (GPT-3), can generate coherent and contextually relevant text based on input prompts, which can be utilized for content creation, chatbots, or even coding.

One of the challenges in NLP is understanding the nuances of human language, including slang, irony, and context-dependent meanings. Additionally, languages continuously evolve, requiring NLP systems to adapt and learn over time.

To create efficient NLP systems, data scientists use various techniques, including tokenization (breaking text into words or phrases), part-of-speech tagging, syntactic parsing, and semantic analysis. The advent of deep learning has further advanced the capabilities of NLP, enabling more accurate and context-aware language processing.

2.5 Understanding computer vision

Computer Vision is another critical field in AI [11], where machines are equipped to interpret and analyze visual data from the world, akin to how human vision operates. By processing and understanding visual information, AI systems can perform a variety of complex tasks that were once considered challenging or impossible for machines.

This technology involves several key processes:

- Image recognition: Identifying objects and features within images, which can be applied to areas like security systems.

- Medical image analysis: Assisting in the diagnosis and research of various conditions through the analysis of medical imagery, which might indirectly contribute to understanding neurological disorders, including aspects of schizophrenia.

- Pattern recognition: Essential for facial recognition and analyzing visual patterns, which could have peripheral applications in patient monitoring or behavioral studies related to schizophrenia.

While Computer Vision is less directly involved in schizophrenia research, its advancements in pattern recognition and image analysis can provide supportive tools in broader medical research and diagnostics.

Artificial Intelligence (AI) systems require data to learn and make decisions. The quality, quantity, and diversity of these data significantly impact the performance of AI systems. Data ethics, including how data are collected, used, and shared, is a critical consideration in AI.

Despite its rapid advancement, AI still faces significant challenges. These include understanding the decision-making processes of AI systems (often referred to as the "black box" problem), ensuring fairness and avoiding bias in AI decisions, and managing the societal and ethical implications of AI.

In healthcare, AI has the potential to transform many aspects, from diagnostics and treatment plans to drug development and patient care. However, the integration of AI in healthcare must be done with consideration for accuracy, privacy, and ethical use of patient data.

For professionals in fields like psychiatry, understanding the fundamentals of AI can provide insights into how this technology might shape future research and practice in mental health care.

3. Artificial intelligence (AI) applications in schizophrenia care

If there is one takeaway message that is important to learn from this chapter, it is that AI's potential in healthcare stems from its ability to process large volumes of data quickly and accurately, uncovering patterns and insights that might elude traditional analysis. This capability is crucial for schizophrenia, when we consider this disorder's multifaceted nature, encompassing a wide spectrum of cognitive, behavioral, and emotional symptoms, which often pose a diagnostic and therapeutic challenge for clinicians.

As AI continues to evolve, its applications in schizophrenia care are expected to expand, potentially leading to groundbreaking changes in how this condition is understood, diagnosed, and treated. The upcoming subsections will delve into the main areas where AI is making an impact, reflecting a potential paradigm shift in the management of schizophrenia.

3.1 Early detection in at-risk individuals

The importance of early detection and intervention in schizophrenia has long been recognized by psychiatrists, with the main objective of reducing the duration of untreated psychosis [12]. AI is also being explored with this goal in mind, aiding in the prediction of early symptoms of schizophrenia in individuals who are at a higher risk for the disease. This early detection can be crucial in initiating timely interventions and possibly mitigating the severity of the disorder. Recent scientific studies [13–14] have made significant advancements in this area. These leverage AI to understand and predict the onset of schizophrenia.

Significant progress has also been made in identifying high-risk polymorphisms associated with schizophrenia [15], and efforts are ongoing to translate these into identifiable biomarkers for the disease. Although the clinical translation of these biomarkers has not happened yet, it is possible that these susceptibility polymorphisms could be important in specific at-risk populations with a family history of schizophrenia or exposure to childhood trauma. As an example, NEDD4 (neuronal precursor cell-expressed developmentally downregulated 4) single-nucleotide polymorphisms and childhood trauma are associated with increased morbidity for this disease, especially in people with a family history of psychoses [16].

Artificial Intelligence (AI) can aid in the clinical translation of these biomarkers, particularly through bioinformatics and computational biology. As previously explained, AI algorithms are adept at analyzing complex genetic data, identifying patterns, and establishing correlations that might be obscure through traditional analysis methods. This includes the analysis of genetic polymorphisms and RNA expressions related to schizophrenia.

It is also important to note that, although AI's predictive modeling capabilities can contribute to the early intervention by forecasting the onset of schizophrenia in at-risk individuals, the performance of machine learning methods is still highly varied, as recently documented in a meta-analysis [17], with the area under the curve (AUC) varying from 0,48 to 0,95. AUC is a measure used in statistics to evaluate the performance of a classification model. AUC scores range from 0 to 1, with higher scores indicating better performance. This means that recent studies report varying success rates in predicting the onset of schizophrenia in at-risk individuals, ranging from 48–95% success rate.

To illustrate the challenges inherent in psychiatric diagnosis, the Rosenhan experiment [18] offers a striking example of the difficulties faced by psychiatrists in accurately diagnosing schizophrenia. In this landmark study, "normal" individuals who feigned auditory hallucinations were all admitted to psychiatric hospitals and diagnosed with schizophrenia, despite having no history of mental illness. This experiment underscored the subjective nature of psychiatric diagnoses and highlighted the potential for misdiagnosis. It serves as a reminder of the importance of developing more reliable diagnostic methods, such as those AI might provide, to complement the clinical expertise of psychiatrists.

Several researchers have also been developing specific machine learning algorithms with a purpose in mind. For example, EMPaSchiz [19] was created for predicting schizotypy in first-degree relatives of schizophrenia patients. This innovative approach demonstrates how AI can be utilized to identify individuals who may be at risk of developing schizophrenia but do not yet show active symptoms. By analyzing features extracted from resting-state functional magnetic resonance imaging (fMRI), the EMPaSchiz algorithm was able to distinguish between individuals with higher schizotypal personality scores and those without, underlining the potential of AI in preemptively identifying vulnerability to schizophrenia. This new type of research marks a significant step in early detection and intervention strategies, highlighting the role of AI in transforming psychiatric diagnostics.

3.2 AI-driven technologies for diagnosis of schizophrenia

Every psychiatrist is aware of how complex and difficult the diagnosis of schizophrenia can be. The clinician must rely mainly on his observation and clinical judgment, leading to subjectivity and heterogeneity. The fact that the information the clinician receives to ascertain this diagnosis can also be subjective and unreliable, being based mainly on patient and relatives' reports, further contributes to this problem. AI-driven technologies can theoretically help bring some objectivity to the diagnosis of this condition and help redefine the concept of schizophrenia itself [20].

One key area of interest is the use of deep learning in schizophrenia research since this is the newest frontier in AI technology. Deep learning algorithms inspired by the nervous system (see Section 2) can potentially assist in classifying and predicting outcomes related to schizophrenia [5]. These methods may offer a new approach to model and analyze the complex, nonlinear systems inherent in schizophrenia. In general, existing studies about deep learning methods applied to schizophrenia [5] have yielded impressive results in terms of accuracy in classification and outcome prediction tasks, justifying the increasing interest in this area. However, methodological issues affecting the generalizability of the results in several of these studies have been identified—namely the small sample sizes and the lack of independency between the training and validation dataset and the testing dataset.

One promising avenue within this field is the use of clinical electroencephalography (EEG) in conjunction with interpretable graph neural networks. Recent research [21–22] has shown that clinical EEG can be effective in capturing abnormal schizophrenia neuropathology, while highlighting the problems the studies in this field face. While these two studies (both with 84 participants) showed an impressive accuracy in distinguishing healthy controls from individuals with schizophrenia, with both sensitivity and specificity above 90%, studies [4] that involve larger samples with cross-site validation tend to show a more realistic performance, with area under the curve (AUC) scores ranging from 0.793 to 0.852 and accuracies between 0.786 and 0.858 for varying schizophrenia prevalence. Feature visualization indicated that EEG theta and alpha band powers are significant biomarkers of schizophrenia pathology, highlighting their translational potential in multiple clinical settings.

While the results of studies employing advanced technologies like deep learning and EEG in distinguishing schizophrenic patients from healthy controls are indeed promising, it's important to recognize that these findings do not directly translate into immediate clinical application. One key reason for this is the fact that when psychiatrists see a new patient, they are not just deciding whether this person is healthy or has schizophrenia, but instead have a multitude of factors to consider, including the patient's premorbid personality, comorbid conditions, and differentiating between multiple psychiatric conditions (for example, between schizophrenia and delusional disorder).

However, while AI models are adept at identifying one condition against a healthy control, their accuracy tends to diminish when required to differentiate between two or more psychiatric conditions [6]. This decline in performance can be attributed to the increased complexity and subtleties involved in distinguishing disorders with similar symptomatology. The role of AI might be then to assist doctors in cases of diagnostic uncertainty, especially in dichotomous situations, thereby serving a complementary rather than a substitutive function.

Moreover, the datasets used in research are often more controlled and less varied than the patient populations seen in real-world clinical settings, due to the inclusion and exclusion criteria of these studies. In practice, patient presentations are more diverse, and other factors, such as comorbid conditions, varying stages of the disorder, and individual patient histories, play a significant role. These real-world complexities can affect the performance of AI models that were trained on more homogenous or specific datasets.

The use of AI to interpret functional magnetic resonance imaging (fMRI) and detect new patterns of structural and functional brain abnormalities in schizophrenia has also been extensively studied [23–26]. This application of AI in magnetic resonance imaging (MRI) has shown potential in identifying abnormalities in the temporal and anterior lobes of the hippocampal regions, which are affected in schizophrenia [27–28]. However, this field faces the same previously discussed challenges, such as the need for large and diverse datasets to train these AI models effectively.

As with different areas in AI, researchers are developing new models to accomplish certain goals. As an example, a new deep learning model [29] was developed that aimed to detect disease-related alterations in the brain's structure and enhance the accuracy of schizophrenia diagnosis. This model was then evaluated using three open datasets, which included MRI scans of patients with schizophrenia. Impressively, the model demonstrated an almost perfect ability to distinguish between schizophrenia patients and healthy controls, achieving an area under the receiver operating characteristic (ROC) curve of 0.987. As previously stated, we should keep in mind that these results may not have a direct translation to clinical practice, where clinicians, to diagnose a patient, do not just choose between two possibilities, but must instead consider a myriad of different options and other factors related to the individual.

3.3 Guiding schizophrenia treatment with AI

A provocative psychopharmacology study published in 2006 [30] discussing bias in schizophrenia clinical trials pointed to a disconcerting conclusion: it implied that treating schizophrenia often resorts to a hit-or-miss method for each patient and each medication. It also noted that we can call psychiatric treatments "individualized" or "personalized" only to the extent that these treatments (and lesser so their adverse effects) are highly variable across each patient, and fall significantly short of the advanced, genetically informed immunotherapies and custom-tailored cancer treatments that signify the maturity of personalized medicine in modern healthcare and scientific research [31].

Although much has changed since then in the field of psychiatry, the method psychiatrists currently use to choose which medication will be given to each patient is mostly through trial and error [32]. Personalized treatment plans could lead to improved outcomes and better quality of life for patients with schizophrenia, but finding a method that correctly predicts which patient will respond to each antipsychotic has proven to be a difficult challenge in research. AI models are then being designed to analyze enormous quantities of genetic and clinical data, in the hope they can help create new personalized treatment plans for individuals with schizophrenia, similarly to what is being developed for other chronic conditions [33].

The idea is that by inserting large amounts of data about a certain patient in an AI model (such as neuroimaging results and genetic samples), it will be able to predict treatment outcomes for that individual [34]. There are some interesting results to report, as some studies [35] showed 86% accuracy in distinguishing between treatment responders and nonresponders.

Artificial Intelligence (AI)-created clinical predictive models may indeed be accurate, but we must also consider that their effectiveness is largely confined to the specific trials for which they were developed [36]. In fact, when these models are applied outside of their original trial environments, their performance varies significantly [36]. This finding highlights the need for further development to enhance the models' generalizability and reliability in diverse clinical settings.

In conclusion, AI in healthcare is witnessing continuous growth and innovation, with its applications ranging from diagnostic accuracy to operational efficiency. The integration of AI promises a healthcare future that is more efficient, accessible, and patient-centric. However, the full realization of AI's potential in healthcare requires ongoing research, development, and careful consideration of ethical and privacy concerns, which leads us to the next section of our chapter.

4. Limitations and ethical concerns of AI in healthcare contexts

In this last section, various crucial aspects need to be addressed to fully grasp the implications of AI in this sensitive and critical area. We decided to divide these into small subsections.

4.1 The "black-box" problem

This concept has recently gained popularity in the media, sometimes being used with a quite hyperbolic meaning, and yet few people truly understand the meaning of this expression. The "Black-Box" problem refers to the opacity or lack of transparency in the decision-making processes of AI systems. At its core, this issue revolves around the difficulty in understanding how AI models, particularly those based on complex algorithms like deep learning, arrive at their conclusions or recommendations. This opacity can be particularly concerning in healthcare, where decisions have significant implications for patient care and outcomes.

As was previously explained, AI systems are trained on large datasets, using algorithms that can identify patterns and correlations within the data to make predictions or decisions. In many cases, especially with deep learning, the internal workings of these algorithms are not easily interpretable by humans. This means that clinicians or even the people who designed that particular AI model may not understand the basis on which an AI system has made a particular recommendation. The "Black-Box" problem thus raises several critical concerns:

- Accountability: If an AI system's decision-making process is not transparent, determining responsibility for any errors or adverse outcomes becomes a significant legal challenge. This ambiguity complicates medical malpractice considerations and undermines trust in AI-assisted healthcare [37].

- Bias and fairness: Without clear insight into how decisions are made, there's a risk that AI systems may perpetuate or even exacerbate biases present in the training data. This can lead to unfair treatment recommendations or diagnoses that disproportionately affect certain groups of patients [38]. A good example of this problem is the famous "ruler incident" [39], where a neural network that famously had reached a level of accuracy comparable to human dermatologists at diagnosing malignant skin lesions. However, a closer examination of the model's saliency methods revealed that the single most influential thing this model was looking for in a picture of someone's skin was the presence of a ruler. Because medical images of cancerous lesions include a ruler for scale, the model learned to identify the presence of a ruler as a marker of malignancy.

- Informed consent: Part of obtaining informed consent involves explaining the risks and benefits of treatment options. The inability to elucidate how an AI system works complicates this process, potentially impacting patient autonomy and trust. Moreover, gaps in policies governing patient data protection and the use of technologies like facial recognition can further exacerbate this problem. This necessitates a nuanced approach to policymaking, balancing the benefits of AI with the need to safeguard patient rights and trust in the healthcare system [37].

Thus, addressing the "Black-Box" problem will require concerted efforts from researchers, policymakers, and practitioners.

4.2 Confidentiality and data privacy

Another issue raised by AI technology concerns confidentiality and data privacy. The transformative shift toward AI-integrated healthcare systems underscores the paradox of relying on extensive patient data while needing to maintain confidentiality and privacy. Issues, such as data ownership in technologies like robotic surgery, where manufacturers may own the data, highlight the complex interplay between the need for enormous amount of personal data in AI development and the ethical obligation to protect patient privacy. Addressing these challenges involves a comprehensive exploration of privacy risks, focusing on large-scale data processing, anonymization techniques, and developing balanced strategies and policies that optimize AI's benefits while protecting patient rights and privacy [40].

4.3 Intersubjectivity of psychiatric symptoms

It is important to mention that the recognition and diagnosis of psychiatric disorders rely heavily on subjective symptom reporting, which poses a unique set of challenges for AI applications in mental health care. This intersubjectivity of symptoms—where patients' experiences and descriptions of their symptoms vary widely—underscores the complexity of developing AI tools that can accurately interpret and diagnose mental health conditions.

Psychiatric symptoms often lack the objective biomarkers or clear-cut diagnostic tests available in other branches of medicine. Instead, diagnoses are based on clinical interviews, patient self-reports, and behavioral observations. This reliance on subjective information introduces variability and potential biases in diagnosis, complicating the training of AI systems. For AI to be effectively integrated into psychiatric care, it must navigate these nuanced subjective experiences, ensuring that systems do not oversimplify the diversity of patient experiences or reinforce existing diagnostic biases.

Moreover, the interpretation of psychiatric symptoms is influenced by cultural, social, and individual factors, adding another layer of complexity to AI's role in mental health diagnosis and treatment. AI systems must be designed to recognize and adapt to these nuances, requiring a sophisticated understanding of the cultural and individual contexts in which symptoms are expressed.

To address these challenges, multidisciplinary collaboration among AI developers, mental health professionals, ethicists, and patients is crucial. Together, they can develop AI tools that are sensitive to the intersubjective nature of psychiatric symptoms, ethical considerations, and the diverse needs of patients. This approach will ensure that AI contributes positively to psychiatric care, enhancing diagnostic accuracy and treatment effectiveness while respecting the complexities and nuances of mental health disorders.

4.4 The European Union's artificial intelligence act (EU AI act)

We would also like to add a note about the recently created EU AI Act, since the official draft was recently released to the public (January 21, 2024), and will likely enter into force soon [41]. This document stands as a pioneering regulation, setting a global precedent for the governance of AI technologies. It applies to AI systems marketed, deployed, or used within the EU, encompassing a wide range of stakeholders from local developers to global vendors. Notably, the Act exempts AI systems developed for military purposes, scientific research, and certain open-source AI components, and introduces a risk-based regulatory approach. This approach categorizes AI systems into four levels of risk—unacceptable, high, limited, and minimal—tailoring regulatory oversight accordingly. Unacceptable risk AI systems, such as those capable of significant manipulation or social scoring, are outright prohibited, whereas high-risk systems are subject to stringent regulation, including comprehensive risk management, data governance, and transparency requirements. The Act also addresses the challenges posed by generative AI systems and foundation models, indicating the EU's commitment to ensuring AI's safe, ethical, and rights-respecting use. As healthcare continues to evolve with AI integration, the EU AI Act exemplifies the kind of forward-thinking policy that can guide the responsible development and application of AI technologies, ensuring they serve the public good while addressing critical ethical and legal challenges.

In conclusion, the integration of AI in healthcare represents a significant milestone with the promise of vastly improved patient care. However, it also brings forth complex ethical, legal, and privacy challenges that must be meticulously addressed. The development and implementation of AI in healthcare necessitate transparent communication, robust ethical guidelines, and strategic policies that ensure the equitable and just use of this technology, safeguarding patient welfare and maintaining the human element in healthcare decision-making.

5. Conclusion

This chapter provides a comprehensive examination of the intersection between AI and schizophrenia care. This work highlights the transformative potential of AI in enhancing diagnostic accuracy, enabling personalized treatment, and improving management strategies in schizophrenia, a complex and multifaceted mental health condition.

Artificial Intelligence's (AI's) integration into healthcare, particularly in schizophrenia, is marked by its ability to process and analyze vast amounts of data, thereby uncovering patterns that may elude traditional methods. This capability proves invaluable in early detection, especially in high-risk individuals, and in aiding accurate diagnoses through advanced technologies like deep learning and EEG analysis. However, challenges remain in translating these findings into clinical practice, particularly in distinguishing between multiple psychiatric conditions with overlapping symptoms.

The chapter also delves into the guiding role of AI in treatment. It discusses the use of predictive models to tailor antipsychotic treatments, emphasizing the emergence of precision psychiatry. Despite the accuracy of these models in specific trials, challenges in generalizability and reliability in diverse clinical settings are noted, underscoring the need for ongoing development.

As AI continues to evolve in healthcare, its applications extend from improving operational efficiencies to reshaping patient care approaches. However, this rapid advancement brings forth critical ethical, legal, and privacy concerns. The chapter addresses issues such as the "black-box" nature of AI algorithms, the potential for bias and discrimination, and the complexities surrounding data privacy and confidentiality. These challenges highlight the necessity for balanced strategies and policies that not only harness AI's benefits but also protect patient rights and ensure equitable healthcare.

In summary, this chapter offers an exploration of AI's potential role in enhancing schizophrenia care. It presents a nuanced understanding of the technology's potential and limitations, emphasizing the need for continued research, ethical considerations, and policy development to fully realize AI's promise in healthcare.

Acknowledgements

We would also like to acknowledge Dr. Pedro Câmara Pestana, who was a guide for our team, and helped refine the vision of our script.

Conflict of interest

The authors declare no conflict of interest.

Author details

António Melo[1*], Joana Romão[2] and Tiago Duarte[2]

1 Hospital of Vila Franca de Xira, Vila Franca de Xira, Portugal

2 Hospital Santa Maria, Lisbon, Portugal

*Address all correspondence to: antonio.melo@hvfx.min-saude.pt

References

[1] Rajpurkar P, Chen E, Banerjee O, Topol EJ. AI in health and medicine. Nature Medicine. 2022;**28**(1):31-38

[2] Alowais SA, Alghamdi SS, Alsuhebany N, Alqahtani T, Alshaya AI, Almohareb SN, et al. Revolutionizing healthcare: The role of artificial intelligence in clinical practice. BMC Medical Education. 2023;**23**(1):689

[3] Organization WH. How Will AI Transform Healthcare in 2024 and beyond 2023. Available from: https://www.worldhealth.net/news/how-will-ai-transform-healthcare-2024-and-beyond/

[4] Jiang H, Chen P, Sun Z, Liang C, Xue R, Zhao L, et al. Assisting schizophrenia diagnosis using clinical electroencephalography and interpretable graph neural networks: A real-world and cross-site study. Neuropsychopharmacology. 2023;**48**(13):1920-1930

[5] Cortes-Briones JA, Tapia-Rivas NI, D'Souza DC, Estevez PA. Going deep into schizophrenia with artificial intelligence. Schizophrenia Research. 2022;**245**:122-140

[6] Abd-alrazaq A, Alhuwail D, Schneider J, Toro CT, Ahmed A, Alzubaidi M, et al. The performance of artificial intelligence-driven technologies in diagnosing mental disorders: An umbrella review. NPJ Digital Medicine. 2022;**5**(1):87

[7] Bertagnolli MM. Advancing health through artificial intelligence/machine learning: The critical importance of multidisciplinary collaboration. PNAS Nexus. 2023;**2**(12):pgad356

[8] Trappenberg TP. Fundamentals of Machine Learning. Oxford University Press; 2019. DOI: 10.1093/oso/9780198828044.001.0001

[9] Goodfellow I, Bengio Y, Courville A. Deep Learning. MIT Press; 2016

[10] Jurafsky D, Martin JH. Speech and Language Processing. Pearson; 2020

[11] Atkins MS, Ayache N, Bankman IN, Barr AH, Bezdek JC, Blu T, et al. Contributors. In: Bankman IN, editor. Handbook of Medical Image Processing and Analysis. Second ed. Burlington: Academic Press; 2009. pp. xvii-xx

[12] Albert N, Weibell MA. The outcome of early intervention in first episode psychosis. International Review of Psychiatry. 2019;**31**(5-6):413-424

[13] Sun J, Cao R, Zhou M, Hussain W, Wang B, Xue J, et al. A hybrid deep neural network for classification of schizophrenia using EEG data. Scientific Reports. 2021;**11**(1):4706

[14] Chilla GS, Yeow LY, Chew QH, Sim K, Prakash KNB. Machine learning classification of schizophrenia patients and healthy controls using diverse neuroanatomical markers and ensemble methods. Scientific Reports. 2022;**12**(1):2755

[15] Giakoumaki SG, Sidiropoulou K, Stamatakis A. Editorial: Understanding early detection markers in schizophrenia. Frontiers in Behavioral Neuroscience. 2021;**15**

[16] Bi X-J, Hu L, Qiao D-D, Han C, Sun M-M, Cui K-Y, et al. Evidence for an interaction between NEDD4 and childhood trauma on clinical characters of schizophrenia with family history

of psychosis. Frontiers in Psychiatry. 2021;**12**

[17] Bracher-Smith M, Crawford K, Escott-Price V. Machine learning for genetic prediction of psychiatric disorders: A systematic review. Molecular Psychiatry. 2021;**26**(1):70-79

[18] Rosenhan DL. On Being Sane in Insane Places. Science. 1973;**179**(4070):250-258

[19] Kalmady SV, Paul AK, Greiner R, Agrawal R, Amaresha AC, Shivakumar V, et al. Extending schizophrenia diagnostic model to predict schizotypy in first-degree relatives. NPJ Schizophrenia. 2020;**6**(1):30

[20] Sun J, Dong Q-X, Wang S-W, Zheng Y-B, Liu X X, Lu T S, et al. Artificial intelligence in psychiatry research, diagnosis, and therapy. Asian Journal of Psychiatry. 2023;**87**:103705

[21] Calhas D, Romero E, Henriques R. On the use of pairwise distance learning for brain signal classification with limited observations. Artificial Intelligence in Medicine. 2020;**105**:101852

[22] Phang CR, Noman F, Hussain H, Ting CM, Ombao H. A multi-domain connectome convolutional neural network for identifying schizophrenia from EEG connectivity patterns. IEEE Journal of Biomedical and Health Informatics. 2020;**24**(5):1333-1343

[23] Pinaya WHL, Gadelha A, Doyle OM, Noto C, Zugman A, Cordeiro Q, et al. Using deep belief network modelling to characterize differences in brain morphometry in schizophrenia. Scientific Reports. 2016;**6**(1):38897

[24] Pinaya WHL, Mechelli A, Sato JR. Using deep autoencoders to identify abnormal brain structural patterns in neuropsychiatric disorders: A large-scale multi-sample study. Human Brain Mapping. 2019;**40**(3):944-954

[25] Vieira S, Gong Q-y, Pinaya WHL, Scarpazza C, Tognin S, Crespo-Facorro B, et al. Using machine learning and structural neuroimaging to detect first episode psychosis: Reconsidering the evidence. Schizophrenia Bulletin. 2020;**46**(1):17-26

[26] Oh J, Oh B-L, Lee K-U, Chae J-H, Yun K. Identifying schizophrenia using structural MRI with a deep learning algorithm. Frontiers in Psychiatry. 2020;**11**

[27] Sone M, Koshiyama D, Zhu Y, Maikusa N, Okada N, Abe O, et al. Structural brain abnormalities in schizophrenia patients with a history and presence of auditory verbal hallucination. Translational Psychiatry. 2022;**12**(1):511

[28] Howes OD, Cummings C, Chapman GE, Shatalina E. Neuroimaging in schizophrenia: An overview of findings and their implications for synaptic changes. Neuropsychopharmacology. 2023;**48**(1):151-167

[29] Zhang J, Rao VM, Tian Y, Yang Y, Acosta N, Wan Z, et al. Detecting schizophrenia with 3D structural brain MRI using deep learning. Scientific Reports. 2023;**13**(1):14433

[30] Heres S, Davis J, Maino K, Jetzinger E, Kissling W, Leucht S. Why olanzapine beats risperidone, risperidone beats quetiapine, and quetiapine beats olanzapine: An exploratory analysis of head-to-head comparison studies of second-generation antipsychotics. The American Journal of Psychiatry. 2006;**163**(2):185-194

[31] Lyman GH, Moses HL. Biomarker tests for molecularly targeted therapies — The key to unlocking precision medicine. New England Journal of Medicine. 2016;**375**(1):4-6

[32] Buckley PF, Miller BJ. Personalized medicine for schizophrenia. NPJ Schizophrenia. 2017;**3**(1):2

[33] Ng K, Kartoun U, Stavropoulos H, Zambrano JA, Tang PC. Personalized treatment options for chronic diseases using precision cohort analytics. Scientific Reports. 2021;**11**(1):1139

[34] Patrinos GP, Sarhangi N, Sarrami B, Khodayari N, Larijani B, Hasanzad M. Using ChatGPT to predict the future of personalized medicine. The Pharmacogenomics Journal. 2023;**23**(6):178-184

[35] Wang M, Hu K, Fan L, Yan H, Li P, Jiang T, et al. Predicting treatment response in schizophrenia with magnetic resonance imaging and polygenic risk score. Frontiers in Genetics. 2022;**13**

[36] Chekroud AM, Hawrilenko M, Loho H, Bondar J, Gueorguieva R, Hasan A, et al. Illusory generalizability of clinical prediction models. Science. 2024;**383**(6679):164-167

[37] Rigby MJ. Ethical dimensions of using artificial intelligence in health care. AMA Journal of Ethics. 2019

[38] AlHasan A. Bias in medical artificial intelligence. The Bulletin of the Royal College of Surgeons of England. 2021;**103**(6):302-305

[39] Staff V. When AI Flags the Ruler, Not the Tumor — And Other Arguments for Abolishing the Black Box (VB Live). 2021. Available from: https://venturebeat.com/business/when-ai-flags-the-ruler-not-the-tumor-and-other-arguments-for-abolishing-the-black-box-vb-live/

[40] Williamson SM, Prybutok V. Balancing privacy and Progress: A review of privacy challenges, systemic oversight, and patient perceptions in AI-driven healthcare. Applied Sciences [Internet]. 2024;**14**(2)

[41] Proposal for a Regulation of the European Parliament and of the Council Laying Down Harmonised Rules on Artificial Intelligence (Artificial Intelligence Act) and Amending Certain Union Legislative Acts

Chapter 6

Navigating Schizophrenia Treatment: Balancing Symptom Relief and Long-Term Needs

Agota Barabassy, Zsófia B. Dombi, Réka Csehi and Darko Djuric

Abstract

Schizophrenia is a long-term disease that needs to account for acute symptom control and long-term treatment needs such as relapse prevention, remission, and safety. The aim of the present book chapter was to summarize available literature data and guidelines on how to treat specific symptoms of schizophrenia and what aspects to consider long term. Looking at single symptoms, clozapine was better than all other antipsychotics in addressing positive and hostility symptoms of schizophrenia: however, it is not first-line treatment. Cariprazine showed superior efficacy in treating primary negative symptoms and is treatment of choice for these symptoms. Additionally, partial agonists (aripiprazole, brexpiprazole, cariprazine) were better in addressing comorbid substance use, while quetiapine, cariprazine, and olanzapine/fluoxetine showed advantages in treating mood disorders. In long term, there was no difference between antipsychotics in addressing relapse and remission; however, distinct differences in safety aspects are seen; overall, newer generation antipsychotics (aripiprazole, brexpiprazole, cariprazine, and lurasidone) are favored over other antipsychotics. In summary, careful consideration should be applied when choosing the right treatment for schizophrenia, accounting for prevalent symptoms, longitudinal aspects, psychiatric and somatic comorbidities as well as preference of patients.

Keywords: schizophrenia, acute symptoms, long-term symptoms, symptom-based treatment, patient-centered treatment, antipsychotics

1. Introduction

Schizophrenia, a complex mental disorder, historically condemned patients to perpetual institutionalization. The absence of targeted therapies resulted in prolonged stays within psychiatric facilities and devoid of hope for reintegration into society [1]. The advent of antipsychotic medications (AP) revolutionized psychiatric care, aiming to alleviate positive symptoms and allow for a more humane life for patients. Despite their adverse effects, they offered a glimmer of hope for patients who had long been locked away; hence, these side effects were tolerated. Subsequent generations of antipsychotics expanded their scope, addressing additional unmet needs beyond positive symptom control [2].

While all medicines of the antipsychotic class can address symptoms of psychosis, AKA positive symptoms [3], they vary in the way they can address other symptoms of schizophrenia, including negative [4], cognitive [5], mood symptoms [6], hostility and anxiety, but also comorbidities with substance use [7] or mood disorders. Additionally, considerations extend to relapse prevention, remission, and overall functional outcomes. As a result, psychopharmacological treatment today is rather focused on remission and reintegration than just purely symptom control [8]. So, to choose an effective holistic treatment for schizophrenia patients addressing their symptoms along with accounting for longitudinal outcomes must be considered.

A symptom-based approach considers the various symptoms of schizophrenia and identifies the most suitable treatment for each specific symptom. It is a case-by-case approach always addressing the prominent symptom first. This is especially needed in acute patient care where severe positive symptoms, hostility, or self-harm need to be addressed immediately [9]. The longitudinal approach recognizes schizophrenia as a chronic condition, necessitating long-term management [10]. While addressing the prevailing symptom is essential, it is not the sole focus. Instead, treatment aims for sustained stability, functional improvement, and quality of life. Factors, such as relapse prevention, maintaining remission, and promoting recovery, become paramount [8]. The patient-centered approach combines both approaches and hence ensures holistic care for individuals navigating the complexities of schizophrenia. Clinicians collaborate with patients to find the most suitable treatment regimen over the long haul, balancing symptom control with minimizing side effects and optimizing functioning [11].

This review aims at examining symptom-based treatment strategies and summarizing available evidence, along with longitudinal treatment aspects, which consider safety and long-term functioning/quality of life of patients.

2. Symptom-based treatment strategies

Generally, three major symptom clusters are distinguished in schizophrenia, which are positive, negative, and cognitive symptoms; however, other symptoms, such as hostility, affective symptoms, or catatonic symptoms, are also described [12]. Newer guidelines also raise awareness about comorbidities, specifically substance use disorder [13] or other mental disorders along with psychical disorders when choosing a symptom-based treatment.

2.1 Positive symptoms

Positive symptoms of schizophrenia include hallucinations, delusions, disorganized thoughts, and bizarre behaviors [14, 15]. All antipsychotic medications (first, second, and newer generation antipsychotics) address positive symptoms of schizophrenia, hence the name antipsychotic.

Previously, most schizophrenia guidelines suggested second (SGA) or newer generation antipsychotics to manage positive symptoms because first-generation antipsychotics are more likely to cause severe and irreversible extrapyramidal side effects and more often lead to discontinuation than SGA [16]. However, newer studies debate whether there is a real advantage of SGA over first-generation antipsychotics.

Hence, guideline recommendations today [17] do not differentiate among antipsychotics to address positive symptoms. Treatment choices should rather consider aspects of other symptom domains, adherence, long-term functioning along with formulation, dosing, onset of effect, and half-life.

Among the antipsychotics clozapine stands out as showing better efficacy in the treatment of positive symptoms than all other antipsychotics; however, due to severe side effects, such as agranulocytosis, it is not used as first-line treatment [17]. In fact, guidelines suggest to first try two other antipsychotics before initiating treatment with clozapine. In clinical practice, this means that doctors are left with choosing any antipsychotic they prefer to address positive symptoms of schizophrenia.

2.2 Hostility

Hostility, irritability, aggressive behavior, and impulsivity are often observed in individuals with schizophrenia [18]. These behaviors can occur during both the acute and the chronic phases of the illness [18]. Hostility, broadly defined, encompasses unfriendly attitudes that manifest through overt behaviors such as irritability, anger, resentment, or aggression [18]. Clinically, it is operationalized using rating scales, such as the Positive and Negative Syndrome Scale (PANSS), which classifies hostility as a positive symptom [18].

The impact of hostility on the quality of life in individuals with schizophrenia is noteworthy; studies have consistently shown a negative correlation between hostility and overall quality of life [18]. Consequently, pharmacological treatments targeting hostility as a primary focus in managing schizophrenia have been extensively investigated in the past [18].

Multiple reviews have consistently highlighted clozapine as an effective choice for managing aggression in schizophrenia [17]. This nicely taps into the notion of hostility being regarded as a positive symptom, where clozapine has also advantages compared to other antipsychotics. Nevertheless, in clinical practice doctors are once again faced with the issue of having to try other treatments before choosing clozapine. Efficacy on hostility has been described for various treatments, including haloperidol [19], risperidone [20], olanzapine [21], cariprazine [22], asenapine, brexpiprazole, aripiprazole, lurasidone, loxapine, ziprasidone, quetiapine, iloperidone, and paliperidone. The evidence comes from post hoc analyses of clinical trials, initially conducted for regulatory purposes as well as analyses of large effectiveness trials [23, 24]. However, the generalizability of these studies may be limited since participants in these trials were not specifically selected for aggressive or hostile behavior [23, 24].

2.3 Negative symptoms

Negative symptoms play a crucial role in schizophrenia [25]. Persistent primary negative symptoms are believed to be core symptoms of schizophrenia, which are difficult to address with treatment strategies [25]. Recently, a consensus on describing negative symptoms using five key constructs, known as the "5 A's," has been reached [25]:

- Affect (blunted): Refers to the diminished emotional expression.
- Alogia: Characterized by reduced speech output or poverty of speech.

- Anhedonia: The inability to experience pleasure or interest in previously enjoyable activities.

- Asociality: Social withdrawal and disinterest in forming relationships.

- Avolition: A lack of motivation or initiative to pursue goals or engage in purposeful activities.

Clinically, negative symptoms are operationalized using rating scales, such as the Brief Negative Symptom Scale (BNSS) or the older Positive and Negative Syndrome Scale (PANSS) [25].

The advent of SGA initially sparked hope in addressing not only the positive symptoms of schizophrenia but also the negative and cognitive symptoms. However, therapeutic guidelines remain divided on whether SGAs truly outperform first-generation antipsychotics (FGAs) in addressing these symptoms [26]. In a recent meta-analysis [27] examining efficacy of antipsychotics on prominent and predominant negative symptoms, the authors have shown that amisulpride is better than placebo, and cariprazine is better than risperidone in addressing primary negative symptoms of schizophrenia. Amisulpride failed to show superior efficacy over other antipsychotics; so although it might address negative symptoms in untreated patients, in patients already treated with an antipsychotic it has no proven efficacy so far [27].

Cariprazine, on the other hand, has shown efficacy on primary negative symptoms in a well-designed study against risperidone [28], in another study against aripiprazole, in two real-world evidence studies [29, 30], and in several single case reports [31]. Hence, it is considered by Cerveri et al. [32] as first-line treatment for negative symptoms of schizophrenia (**Figure 1**) and is also endorsed as a treatment option in the EPA treatment guideline for negative symptoms [25].

2.4 Cognitive symptoms

Cognitive symptoms in schizophrenia are usually present from the onset of psychosis and are not merely side effects of antipsychotic medication [33]. Research shows that people with schizophrenia have altered brain structures, including reduced cortical thickness and gray matter volume [33]. Cognitive symptoms include [33]:

- Processing speed: Processing speed refers to how quickly an individual receives, assesses, and responds to new information. People with schizophrenia may experience slower processing speed due to disruptions in the brain's white matter,

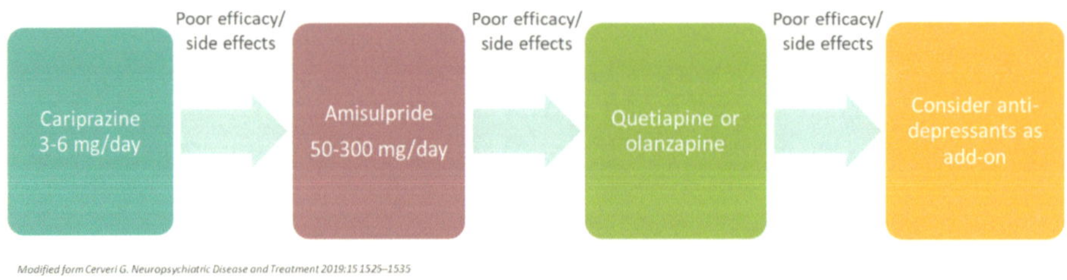

Figure 1.
Treatment algorithm in predominantly negative symptoms.

affecting signal transmission. They might need extra time to respond, feel overwhelmed by excessive information, and require repeated instructions.

- Working memory involves temporarily retaining information to complete immediate tasks. Schizophrenia can impair working memory, affecting learning, problem-solving, and task execution.

- Attention difficulties make it hard to focus on tasks or follow conversations. Individuals may struggle with sustained attention and filtering out distractions.

- Verbal learning pertains to acquiring and retaining new information through language. Schizophrenia can hinder verbal learning, affecting memory recall and comprehension.

- Reasoning and problem-solving: These cognitive abilities involve logical thinking and solving complex problems. Schizophrenia may disrupt reasoning skills, making it harder to navigate daily challenges.

- Social cognition refers to understanding social cues, emotions, and interpersonal interactions. Individuals with schizophrenia might struggle with interpreting others' intentions, leading to social withdrawal.

Just as negative symptoms, cognitive symptoms impact patient's activities of daily living and reduce quality of life when present [12]. Therefore, their potential treatment could be of great benefit. In the 1990s, SGA raised hopes of addressing not only psychotic symptoms but also cognitive impairments in schizophrenia. Initial trials hinted at cognitive benefits alongside symptom control. However, subsequent research revealed that these advantages might have been influenced by trial design rather than true effects. Presently, the literature suggests that all antipsychotics yield similarly modest impacts on cognitive function [34].

2.5 Mood symptoms

Mood symptoms are common in schizophrenia and can affect the quality of life and functioning of people with this disorder [35]. Mood symptoms can include depression, anxiety, mania, or a combination of these [35]. They can occur at any stage of schizophrenia but are more likely to appear during the prodromal phase (before the onset of psychosis), the residual phase (after the acute psychotic episode), or during a relapse [36]. Mood symptoms can also be influenced by factors such as stress, substance use, medication side effects, or co-occurring medical conditions [35].

These symptoms in schizophrenia represent a treatment challenge because they can complicate the diagnosis, increase the risk of suicide, impair the response to antipsychotic medication, and reduce the adherence to treatment [37]. Therefore, it is important to assess and treat them as part of a comprehensive and individualized care plan. Treatment options may include the use of antidepressants, mood stabilizers, or anxiolytics, depending on the type and severity of mood symptoms; but antipsychotic medication that has proven benefits on mood symptoms might be first line. Presently, only quetiapine [38] and cariprazine (US only) [39] have indications in all four major psychiatric disorders: schizophrenia, bipolar mania, bipolar depression, and major depression. Olanzapine [40] alone is effective in schizophrenia and bipolar mania and can address depressed mood symptoms in combination with fluoxetine [41]. All other antipsychotics failed to show efficacy either on mania or bipolar depression of major depression—either because the studies failed or because they did not run any studies.

One of the most dangerous psychiatric symptoms that can occur is suicidality [37]. Suicide is a cause of early mortality in nearly 5% of patients with schizophrenia, and 25–50% of patients with schizophrenia attempt suicide in their lifetime [37]. Research indicates that antipsychotic medications, such as clozapine, risperidone, olanzapine, and quetiapine, may play a role in reducing mortality and suicide risk in individuals with schizophrenia [37]. In 2002, the U.S. Food and Drug Administration (FDA) specifically approved clozapine for decreasing suicide risk in patients with schizophrenia [37].

2.6 Substance use comorbidity

Dual disorder, also known as co-occurring disorder or dual diagnosis, refers to the simultaneous presence of a mental illness and a substance use disorder (SUD) [42]. This condition is associated with a higher likelihood of negative health outcomes, including increased rates of suicide, unplanned hospital admissions, and premature death [43]. The repercussions of dual disorders may extend to violence, homelessness, interactions with the criminal justice system, and the disintegration of personal relationships [43].

A staggering 75% of individuals with a severe mental health disorder are also grappling with a substance use disorder [43]. Similarly, 60% of adults with a substance use disorder are diagnosed with at least one severe mental health disorder [43]. Unfortunately, patients with dual disorders often receive incorrect diagnoses and inadequate treatment, slipping through the gaps in the healthcare system [42]. This is exacerbated by the fact that they may be turned away by both drug treatment and mental health services due to their complex needs [42].

The consequences of this neglect are profound: patients with dual disorders generally experience a diminished quality of life, along with higher mortality and suicide rates [44]. Those with schizophrenia and a substance use disorder are particularly vulnerable, facing an elevated risk of death, suicide, and other health complications [44]. Despite the critical need for comprehensive treatment, only a minority of these patients receive the necessary care [44]. Alarmingly, a mere 7% of patients with dual disorders receive treatment for both conditions, highlighting a significant gap in the current healthcare provision [44].

In terms of prevalence, 42% of individuals with schizophrenia also suffer from a substance use disorder, mostly smoking and cannabis [45]. Addressing the complexities of dual schizophrenia, which encompasses both schizophrenia and substance use disorders, presents a formidable challenge in psychiatric care [44, 46]. Although current clinical guidelines acknowledge the necessity of treating dual disorders, they offer scant direction on how to approach such cases [47]. This gap underscores the urgent need for integrated treatment strategies, which remains an unmet medical need [47].

In the realm of pharmacotherapy, first-generation antipsychotics (FGAs) are generally discouraged for treating dual disorders [48]. This recommendation stems from several detrimental characteristics associated with FGAs [48]. Notably, these drugs have been implicated in increasing cravings and self-administration of substances, such as cocaine in animal studies [48]. The pharmacological action of FGAs, particularly as dopaminergic D2 receptor antagonists, may exacerbate the situation by further diminishing the already reduced dopaminergic tone observed in drug users [48]. This significant blockade could inadvertently prompt individuals to consume greater amounts of psychoactive substances in an attempt to counteract experiences of anhedonia and cognitive deficits [48].

Therefore, contemporary guidelines and scientific literature advocate for the use of second-generation antipsychotics (SGAs) in the treatment of dual disorders [7]. Research focusing on the impact of SGAs on individuals with schizophrenia, who also consume cannabis or alcohol, has identified aripiprazole as the most frequently utilized medication [7]. It is important to recognize that aripiprazole's effectiveness may be indicative of a broader class effect associated with dopamine partial agonists [7].

Dopamine partial agonists or third-generation antipsychotics (TGAs), such as aripiprazole, cariprazine, and brexpiprazole, offer potential therapeutic benefits for treating both psychosis and substance use disorders (SUD) [7]. Among the partial agonists and in fact, among all other antipsychotics, cariprazine has the highest binding affinity to the D3 receptors in the brain [49]. Substance abuse has been linked to the upregulation of D3 receptors, with studies showing that repeated exposure to drugs can lead to a selective increase in D3 receptor expression [50]. This is evident in D3 receptor knockout (D3-KO) mice, which, unlike their wild-type counterparts, exhibit a heightened propensity for self-administering heroin and cocaine, along with an increased motivation for drug-seeking behavior [50]. The role of D3 receptors in addiction is further highlighted by the fact that antagonists or partial agonists targeting these receptors have been found to diminish the motivation for psychostimulant seeking in various animal models of relapse [50]. Cariprazine stands out in this context as it possesses both partial agonist properties and high affinity for D3 receptors [49]. Remarkably, cariprazine's affinity for D3 receptors surpasses that of dopamine itself by three orders of magnitude and all other antipsychotics currently in use [49].

This unique binding profile is theorized to enhance cariprazine's effectiveness in treating negative symptoms and may be beneficial for addressing issues related to cognition, mood, emotions, and reward mechanisms, which are particularly relevant in the context of substance use [49]. Given these pharmacological profiles, Martinotti et al. recommend the use of dopamine partial agonists as the first-line treatment in maintenance settings for dual disorders [7]. Notably, the effectiveness of cariprazine in preventing substance abuse is approximately 20 times greater than that of aripiprazole, underscoring its significant promise as a treatment option in the context of addiction and dual disorders [51].

2.7 Catatonic symptoms

Catatonia is a multifaceted psychomotor syndrome that was once considered a subtype of schizophrenia [52]. However, following revisions in the DSM-5, it can now be categorized as arising from various other mental health conditions [52]. These include brief psychotic, schizophreniform, and schizoaffective disorders or substance use [52]. Its symptoms are a distinct set of behaviors observed in individuals with schizophrenia [52]. These include [52]:

- Stupor: This state resembles near unconsciousness. The person becomes unresponsive, immobile, and lacks awareness of their surroundings.

- Catalepsy: Individuals experience trance-like seizures characterized by rigid body posture. They may hold unusual positions for extended periods.
- Waxy flexibility: A peculiar phenomenon where the limbs remain in the position someone else puts them in. It is as if the person's body is malleable like wax.
- Mutism: Lack of verbal response, catatonic individuals may not speak or communicate effectively.
- Negativism: A tendency to resist or oppose external stimuli or instructions. For instance, they might refuse to move when asked.
- Posturing: Catatonic patients exhibit unusual body postures that defy gravity. These positions can be sustained for extended periods.
- Mannerism: This involves displaying odd and exaggerated movements, gestures, or expressions.
- Stereotypy: Repetitive, purposeless movements without an apparent reason. These actions can persist for minutes, hours, or even days.

Interestingly, although catatonia might be a form of schizophrenia, it is not treated primarily with antipsychotics [52, 53]. Treatment includes the administration of benzodiazepines, such as lorazepam or alternatively electroconvulsive therapy (ECT) [52, 53]. Antipsychotics should be evaluated for their potential to induce catatonic symptoms and discontinued if possible [52, 53]. There is some ambiguity about the role of antipsychotics, but it is generally encouraged to discontinue treatment in patients presenting with catatonia [52, 53].

3. Longitudinal treatment aspects

The longitudinal treatment approach recognizes schizophrenia as a chronic condition, necessitating long-term management. It accounts for schizophrenia management from the prodromal phase to the first occurrence of acute symptoms to sustained stability, functional improvement, rehabilitation, and improvement of quality of life (**Figure 2**). Different stages need different treatment considerations,

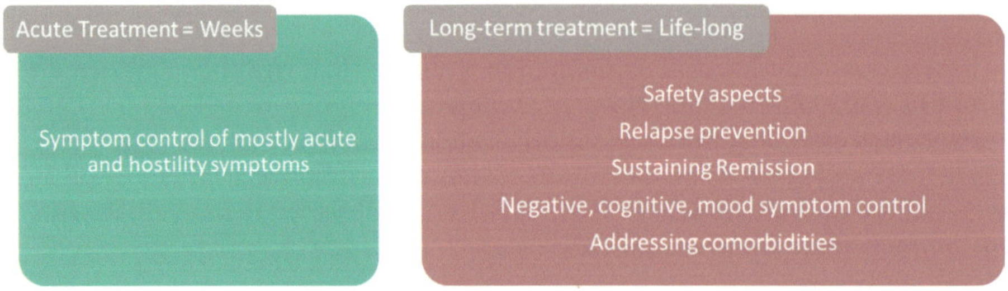

Figure 2.
Aspects of longitudinal treatment in schizophrenia.

and while in the acute phase, the most important is effective symptom control, on long-term safety and quality of life considerations shift more into focus.

Schizophrenia treatment in general starts with the onset of acute symptoms and acute psychosis. While the prodromal phase precedes this acute stage, antipsychotic treatment typically is not initiated this early. However, once acute symptoms appear, swift intervention becomes crucial due to the significant impact of the duration of untreated psychosis (DUP) on overall outcomes [54, 55]. DUP represents the time span between the onset of psychotic symptoms and the commencement of treatment. Prioritizing DUP reduction becomes a critical strategy, especially for managing first-episode psychosis [54, 55]. Detecting and addressing symptoms promptly are essential. Notably, extended DUP has been associated with less favorable prognoses [54, 55]. It serves as a predictor for the likelihood and extent of recovery, while early treatment offers promise for long-term well-being [54, 55]. Research consistently underscores the effects of prolonged DUP on individuals experiencing their initial psychotic episode. Longer DUP correlates with more severe positive symptoms (such as hallucinations and delusions) and lower rates of symptom remission [54, 55]. Furthermore, extended DUP is linked to impaired social cognition, impacting interpersonal relationships and overall functioning [54, 55]. Addressing DUP promptly becomes pivotal in enhancing outcomes and improving the quality of life for individuals navigating the complexities of psychosis [54, 55].

During the acute phase of schizophrenia, managing the prevailing symptoms takes priority [36]. These symptoms primarily involve positive symptoms, alongside potential hostility and self-harm [36]. However, as the course of schizophrenia unfolds, symptomatology evolves [36]. Negative symptoms, cognitive impairments, and mood disturbances become more pronounced, necessitating treatment adjustments [36]. An ideal approach considers both immediate and long-term treatment needs of schizophrenic patients [36]. Notably, altering treatments during stable phases carries a substantial risk of relapse, emphasizing the importance of thoughtful decisions [56]. Therefore, the right treatment choice balances short-term efficacy with long-term symptom control and safety from the start. Taking sedation as an example, antipsychotics' sedative effects during the first stages of treating acute psychosis can be therapeutically beneficial for agitated patients [8, 57]. Patients who are having trouble sleeping may also benefit from bedtime sedation [8, 57]. Unwanted daytime sedation, on the other hand, may have a detrimental influence on recovery, impeding the positive effects of psychosocial training, psychiatric rehabilitation, and other treatments [8, 57]. It is linked to long-term detrimental effects on cognitive function and metabolic changes, including weight gain [8, 57]. Persistent sedation can affect social, recreational, and occupational functioning [8, 57]. It can cause daytime sleepiness, longer sleep durations, and decreased cognitive sharpness [8, 57].

As schizophrenia evolves, relapse, remission, and overall safety considerations move into focus and become a cornerstone of compassionate care. Relapse among patients with schizophrenia carries profound implications. It results in the deterioration of symptoms, compromised functioning, cognitive decline, and a diminished quality of life [58]. This downward trajectory places a substantial burden on both patients and their families, causing emotional distress and financial strain [58]. Consequently, preventing relapse becomes a paramount therapeutic objective [58]. In real-world scenarios, hospitalization often serves as an indirect measure of relapse [58]. When patients require hospital care, it signifies a significant worsening of symptoms [58].

Numerous factors contribute to the risk of relapse, including nonadherence to antipsychotic medications, stress, depression, and substance misuse [58]. The Role of Continuous Antipsychotic Treatment: Consistent use of antipsychotic medications is associated with reduced hospitalization frequency and duration [58]. In summary, relapse remains a recurring challenge in schizophrenia management, transcending mere symptomatology [58]. Timely detection, intervention, and sustained treatment are pivotal for improving outcomes and enhancing the overall well-being of individuals navigating this intricate disorder [58].

A standardized definition of remission criteria was proposed by the International group led by Dr. Nancy Andreasen in 2005 [59]. It involves a low symptom threshold for the eight core symptoms (both positive and negative) on the Positive and Negative Syndrome Scale (PANSS) for at least 6 consecutive months [59]. Remission not only sets a standard for minimal symptom severity (resolution) but also specifies how long symptoms must remain at this minimal level (6 months) [59]. Individuals who achieve remission experience better subjective well-being [59]. Reduced symptoms contribute to an improved quality of life [59]. Remission is associated with better functional outcomes compared to those who do not achieve it [59]. Research suggests that remission can be attained in 20–60% of people with schizophrenia. Remission serves as a useful way to monitor improved health. Clinicians often use the Andreasen Consensus Group criteria to assess remission in clinical practice. Achieving remission involves not only symptom reduction but also maintaining this state over time. Balancing short-term symptom control with long-term stability is crucial. Remission reduces the burden on patients, families, and healthcare systems. It minimizes hospitalizations, improves functioning, and enhances overall well-being. Overall, it is established that remission duration is predicted by negative, positive, and cognitive symptom control, treatment dosage, and duration of illness [60]. Hence, antipsychotics addressing negative and cognitive symptoms might have advantages.

Finally, accounting for safety aspects protects patients from harm, provides a stable foundation for therapeutic interventions, and fosters trust between patients and caregivers [61–64]. This trust is crucial as it encourages adherence to treatment plans and promotes open communication about symptoms, side effects, and concerns [61–64]. Moreover, considering safety aspects is vital in mitigating risks associated with the condition itself, such as vulnerability to self-harm or the potential for unpredictable reactions to medication [61–64]. Especially, since 86–98% of patients report experiencing side effects that are often viewed as being worse than the positive symptoms of psychosis [65–67].

Schizophrenia patients often harbor fears and concerns related to specific side effects of antipsychotic medications [68, 69]. Weight gain is a common worry as it can impact self-esteem, physical health, and overall well-being [68, 69]. Extrapyramidal symptoms (EPS), which encompass tremors, muscle stiffness, and abnormal movements, are also a concern, along with restlessness or an inability to sit still [68, 69]. Although tardive dyskinesia is less frequent with newer antipsychotics, it is still a worry to patients as it is highly stigmatizing [68, 69]. Excessive sleepiness or drowsiness can disrupt daily activities and productivity, hence patients feel very bothered when they occur [68, 69]. Elevated prolactin levels may lead to abnormal breast milk production (galactorrhea) and other hormonal imbalances, including sexual dysfunction [68, 69]. Furthermore, some antipsychotics can cause cognitive dullness or difficulty thinking clearly, which can be distressing for patients [68, 69]. Doctors share similar apprehensions. When making treatment decisions, they aim to prevent relapse while minimizing side effects such as cardio-metabolic symptoms, severe EPS, anticholinergic effects, and cognitive blunting. Prioritizing safety in schizophrenia treatment underscores a commitment to holistic, patient-centered care, recognizing the unique challenges faced by individuals living with this condition.

Two recent large-scale meta-analysis studies, comparing the efficacy and tolerability of 32 oral and long-acting injectable antipsychotics for the acute and maintenance treatment of adults with schizophrenia found no clear differences between antipsychotics in addressing acute symptoms of schizophrenia or in their ability to prevent relapse [3, 70]. Authors, therefore, proposed that the main consideration when choosing an antipsychotic for ongoing treatment should be its tolerability [3, 70]. Authors compared different safety concerns such as EPS, weight gain, sedation, QT prolongation, etc. among antipsychotics and concluded that in most aspects, newer generation antipsychotics such as partial dopamine agonists (aripiprazole, brexpiprazole, cariprazine) and lurasidone performed better on safety parameters [3, 70]. First-generation antipsychotics, primarily antagonists such as haloperidol, often result in noticeable extrapyramidal side effects, while older second-generation antipsychotics frequently lead to weight gain—a concern due to its potential impact on cardiovascular health and diabetes risk [3, 70]. In contrast, aripiprazole and cariprazine were comparable to placebo in their potential to cause weight gain on long term, and all three partial agonists (aripiprazole, brexpiprazole, cariprazine) had no issues with causing hyperprolactinemia [70]. In the past, treatment of hyperprolactinemia was primarily recommended for symptomatic patients [71]. However, recent insights have highlighted that persistent asymptomatic hyperprolactinemia can lead to long-term complications, including osteoporosis and breast cancer [71]. Consequently, it is crucial to manage hyperprolactinemia even if it is asymptomatic at the time of initial detection [71]. This can be done by reducing the dose of antipsychotic medication, switching to a prolactin-sparing antipsychotic, or adding a dopamine partial agonist to the treatment regime [71].

4. Combination strategies

Antipsychotic polytherapy (APP), involving the use of multiple antipsychotic medications, is utilized for approximately 20–30% of patients undergoing antipsychotic therapy [72]. However, APP is not universally applicable for all cases of antipsychotic treatment [72]. The NICE, UK, Clinical Guidelines provide a framework for considering APP, suggesting it as a potential option following the failure of two or more antipsychotic monotherapy (APM) trials and subsequent clozapine (CLZ) monotherapy [72]. The transition to APP should be gradual with careful monitoring at each stage, and should consider the pharmacological profiles of the antipsychotic drugs involved [72]. A key focus is on optimizing dopamine D2 receptor occupancy and leveraging other receptor categories or subtypes to achieve a more favorable balance between efficacy and adverse events (AE) [72].

A review and meta-analysis of the literature indicated that APP may be superior to monotherapy in open-label studies of lower quality [72]. However, this superiority is not consistently supported in high-quality, double-blind, and randomized studies [72]. These studies suggest that enhanced efficacy with APP is limited to specific strategies rather than a general advantage over monotherapy [72]. Notably, the combination of two first-generation or second-generation D2 antagonists did not show superiority, but the addition of partial dopamine agonists did [72].

One possible treatment option to cover the acute and long-term needs of schizophrenia is to combine AP, which is classically perceived as highly effective, dopamine antagonists (haloperidol, olanzapine, risperidone, clozapine or LAI) with a dopamine partial agonist. Thereafter, when the acute symptoms improve a slow down-titration of the antagonist can be evaluated leaving patients with the well tolerable long-term partial agonist medication. The choice of the partial agonist should be based on individual treatment needs and should also consider long-term symptoms such as negative, addiction, and mood symptoms.

5. Conclusion

This review's objective was to examine the literature concerning acute (symptom based) and long-term (safety based) treatment aspects of schizophrenia. In summary, clozapine was superior to all other antipsychotics in addressing positive symptoms of schizophrenia along with hostility, however, is not a first-line treatment drug due to its severe side effects. Besides, clozapine no other antipsychotic differed in its efficacy on positive symptoms, so treatment choices may vary. One way to influence this treatment choice is to look at the other symptom domains. Concerning negative symptoms cariprazine outperformed risperidone. No other antipsychotic could show efficacy on primary negative symptoms in comparison with another antipsychotic. Cariprazine further, along with quetiapine and olanzapine/fluoxetine, can address mood symptoms of various mood disorders such as mania, bipolar depression, and major depression, which makes these drugs a good treatment choice if mood symptoms of schizophrenia are present. Further, if comorbid substance use is present, partial agonists (aripiprazole, brexpiprazole, and cariprazine) are choice of treatment, with an advantage of cariprazine due to its D3 mechanism of action, which also plays an important role in substance use. Although cognition is an important aspect to maintain and not worsen in schizophrenia, evidence suggests no difference between the antipsychotics in their efficacy to improve cognition. A tabulated summary is provided below in **Figure 3**.

Considering long-term aspects, no antipsychotic was better than the other in preventing relapse or achieving remission. Differences were rather modest and treatment choice should be led by considerations of tolerability. Here, first-generation antipsychotics mostly cause severe EPS, while most second-generation antipsychotics cause weight gain, hyperlipidemia, sedation, or prolactin increase. Newer generation antipsychotics, among them also the partial agonists cause less side effects and are often favored by doctors and patients.

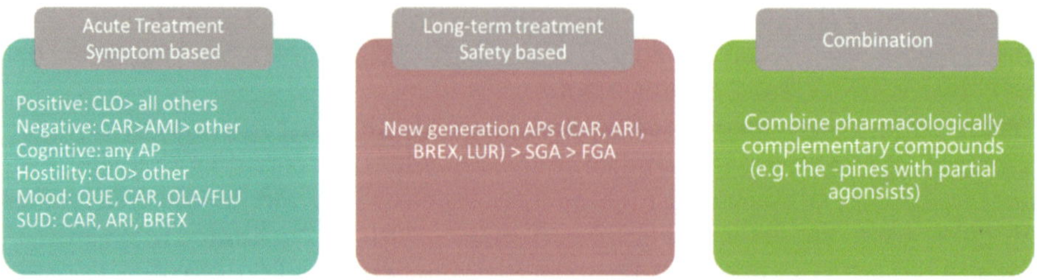

Figure 3.
Tabulated summary of findings.

DOI: http://dx.doi.org/10.5772/intechopen.1005488

Combining different antipsychotics is a well-established practice in psychiatry. Combinations should consider complementary efficacy and reduced safety concerns by, for example, reducing doses.

Overall, a careful consideration should be applied when choosing treatment accounting for prevalent symptoms, longitudinal aspects, along with psychiatric and somatic comorbidities, as well as preference of patients—this is what a patient-centered treatment is all about!

Acknowledgements

Authors would like to thank their mentor Dr. György Németh for his continued support.

Conflict of interest

Authors are all co-workers of Gedeon Richter Plc.

Author details

Agota Barabassy, Zsófia B. Dombi*, Réka Csehi and Darko Djuric
Gedeon Richter Plc, Global Medical Division, Hungary

*Address all correspondence to: dombizsb@richter.hu

References

[1] Kurtz MM. A brief history of the treatment of schizophrenia. In: Schizophrenia and its Treatment: Where Is the Progress? New York: Oxford Academic; 2015

[2] Kane JM, Correll CU. Past and present progress in the pharmacologic treatment of schizophrenia. The Journal of Clinical Psychiatry. 2010;**71**(9):1115-1124

[3] Huhn M, Nikolakopoulou A, Schneider-Thoma J, Krause M, Samara M, Peter N, et al. Comparative efficacy and tolerability of 32 oral antipsychotics for the acute treatment of adults with multi-episode schizophrenia: A systematic review and network meta-analysis. American Psychiatric Publishing; 2019;**18**(4):443-455. DOI: 10.1176/appi.focus.18306

[4] Correll CU, Schooler NR. Negative symptoms in schizophrenia: A review and clinical guide for recognition, assessment, and treatment. Neuropsychiatric Disease and Treatment. 2020;**16**:519-534

[5] Maroney M. Management of cognitive and negative symptoms in schizophrenia. Mental Health Clinician. 2022;**12**(5):282-299

[6] Reynolds GP, Mcgowan OO. Schizophrenia, depressive symptoms, and antipsychotic drug treatment. The International Journal of Neuropsychopharmacology. 2021;**24**(4):253-255

[7] Martinotti G, Chiappini S, Mosca A, Miuli A, Santovito MC, Pettorruso M, et al. Atypical antipsychotic drugs in dual disorders: Current evidence for clinical practice. Current Pharmaceutical Design. 2022;**28**(27):2241-2259

[8] Keepers GA, Fochtmann LJ, Anzia JM, Benjamin S, Lyness JM, Mojtabai R, et al. The American psychiatric association practice guideline for the treatment of patients with schizophrenia. The American Journal of Psychiatry. 2020;**177**(9):868-872

[9] Marder SR, Cannon TD. Schizophrenia. The New England Journal of Medicine. 2019;**381**:1753-1761

[10] Rege S. Short and Long Term Considerations in the Management of Schizophrenia. 2020. Available from: https://psychscenehub.com/psychinsights/short-and-long-term-considerations-in-the-management-of-schizophrenia/

[11] Fiorillo A, Barlati S, Bellomo A, Corrivetti G, Nicolò G, Sampogna G, et al. The role of shared decision-making in improving adherence to pharmacological treatments in patients with schizophrenia: A clinical review. Annals of General Psychiatry. 2020;**19**:1-12. DOI: 10.1186/s12991-020-00293-4

[12] McCutcheon RA, Keefe RSE, McGuire PK. Cognitive impairment in schizophrenia: Aetiology, pathophysiology, and treatment. Molecular Psychiatry. 2023;**28**: 1902-1918

[13] National Collaborating Centre for Mental Health. Psychosis with Coexisting Substance Misuse: Assessment and Management in Adults and Young People [Internet]. 2011. Available from: https://www.ncbi.nlm.nih.gov/books/NBK109783/

[14] American Psychiatric Association. American Psychiatric Association: Diagnostic and Statistical Manual of

Mental Disorders. 5th ed. Arlington: American Psychiatric Association; 2013

[15] The World Health Organisation. WHO | International Classification of Diseases, 11th Revision (ICD-11). World Health Organization (WHO) 2019/2021; 2018. Available from: https://icd.who.int/browse11

[16] Fabrazzo M, Cipolla S, Camerlengo A, Perris F, Catapano F. Second-generation antipsychotics' effectiveness and tolerability: A review of real-world studies in patients with schizophrenia and related disorders. Journal of Clinical Medicine. 2022;**11**:1-28

[17] Remington G, Addington D, Honer W, Ismail Z, Raedler T, Teehan M. Guidelines for the pharmacotherapy of schizophrenia in adults. Canadian Journal of Psychiatry. 2017;**62**(9):604-616

[18] Volavka J, Van Dorn RA, Citrome L, Kahn RS, Fleischhacker WW, Czobor P. Hostility in schizophrenia: An integrated analysis of the combined Clinical Antipsychotic Trials of Intervention Effectiveness (CATIE) and the European First Episode Schizophrenia Trial (EUFEST) studies. European Psychiatry. 2016;**31**:13-19

[19] Powney MJ, Adams CE, Jones H. Haloperidol for psychosis-induced aggression or agitation (rapid tranquillisation). Cochrane Database of Systematic Reviews. 2012;**11**:1-281

[20] Aleman A, Kahn RS. Effects of the atypical antipsychotic risperidone on hostility and aggression in schizophrenia: A meta-analysis of controlled trials. European Neuropsychopharmacology. 2001;**11**:289-293. Available from: http://ovidsp.ovid.com/ovidweb.cgi?T=JS&PAGE=reference&D=emed5&NEWS=N&AN=2001300586

[21] Citrome L, Volavka J. The psychopharmacology of violence: Making sensible decisions. CNS Spectrums. 2013;**19**(5):411-418

[22] Citrome L, Durgam S, Lu K, Ferguson P, Laszlovszky I. The effect of Cariprazine on hostility associated with schizophrenia: Post hoc analyses from 3 randomized controlled trials. The Journal of Clinical Psychiatry. 2016;**77**(1):109-115

[23] Volavka J, Czobor P, Citrome L, Van Dorn RA. Effectiveness of antipsychotic drugs against hostility in patients with schizophrenia in the Clinical Antipsychotic Trials of Intervention Effectiveness (CATIE) study. CNS Spectrums. 2013;**19**(5):374-381

[24] Volavka J, Czobor P, Derks EM, Bitter I, Libiger J, Kahn RS, et al. Efficacy of antipsychotic drugs against hostility in the European First-Episode Schizophrenia Trial (EUFEST). The Journal of Clinical Psychiatry. 2011;**72**(7):955-961

[25] Galderisi S, Mucci A, Dollfus S, Nordentoft M, Falkai P, Kaiser S, et al. EPA guidance on treatment of negative symptoms in schizophrenia. European Psychiatry. 2021;**64**(1):1-23

[26] van Os J, Kapur S. Schizophrenia. Lancet. 2009;**374**(9690):635-645

[27] Krause M, Zhu Y, Huhn M, Schneider-Thoma J, Bighelli I, Nikolakopoulou A, et al. Antipsychotic drugs for patients with schizophrenia and predominant or prominent negative symptoms: A systematic review and meta-analysis. European Archives of Psychiatry and Clinical Neuroscience. 2018;**268**(7):625-639

[28] Németh G, Laszlovszky I, Czobor P, Szalai E, Szatmári B, Harsányi J, et al.

Cariprazine versus risperidone monotherapy for treatment of predominant negative symptoms in patients with schizophrenia: A randomised, double-blind, controlled trial. Lancet. 2017;**389**(10074):1103-1113

[29] Rancans E, Dombi ZB, Mátrai P, Barabaissy A, Sebe B, Skrivele I, et al. The effectiveness and safety of cariprazine in schizophrenia patients with negative symptoms and insufficient effectiveness of previous antipsychotic therapy: An observational study. International Clinical Psychopharmacology. 2021;**36**(3):154-161. DOI: 10.1097/YIC.0000000000000351

[30] Dragasek J, Dombi ZB, Acsai K, Dzurilla V, Barabássy Á. The management of patients with predominant negative symptoms in Slovakia: A 1-year longitudinal, prospective & multicentric cohort study. European Psychiatry.

[31] Csehi R, Dombi ZB, Sebe B, Molnár MJ. Real-life clinical experience with cariprazine: A systematic review of case studies. Frontiers in Psychiatry. 2022;**13**:827744

[32] Cerveri G, Gesi C, Mencacci C. Pharmacological treatment of negative symptoms in schizophrenia: Update and proposal of a clinical algorithm. Neuropsychiatric Disease and Treatment. 2019;**15**:1525-1535

[33] Bowie CR, Harvey PD. Cognitive deficits and functional outcome in schizophrenia. Neuropsychiatric Disease and Treatment. 2006;**2**(4):531-536

[34] Keefe RSE, Bilder RM, Davis SM, Harvey PD, Palmer BW, Gold JM, et al. Neurocognitive effects of antipsychotic medications in patients with chronic schizophrenia in the CATIE trial. Archives of General Psychiatry. 2007;**64**:633-647

[35] Harvey PD. Mood symptoms, cognition, and everyday functioning in major depression, bipolar disorder, and schizophrenia. Innovations in Clinical Neuroscience. 2011;**8**(10):14-18

[36] Fountoulakis KN, Dragioti E, Theofilidis AT, Wikilund T, Atmatzidis X, Nimatoudis I, et al. Staging of schizophrenia with the use of PANSS: An international multi-center study. The International Journal of Neuropsychopharmacology. 2019;**22**(11):681-697

[37] Berardelli I, Rogante E, Sarubbi S, Erbuto D, Lester D, Pompili M. The importance of suicide risk formulation in schizophrenia. Frontiers in Psychiatry. 2021;**12**:1-13

[38] FDA. SEROQUEL XR FDA Label [Internet]. 2020. Available from: https://www.accessdata.fda.gov/drugsatfda_docs/label/2020/022047Orig1s042lbl.pdf

[39] FDA. VRAYLAR FDA Label [Internet]. 2022. Available from: https://www.accessdata.fda.gov/drugsatfda_docs/label/2022/204370s009lbl.pdf

[40] FDA. ZYPREXA FDA Label [Internet]. 2014. Available from: https://www.accessdata.fda.gov/drugsatfda_docs/label/2014/020592s062021086s040021253s048lbl.pdf

[41] FDA. SYMBYAX FDA Label [Internet]. 2009. Available from: https://www.accessdata.fda.gov/drugsatfda_docs/label/2009/021520s022lbl.pdf

[42] Woody G. The challenge of dual diagnosis. Alcohol Research and Health. 1996;**20**(2):76-80

[43] Alsuhaibani R, Smith DC, Lowrie R, Aljhani S, Paudyal V. Scope, quality and inclusivity of international

clinical guidelines on mental health and substance abuse in relation to dual diagnosis, social and community outcomes: A systematic review. BMC Psychiatry. 2021;**21**(1):1-23

[44] Priester MA, Browne T, Iachini A, Clone S, DeHart D, Seay KD. Treatment access barriers and disparities among individuals with co-occurring mental health and substance use disorders: An integrative literature review. Journal of Substance Abuse Treatment. 2016;**61**:47-59

[45] Hernández-Huerta D, Morillo-González J. Dopamine D_3 partial agonists in the treatment of psychosis and substance use disorder comorbidity: A pharmacological alternative to consider? CNS Spectrums. 2021;**26**(5):444-445

[46] Hakobyan S, Vazirian S, Lee-Cheong S, Krausz M, Honer WG, Schutz CG. Concurrent disorder management guidelines. Systematic review. Journal of Clinical Medicine. 2020;**9**(8):2406

[47] Szerman N, Torrens M, Maldonado R, Balhara YPS, Salom C, Maremmani I, et al. Addictive and other mental disorders: A call for a standardized definition of dual disorders. Translational Psychiatry. 2022;**12**:1-6

[48] Indave BI, Minozzi S, Pani PP, Amato L. Antipsychotic medications for cocaine dependence. The Cochrane Database of Systematic Reviews. 2016;**3**(3):CD006306. DOI: 10.1002/14651858.CD006306.pub3

[49] Stahl SM. Drugs for psychosis and mood: Unique actions at D3, D2, and D1 dopamine receptor subtypes. CNS Spectrums. 2017;**22**(5):375-384

[50] Galaj E, Newman AH, Xi ZX. Dopamine D3 receptor-based medication development for the treatment of opioid use disorder: Rationale, progress, and challenges. Neuroscience and Biobehavioral Reviews. 2020;**114**:38-52

[51] Román V, Gyertyán I, Sághy K, Kiss B, Szombathelyi Z. Cariprazine (RGH-188), a D3-preferring dopamine D3/D2 receptor partial agonist antipsychotic candidate demonstrates anti-abuse potential in rats. Psychopharmacology. 2013;**226**(2):285-293

[52] Edinoff AN, Kaufman SE, Hollier JW, Virgen CG, Karam CA, Malone GW, et al. Catatonia: Clinical overview of the diagnosis, treatment, and clinical challenges. Neurology International. 2021;**13**(4):570-586

[53] Sienaert P, Dhossche DM, Vancampfort D, De Hert M, Gazdag G. A clinical review of the treatment of catatonia. Frontiers in Psychiatry. 2014;**5**:181. DOI: 10.3389/fpsyt.2014.00181

[54] Marshall M, Lewis S, Lockwood A, Drake R, Jones P, Croudace T. Association between duration of untreated psychosis and outcome in cohorts of first-episode patients: A systematic review. Archives of General Psychiatry. 2005;**62**(9):975-983

[55] Howes OD, Whitehurst T, Shatalina E, Townsend L, Onwordi EC, Mak TLA, et al. The clinical significance of duration of untreated psychosis: An umbrella review and random-effects meta-analysis. World Psychiatry. 2021;**20**(1):75-95

[56] Bogers JPAM, Hambarian G, Schmidt NW, Vermeulen JM, de Haan L. Risk factors for psychotic relapse after dose reduction or discontinuation of antipsychotics in patients with chronic schizophrenia. A meta-analysis of randomized controlled trials. Schizophrenia Bulletin. 2023;**49**(1):11-23

[57] Stahl SM, Sy S, Maguire GA. How and when to treat the most common adverse effects of antipsychotics: Expert review from research to clinical practice. Acta Psychiatrica Scandinavica. 2021;**143**:172-180

[58] Olivares JM, Sermon J, Hemels M, Schreiner A. Definitions and drivers of relapse in patients with schizophrenia: A systematic literature review. Annals of General Psychiatry. 2013;**12**(1):32. DOI: 10.1186/1744-859X-12-32

[59] Mosolov SN, Potapov AV, Ushakov UV. Remission in schizophrenia: results of cross-sectional with 6-month follow-up period and 1-year observational therapeutic studies in an outpatient population. Annals of General Psychiatry. 2012;**11**(1):1. DOI: 10.1186/1744-859X-11-1

[60] Carpiniello B, Pinna F, Manchia M, Tusconi M, Cavallaro R, Bosia M. Sustained symptomatic remission in schizophrenia: Course and predictors from a two-year prospective study. Schizophrenia Research. 2022;**239**:34-41

[61] Velligan DI, Lam YWF, Glahn DC, Barrett JA, Maples NJ, Ereshefsky L, et al. Defining and assessing adherence to oral antipsychotics: A review of the literature. Schizophrenia Bulletin. 2006;**32**(4):724-742

[62] Byerly MJ, Nakonezny PA, Lescouflair E. Antipsychotic medication adherence in schizophrenia. Psychiatric Clinics of North America. 2007;**30**:437-452

[63] Mitchell AJ, Selmes T. Why don't patients take their medicine? Reasons and solutions in psychiatry. Advances in Psychiatric Treatment. 2007;**13**:336-346

[64] Barnes TRE, Drake R, Paton C, Cooper SJ, Deakin B, Ferrier IN, et al. Evidence-based guidelines for the pharmacological treatment of schizophrenia: Updated recommendations from the British Association for Psychopharmacology. Journal of Psychopharmacology. 2020;**34**(1):3-78

[65] DiBonaventura M, Gabriel S, Dupclay L, Gupta S, Kim E. A patient perspective of the impact of medication side effects on adherence: Results of a cross-sectional nationwide survey of patients with schizophrenia. BMC Psychiatry. 2012;**12**(20):1-7

[66] Doane MJ, Sajatovic M, Weiden PJ, O'sullivan AK, Maher S, Bjorner JB, et al. Antipsychotic treatment experiences of people with schizophrenia: Patient perspectives from an online survey. Patient Preference and Adherence. 2020;**14**:2043-2054

[67] Awad AG, Voruganti LNP. Antipsychotic medications, schizophrenia and the issue of quality of life. In: Quality of Life Impairment in Schizophrenia, Mood and Anxiety Disorders: New Perspectives on Research and Treatment. Dordrecht: Springer; 2007

[68] Achtyes E, Simmons A, Skabeev A. et al. Patient preferences concerning the efficacy and side-effect profile of schizophrenia medications: A survey of patients living with schizophrenia. BMC Psychiatry. 2018;**18**:292. DOI: 10.1186/s12888-018-1856-y

[69] Tandon R, Lenderking WR, Weiss C, Shalhoub H, Barbosa CD, Chen J, et al. The impact on functioning of second-generation antipsychotic medication side effects for patients with schizophrenia: A worldwide, cross-sectional, web-based survey. Annals of General Psychiatry. 2020;**19**:42. DOI: 10.1186/s12991-020-00292-5

[70] Schneider-Thoma J, Chalkou K, Dörries C, Bighelli I, Ceraso A, Huhn M, et al. Comparative efficacy and tolerability of 32 oral and long-acting injectable antipsychotics for the maintenance treatment of adults with schizophrenia: A systematic review and network meta-analysis. Lancet. 2022;**399**(10327):824-836

[71] Tewksbury A, Olander A. Management of antipsychotic-induced hyperprolactinemia. Mental Health Clinician. 2016;**6**:185-190

[72] Hjorth S. The more, the merrier...? Antipsychotic polypharmacy treatment strategies in schizophrenia from a pharmacology perspective. Frontiers in Psychiatry. 2021;**12**:760181

Chapter 7

Role of Phytochemicals in Management of Schizophrenia

Shazia Perveen, Sumaria Kanwal, Ali S. Alqahtani, Faiza Rao, Ayesha Asghar, Ali Irfan, Mahtab Ahmad Khan and Riaz Ullah

Abstract

Bioactive substances derived from plants, created by them for defense, are known as phytochemicals. Alkaloids, glycosides, polyphenols, terpenes and terpenoids, phytosterols, cannabinoids and carotenoids are the different categories of phytochemicals. Schizophrenia is associated with changes in the structure of the brain, decrease of dendritic spines from pyramidal neurons in the cortex, loss of gray matter and enlarged ventricles. Hallucinations, delusions, disorganized behavior and amotivation are some symptoms of schizophrenia. Phytochemicals are a key component of the management of schizophrenia. Alkaloids can operate as cholinergic agonists on muscarinic receptors and improve memory deficits. Glycosides target ErbB signaling, inhibit D3/D4 receptors and change dopamine and serotonin metabolism. Because of their anti-inflammatory, antioxidant and anti-apoptotic properties, polyphenols display neuroprotective and anti-schizophrenic activity. Terpenes and terpenoids act on the glutamate and dopamine pathways and inhibit glycinergic action. Cannabinoids have an anti-schizophrenic effect plus boost GABAergic activity and prevent serotonin uptake. Phytosterols have antipsychotic potential by blocking ketamine-induced biochemical, histological and behavioral changes. Because they regulate brain-derived neurotrophic factor (BDNF), carotenoids show significant potential for treating a variety of central nervous system problems. They are also an excellent antipsychotic medication.

Keywords: phytochemicals, schizophrenia, disorder, polyphenols, management

1. Introduction

Phytochemicals are plant-based bioactive compounds produced by plants for their protection. There are many different sources of phytochemicals, including whole grains, fruits, vegetables, nuts and herbs. To date, over a thousand phytochemicals have been identified. Carotenoids, polyphenols, isoprenoids, phytosterols, saponins, dietary fibers and certain polysaccharides are a few of the important phytochemicals. In besides having potent antioxidant properties, these phytochemicals have antiviral, antibacterial, anthelmintic, antiallergic and antidiarrheal properties. Additionally, they support immunology, gap junction communication, gene transcription regulation and protection against lung and prostate malignancies. The properties of functional foods have been broadened by a greater focus on translational research. Following their extraction from a variety of sources, phytochemicals are widely used in the development of nutraceuticals and functional foods. The affinity of phytochemicals for solvents and their heat tolerance vary. The quality of the recovered phytochemical and its use in the creation of food and nutraceutical products are also influenced by the solvent choice [1].

The purpose of the study is to describe the role of phytochemicals in management of schizophrenia which could be beneficial in the improvement of symptoms of schizophrenia in patients, reduction of health issues regarding schizophrenia and maintenance of healthy life style.

1.1 Sources of phytochemicals

Our regular diet We first discuss a few terminologies:

Designer food: processed meals enriched with naturally occurring foods high in compounds that prevent disease.

Functional food: Any food or ingredient that has been improved and may have health benefits in addition to the usual nutrients it contains.

Nutraceutical: Certain substances found in food, such as vitamins and chemicals that may help prevent illness.

Pharmafood: Food or nutrient that claims medical or health benefits, including the prevention and treatment of disease [2].

1.2 Classification of phytochemicals

Phytochemical compounds have primary as well as secondary constituents. Phytochemicals can be classified into various groups. Alkaloids, glycosides, polyphenols, terpenes and terpenoids, phytosterols, cannabinoids and carotenoids are the different categories of phytochemicals (**Figure 1**) [2].

1.2.1 Alkaloids

Alkaloids are a vast group of chemicals that are based on the amino acids that supply their nitrogen atom and a portion of their skeleton; this heterogeneous chemical group is divided into groups. Alkaloids with distinct biosynthesis processes

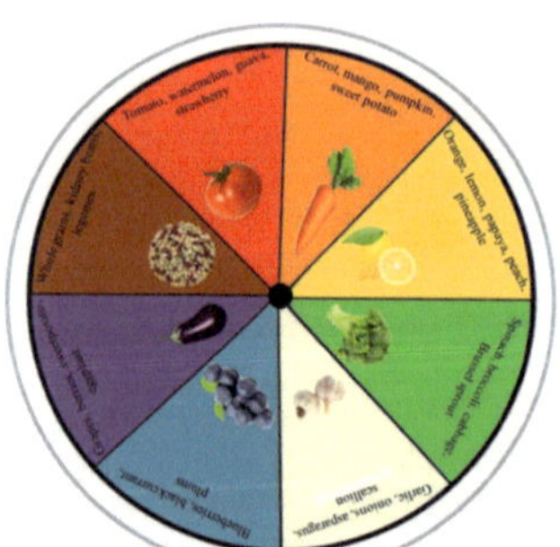

Figure 1.
The color wheel of phytochemicals [2].

and varying biological activities might arise from alkaloids with comparable origins or sharing an identical basic nucleus. L-phenylalanine, L-tyrosine, L-histidine, L-ornithine, nicotinic acid, anthracitic acid or acetate and L-lysine are the sources of these. They are used in daily life by people from all over the world. Animals can also be the source of alkaloids, either endogenously or exogenously [3].

1.2.2 Glycosides

A broad class of secondary metabolites is made up of glycosides. Glycosides have a variety of structural forms, and because of their established bioactivities and historical applications, they are crucial to the pharmacognosy regime. It is composed of two parts, a hydrophilic glycone unit made up of one or more sugar components and an aglycone (genin) unit that is mostly lipophilic [4].

1.2.3 Polyphenols

A class of naturally occurring substances with phenolic structures is called polyphenols. There are four main subclasses within this family which are lignans, flavonoids, stilbenes and phenolic acids. Anthocyanidins, flavanones, flavones and flavonols are other classifications of flavonoids. Artichokes, spinach, broccoli, chicory, apples, plums, pears, grapes and cherries are rich in polyphenols. Red wine, tea and olive oil are regarded as excellent sources of polyphenols [5]. About 350 aglycones and 100 glycosylate forms make up flavanones, which have a flavan nucleus made up of two aromatic rings connected by a dihydropyrone ring [6]. The presence of a double bond between C-2 and C-3, along with the attachment of the B-ring to C-2, characterizes flavones, a vast class of flavonoids [7]. The hydroxyl group at position three sets flavonols apart from flavanones and creates a double bond between C-2 and C-3. The majority of anthocyanidins in nature are found as their sugar-conjugated derivatives or anthocyanins, which gives fruit and flower tissues their characteristic red, blue and purple hues. Polyphenols have been found to provide health benefits such as scavenging free radicals, guarding against cancer, heart disease and other age-related illnesses and preventing allergies and inflammation. Additionally, flavonoids have been shown to help with gastrointestinal disorders, diabetes, rhinitis, angina pectoris, cervical lesions, chronic venous insufficiency, dermatopathy, lymphocytic leukemia, menopausal symptoms and traumatic cerebral infarction [1].

1.2.4 Terpenes and terpenoids

Terpenes are the largest class of secondary metabolites. They are simply made up of five carbon isoprene units that may be put together in thousands of different ways to form multiple isoprene units. Terpenoids are a modified class of terpenes with distinct functional groups and an oxidized methyl group that is relocated or deleted at different places. Terpenes are simple hydrocarbons. Depending on the number of carbon units, terpenoids are classified as monoterpenes, sesquiterpenes, diterpenes, sesterpenes and triterpenes. With their diverse structural variations, the majority of terpenoids are physiologically active and utilized globally to treat a wide range of illnesses. Many terpenoids, including Taxol and its variants utilized as anticancer medications because they suppress certain human cancer cells. Terpenes have a pleasant scent which is why many flavorings and fragrances contain them. Antimalarial medications like artemisinin and similar substances are made from terpenes and their derivatives. In the meantime, terpenoids are used in a variety of products, including hormones, vitamins, medications, meals and cosmetics [8].

1.2.5 Cannabinoids

Cannabis is the first illegal drug as well as the third one if tobacco and alcohol are taken into account. Cannabis is becoming more and more common in our culture, both for medicinal and recreational purposes. An estimated 183.3 million adults between the ages of 15 and 64 smoked cannabis in 2015 (3.8% of the world's population). Young adults between the ages of 15 and 34 are the most likely to consume cannabis (13.9 percent in the previous year). Cannabis use among students in Europe and the United States between the ages of 15 and 16 was 8 and 15%, respectively [9].

1.2.6 Phytosterols

The collective term for the sterols and stanols found in plants that control their physiological processes is called phytosterol. Olive oil and the oils of corn, sesame, sunflower, peanuts, macadamia, nuts, beans and almonds are abundant in them. Plant stanols include campestanol, sitostanol and stigmastanol, whereas some plant sterols include campesterol, stigmasterol and sitosterol. Campesterol is the most basic sterol, with the exception of the five or six double bonds in the B-ring. Generally speaking, phytosterols have several health advantages, such as increased antioxidant activity, decreased low-density lipoprotein (LDL) cholesterol and support for prostate health and hair development [1].

1.2.7 Carotenoids

Carotenoids are pigments that are found in plants, algae and photosynthetic bacteria. They are vivid yellow, red, and orange. Carotenoids are found in abundance in fruits, but they are also abundant in vegetables. According to reports, fucoxanthin has anti-inflammatory, antihypertensive, anticancer, radioprotective and anti-obesity properties [1].

1.3 Schizophrenia

Schizophrenia, as a long-term mental disorder, affects about one percent of the world's total population. Early environmental and genetic variables appear to be the primary contributors to this disease, while the existence of other mental diseases may also be involved. It is unclear if schizophrenia is a single condition or a collection of several syndromes due to the wide range of symptom combinations that might occur. There may be a connection between the pathophysiology of schizophrenia and increased oxidative stress. Changes in the structure of the brain associated with this illness include a reduction in dendritic spines from pyramidal neurons in the cortex, an expansion of ventricles and a loss of gray matter. Further potential links between schizophrenia and the prefrontal brain include elevated phospholipid metabolism and decreased dopaminergic function [10].

1.3.1 Symptoms of schizophrenia

A mental illness known as heterogeneous syndrome, schizophrenia can present with a variety of symptoms, including delusions, hallucinations, very disordered thinking or speech, disorganized behavior, flat affect and amotivation. The pathophysiology of the onset and progression of schizophrenia and sensitive and specific biomarkers have not yet been reliably identified [11].

2. Phytochemicals and their role in management of schizophrenia

Approximately 80% of people in Asia and Africa rely on complementary and alternative medicine. Antipsychotic medications that are often used have a number of side effects. Thus, in animal and cell culture models of central nervous system (CNS) diseases, a number of phytochemicals have been studied for their potential to preserve neurons and have antipsychotic properties. The overwhelming majority of research has shown that phytochemicals' antioxidant activity is what gives them their antipsychotic and neuroprotective properties. Since oxidative stress in the brain is clearly depicted in the pathophysiology of schizophrenia, natural antioxidants in the form of extracts or specific phytochemicals are useful in the treatment of schizophrenia. These phytochemicals' medicinal usefulness, low side effect rate, improved safety profile and excellent efficacy have drawn attention [12]. Phytochemicals demonstrate efficacy against schizophrenia and are associated with different phytochemical classes such as alkaloids, tannins, glycosides, phenolic acids, flavonoids, terpenes, terpenoids and essential oils [13].

2.1 Role of alkaloids in management of schizophrenia

Alkaloids are present in all plant parts especially in flowers. These are mostly helpful in the treatment of various neurodegenerative illnesses. These phytochemicals are beneficial against schizophrenia via changing acetylcholine concentration, boosting GABA, antagonizing N-methyl-D-aspartate (NMDA) receptors, antioxidant action, anti-amyloid activity and reducing neuro-inflammation [14]. Stepholidine, a protoberberine alkaloid, has a special feature of combined D1 agonist and D2 antagonist effect and is useful in improving memory deficit in schizophrenia [15]. Aporphine alkaloids, including apomorphine, reportedly cause amelioration of schizophrenic symptoms in patients by potently antagonizing dopamine at its receptor site [16]. Anti-schizophrenia studies have also been conducted using isoquinoline alkaloids. The NMDA current in the cortical neurons of rats is increased by galantamine. Additionally, it strengthened the benefits of Ach by positively modulating nAchR, which reduced attention deficit and improved short-term memory and focus [17, 18]. A combination of galantamine and memantine was effective in enhancing cognition in schizophrenic patients [19]. Reticuline has also demonstrated antipsychotic activity through anti-dopaminergic actions [20].

As an alpha nicotinic receptor agonist, nicotine, a pyridine alkaloid, was found to be beneficial in treating attention deficit disorder in people with schizophrenia [21]. Geissoschinzine methyl ether's partly antagonistic action against NMDA receptors and regulation of dopamine receptors both contributed to its ameliorative effects against schizophrenia [13].

2.2 Role of glycosides in management of schizophrenia

Glycosidic bonding is the process by which a sugar moiety is joined to a non-sugar molecule in glycosides. Plants have glycosides as secondary metabolites; they are the parts of their "offense and defense" [22, 23]. By enhancing vesicular glutamate transporter 2 in the cingulate gyrus region, a study investigating the effects of bacoside A and B isolated from *Bacopa monnieri* demonstrated improvement in cognitive deficits in a schizophrenic model [24]. Isothiocyanates, like sulforaphane, shown antioxidant activity by boosting electrophilic response elements, detoxifying phase 2 enzymes and activating the Nrf2 pathway to exhibit antipsychotic activity [25]. Nephthodianthrone or hypericin has antioxidant qualities. Inhibiting D3/D4 receptors, it is a potential medication for the treatment of schizophrenia [26, 27]. Emodin targets ErbB signaling and modifies the metabolism of dopamine and serotonin to reduce symptoms of schizophrenia [28, 29]. Polygala saponin, a saponin glycoside, has anti-schizophrenic activity due to its dopamine and serotonin antagonist activities. Cardenolides and iridoid glycosides are also shown to be useful in treating psychotic symptoms that need more research. Docking experiments also showed that beta-sitosterol blocked NMDA receptors that included GluN2B. Additionally, picroside II demonstrated antipsychotic activity potential in vitro [30, 31].

2.3 Role of polyphenols in management of schizophrenia

Plant secondary metabolites known as polyphenols have been shown to have neuroprotective and anti-schizophrenic properties. These appear to be effective against neurologic and psychotic diseases, according to several studies [32]. Because of its anti-inflammatory, antioxidant and anti-apoptotic properties, kaempferol has shown neuroprotective effects against schizophrenia [33]. It has been observed that baicalin improves cognitive dysfunction and unpleasant symptoms in psychosis. Its anti-inflammatory, antioxidant and anti-prolyl-oligopeptidase properties may be responsible for this psychotic impact [13, 34].

Quercitin is a bioflavonoid that has the ability to alleviate symptoms of schizophrenia by scavenging free radicals [35]. Protein kinase C and nitric oxide are both inhibited by myricitrin. Its antioxidant action is responsible for its anti-schizophrenic properties [36]. Scopoletin and rutin's inhibitory interaction with the D2 receptor makes them beneficial for reducing positive symptoms of schizophrenia [37]. The anti-schizophrenic properties of xanthones, like magniferin and α-mangostin, have also been investigated. α-mangostin possesses anti-inflammatory and antioxidant properties. In rodent models of schizophrenia, it was also demonstrated to be efficacious and to inhibit phosphodiesterases and 5HT2A receptors. Magniferin's antioxidant mechanism, preservation of mitochondrial capabilities, anti-inflammatory activity and dopamine decrease all contributed to its better cognitive effects [38, 39]. One cholesterol that has demonstrated neuroprotection against a variety of neurological and psychological conditions is hydroxytyrosol. By activating the Nrf2 pathway, it reduced oxidative stress and improved mitochondrial functioning. When given during pregnancy, it improved learning and memory in fetuses of stressed animals and humans, demonstrating the importance of maintaining neurogenesis and cognitive abilities in offspring [40, 41].

Because curcumin can increase decreased glutathione levels, it has a number of advantageous benefits on the neurological system [42]. In patients with persistent schizophrenia, curcumin enhanced the effectiveness of regular antipsychotic medications. These therapies have improved the negative symptoms associated with schizophrenia. Curcumin modulates NMDA activity and controls the production of genes linked to inflammation, both of which are linked to symptoms of schizophrenia. By increasing GABA activity, Morin also showed antipsychotic-like effects without having an extrapyramidal side effect [43]. The flavonoid nobiletin reduces the cognitive symptoms of schizophrenia by enhancing the hypo-functioning of NMDA receptors through its action on extracellular signal-regulated kinases (ERK) signaling [44].

Diosmin, a flavone, enhances GABA transmission to treat symptoms of schizophrenia [45]. Isoflavone [46], luteolin and apigenin have also shown a great deal of promise in reducing the symptoms of schizophrenia [46].

2.4 Role of terpenes and terpenoids in management of schizophrenia

Tutin is a sesquiterpene that inhibits glycinergic activity and blocks GABA-A receptors. In addition, 1, 8 cineole is a monoterpenoid that influences the glutamate and dopamine pathways. Sesquiterpene caryophylline, which is extracted from essential oils and functions as a phytocannabinoid, has been successfully studied in a clinical study on schizophrenia [47].

2.5 Role of cannabinoids in management of schizophrenia

As members of the terpenoid class, cannabinoids are useful in the management of neurodegenerative illnesses. A meta-analysis's findings indicate that people with schizophrenia have higher levels of the endocannabinoid anandamide in their blood, CSF fluids and immune cells' cannabinoid 1 receptor (CB1) [48]. Using cannabinoids has been shown to improve cognition and reduce disease-positive symptoms in three randomized trials [49].

In order to have an anti-schizophrenic effect, cannabinoids, a kind of cannabinoid, boost GABAergic activity and prevent serotonin uptake. Cannabis-using schizophrenic individuals also showed this effect. Furthermore, compared to other antipsychotics, cannabinoids have demonstrated a definite advantage in clinical trials because they did not cause any movement-related side effects [50].

Another cannabinoid, tetrahydrocannabinol, also improved the symptoms of schizophrenia due to its effect on the endocannabinoid receptors [51]. However, some investigations claimed that the administration of 9-tetrahydrocannabinol had exacerbated psychotic symptoms. However, tetrahydrocannabinol may have effects that vary in dose, according to the study. When taken in large quantities, it caused disturbance to brain circuits that exacerbated psychotic symptoms, while at modest dosages, it alleviated the symptoms of psychosis [51].

2.6 Role of phytosterols in management of schizophrenia

Many plants naturally produce phytosterols and oxyphytosterols, which are the byproducts of phytosterol oxidation. Due to a rise in the consumption of plant-based foods enhanced with phytosterol and oxyphytosterol, exposure to these natural agents is increasing [52]. One type of phytosterol found in vegetables, legumes, nuts, herbs and seeds is stigmasterol. It has been demonstrated to suppress the biochemical, histological and behavioral changes brought on by ketamine in mice, suggesting that it may have antipsychotic potential [52].

2.7 Role of carotenoids in management of schizophrenia

The active ingredients of saffron (*Crocus sativus* L.), such as crocins and safranal, have demonstrated great promise in the treatment of a number of illnesses affecting the central nervous system, including anxiety, depression and memory loss [53]. A carotenoid called crocin has demonstrated efficacy as an antipsychotic medication by controlling brain-derived neurotrophic factor (BDNF) in the hippocampal tissues [54]. Growing preclinical data shows that crocins, at doses of 15–50 mg/kg, alleviated the memory impairment, hypermotility and social isolation that ketamine generated in rats [55]. Additionally, it was discovered that crocins prevented rats' apomorphine-induced impairment in a novel object identification test linked to dopaminergic dysfunction [56]. Based on a better safety profile and the preclinical evidence of efficacy against psychosis, there is a strong need for controlled clinical studies of these agents against schizophrenia [57].

2.8 Role of other phytochemicals in management of schizophrenia

Dopamine D2 and/or D1 receptor antagonistism is the mechanism via which alpha asarone, an essential oil from the polypropanoid class, exhibits anti-schizophrenic effects [58]. In a human open trial, the amino acid glycine reduced the unpleasant symptoms associated with schizophrenia. This effect is attributed to its potentiating effect on NMDA receptors. When used as an adjuvant to other medical therapy, it has been shown to be beneficial against treatment-resistant schizophrenia, negative symptoms and cognitive issues. Another amino acid that reduces the symptoms of schizophrenia is leucine, which works on dopaminergic receptors [59].

Because kava contains kavapyrone, which has been shown to have efficacy against a number of neurological illnesses, kava is a well-known herb. Because kavapyrone inhibits glutamate release and increases the density of GABA-A receptors, it may be used to treat schizophrenia. Withaferin A, Withanolide A, Withanolide B and Withanolide D are steroidal lactones that have shown favorable effects on NMDA receptors through docking studies and can be useful in schizophrenia following further examination [31]. The effect of various phytochemicals on positive, negative and cognitive symptoms is summarized in **Figure 2** [13].

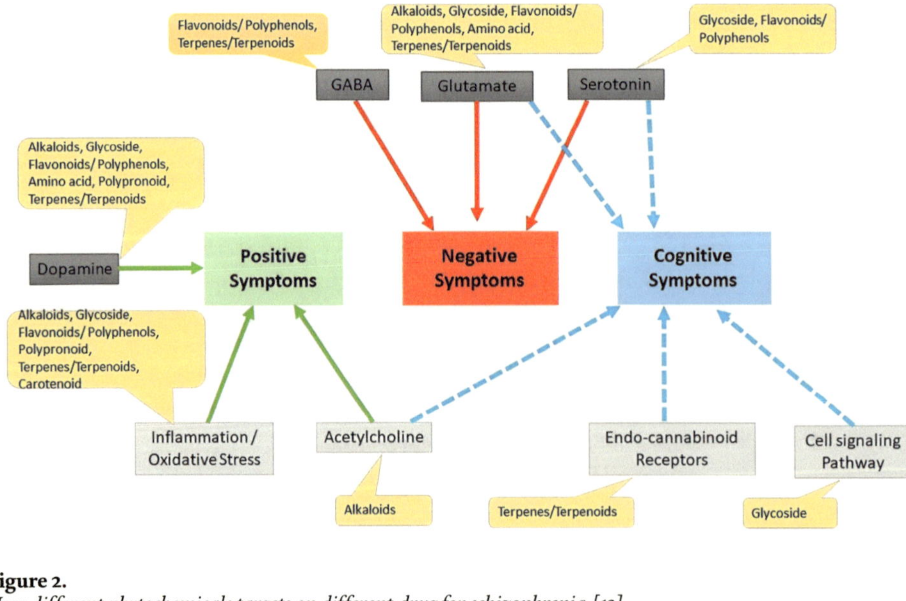

Figure 2.
How different phytochemicals targets on different drug for schizophrenia [13].

3. Importance of vitamins in treatment of schizophrenia

Vitamins are often obtained through diet because many of them cannot be produced by the human body at sufficient levels. Many researchers have linked vitamin deficits to schizophrenia, either in the early stages of the condition or after diagnosis [60]. Vitamin B is necessary for cellular metabolism, which includes oxidation-reduction and trans-methylation [61]. Antioxidants like vitamins C and E guard against cellular damage brought on by highly reactive oxygen-containing molecules or inflammation. Schizophrenia Patients showed decreased fasting vitamin C levels and poorer urinary vitamin C excretion following 1.0 g oral vitamin C load in a small cross-sectional research with 20 schizophrenia patients and 15 controls [62]. Retinoic acid, produced from vitamin A and essential for neuronal migration and differentiation, is thought to be part of the pathophysiology of schizophrenia. Within some subgroups, vitamin supplementation, especially with folic acid, vitamin B12 and vitamin D, may be crucial to the management of schizophrenia [63]. Vitamin D supplementation may be protective against psychosis in patients who are deficient in vitamin D (darker skin, living in a latitude with less sunlight). Supplementing patients with particular genetic variations in the folate metabolic pathway with both folate and vitamin B12 can be helpful, particularly when it comes to alleviating bad symptoms [64].

4. Conclusions

More than a thousand phytochemicals have been discovered to date and can be derived from various sources such as whole grains, fruits, vegetables, nuts and herbs. Some of the significant phytochemicals are carotenoids, polyphenols, isoprenoids, phytosterols, saponins, dietary fibers and certain polysaccharides. These phytochemicals possess strong antioxidant activities and exhibit antimicrobial, antidiarrheal, anthelmintic, antiallergic, antispasmodic and antiviral activities. Schizophrenia is a condition that is related to alterations in brain structures involving loss of gray matter, expanded ventricles and reduction of dendritic spines from pyramidal neurons of the cortex and can manifest with delusions, hallucinations, extremely disordered thinking, disorganized behavior, flat affect, amotivation, energy and failure to maintain hygiene along with many more symptom domains. Alkaloids are effective against schizophrenia by affecting acetylcholine concentration, increasing GABA, antagonizing NMDA receptors, antioxidant action, anti-amyloid activity and preventing neuro-inflammation. Glycosides target ErbB signaling and alter dopamine and serotonin metabolism to exhibit ameliorating effects against schizophrenia symptoms. Polyphenols demonstrate neuroprotective effects against schizophrenia due to their anti-inflammatory, antioxidant and anti-apoptotic effects. Terpenes and Terpenoids inhibit glycinergic activity and block GABA-A receptors. Cannabinoids is a cannabinoid that blocks serotonin uptake and increases GABAergic activity to exert anti-schizophrenic effect. Cannabinoids is a cannabinoid that blocks serotonin uptake and increases GABAergic activity to exert anti-schizophrenic effect. Phytosterols manage psychosis by ameliorating inflammation and oxidative stress and by altering dopaminergic, acetylcholinergic and GABAergic neurotransmission. Carotenoids have shown high potential for treatment of various central nervous system disorders such as anxiety, depression and memory deficit. Hence, phytochemicals play a vital role in management of schizophrenia.

Acknowledgements

The authors wish to thank the Research Centre College of Pharmacy and Deanship of Scientific Research at King Saud University Riyadh, Saudi Arabia.

Conflict of interest

The authors declare no conflict of interest.

Acronyms and abbreviations

BPH	benign prostatic hyperplasia
CNS	central nervous system
NMDA	N-methyl-D-aspartate
Nrf2	nuclear factor E2-related factor 2
GABA	gamma-aminobutyric acid
ERK	extracellular signal-regulated kinases

Author details

Shazia Perveen[1], Sumaria Kanwal[2*], Ali S. Alqahtani[3], Faiza Rao[4], Ayesha Asghar[1], Ali Irfan[5*], Mahtab Ahmad Khan[6] and Riaz Ullah[3*]

1 Department of Zoology, The Women University Multan, Pakistan

2 Department of Biosciences, COMSATS University Islamabad, Sahiwal Campus, Pakistan

3 Medicinal Aromatic and Poisonous Plants Research Center, College of Pharmacy King Saud University, Riyadh, Saudi Arabia

4 Center to Advance level Research and Development (SMC-PVT) Ltd., Pakistan

5 Department of Chemistry, Government College University Faisalabad, Faisalabad, Pakistan

6 Faculty of Pharmaceutical Sciences, University of Central Punjab (UCP), Lahore, Pakistan

*Address all correspondence to: sumaira.kanwal@cuisahiwal.edu.pk, raialiirfan@gmail.com and rullah@ksu.edu.sa

References

[1] Kumar A, Kumar M, Jose A, Tomer V, Oz E, et al. Major phytochemicals: Recent advances in health benefits and extraction method. Molecules. 2023;**28**(2):887

[2] Roy M, Datta A. Cancer Genetics and Therapeutics: Focus on Phytochemicals. Berlin, Germany: Springer Nature; 2019. Available from: https://www.google.com/search?sca_esv=c73958766a138815&rlz=1C1SQJL_en-GBPK1082PK1082&sxsrf=ACQVn08HP6KTc14hGelvVLcB7suR_ceWXQ:1712093497701&q=Berlin&si=AKbGX_paaCugDdYkuX2heTJMr0_FGRox2AzKVmiTg2eQr2d-ro-XRLQqwEMSE5FdJv59BGmSKBYk0RauVT8kKGiSpQiIbcfM6-iosnsygATIAJYznt06PMHVFzkmwQ04zgT-Tfjqlv6n_LMLTlwOOjozpbmOVBJNfUcKi09irT-SpYyWFupJvAw-SDoU2-JMqMMEDfWAfIKZ&sa=X&ved=2ahUKEwjEtIKmvaSFAxUvS_EDHcIBDEsQmxMoAXoECFYQAw

[3] Dey P, Kundu A, Kumar A, Gupta M, Lee BM, Bhakta T, et al. Analysis of alkaloids (indole alkaloids, isoquinoline alkaloids, tropane alkaloids). In: Recent Advances in Natural Products Analysis. Amsterdam, Netherlands: Elsevier; 2020. pp. 505-567

[4] Bartnik M, Facey P. Glycosides. In: Pharmacognosy. United States: Academic Press; 2024. pp. 103-165

[5] D'Archivio M, Filesi C, Di Benedetto R, Gargiulo R, Giovannini C, Masella R. Polyphenols, dietary sources and bioavailability. Annali-Istituto Superiore di Sanita. 2007;**43**(4):348

[6] Barreca D, Gattuso G, Bellocco E, Calderaro A, Trombetta D, Smeriglio A, et al. Flavanones: Citrus phytochemical with health-promoting properties. BioFactors. 2017;**43**(4):495-506

[7] Jiang N, Doseff AI, Grotewold E. Flavones: From biosynthesis to health benefits. Plants. 2016;**5**(2):27

[8] Perveen S, Al-Taweel A, editors. Terpenes and Terpenoids. BoD–Books on Demand. London, UK: Intechopen; 2018

[9] Papaseit E, Pérez-Mañá C, Pérez-Acevedo AP, Hladun O, Torres-Moreno MC, Muga R, et al. Cannabinoids: From pot to lab. International Journal of Medical Sciences. 2018;**15**(12):1286

[10] Rabiee R, Hosseini Hooshiar S, Ghaderi A, Jafarnejad S. Schizophrenia, curcumin and minimizing side effects of antipsychotic drugs: Possible mechanisms. Neurochemical Research. 2023;**48**(3):713-724

[11] Fišar Z. Biological hypotheses, risk factors and biomarkers of schizophrenia. Progress in Neuro-Psychopharmacology and Biological Psychiatry. 2023;**120**:110626

[12] Snyder MA, Gao WJ. NMDA hypofunction as a convergence point for progression and symptoms of schizophrenia. Frontiers in Cellular Neuroscience. 2013;**7**:31. DOI: 10.3389/fncel.2013.00031

[13] Saleem A, Qurat-ul-Ain, Akhtar MF. Alternative therapy of psychosis: Potential phytochemicals and drug targets in the management of schizophrenia. Frontiers in Pharmacology. 2022;**13**:895668. DOI: 10.3389/fphar.2022.895668

[14] Dey A, Mukherjee A. Plant-derived alkaloids. In: Discovery and Development

of Neuroprotective Agents from Natural Products. Amsterdam, Netherlands: Elsevier; 2018. pp. 237-320. DOI: 10.1016/b978-0-12-809593-5.00006-9

[15] Ellenbroek BA, Zhang X, Jin G. Effects of stepholidine in animal models for schizophrenia. Acta Pharmacologica Sinica. 2006;**27**:1111-1118. DOI: 10.1111/j.1745-7254.2006.00365.x

[16] Smith R, Tamminga C, Davis J. Effect of Apomorphine on schizophrenic symptoms. Journal of Neural Transmission. 1977;**40**:171-176. DOI: 10.1007/BF01250567

[17] Moriguchi S, Zhao X, Marszalec W, Yeh JZ, Narahashi T. Modulation of N methyl-D-aspartate receptors by donepezil in rat cortical neurons. The Journal of Pharmacology and Experimental Therapeutics. 2005;**315**:125-135. DOI: 10.1124/jpet.105.087908

[18] Schubert MH, Young KA, Hicks PB. Galantamine improves cognition in schizophrenic patients stabilized on risperidone. Biological Psychiatry. 2006;**60**:530-533. DOI: 10.1016/j.biopsych.2006.04.006

[19] Koola MM, Buchanan RW, Pillai A, Aitchison KJ, Weinberger DR, Aaronson ST, et al. Potential role of the combination of galantamine and memantine to improve cognition in schizophrenia. Schizophrenia Research. 2014;**157**:84-89. DOI: 10.1016/j.schres.2014.04.037

[20] Morais LC, Barbosa-Filho JM, Almeida RN. Central depressant effects of reticuline extracted from Ocotea Duckei in rats and mice. Journal of Ethnopharmacology. 1998;**62**:57-61. DOI: 10.1016/s0378-8741(98)00044-0

[21] Levin ED, Conners CK, Silva D, Hinton SC, Meck WH, March J, et al. Transdermal nicotine effects on attention. Psychopharmacology. 1998;**140**:135-141. DOI: 10.1007/s002130050750

[22] Shadkami F, Jones AD. Nontargeted profiling of specialized metabolites of digitalis Purpurea with a focus on cardiac glycosides. In: Emerging Trends in Dietary Components for Preventing and Combating Disease. ACS Publications; 2012. pp. 185-205. DOI: 10.1021/bk-2012-1093.ch011

[23] Wang Y, Singh AP, Nelson HN, Kaiser AJ, Reker NC, Hooks TL, et al. Urinary clearance of cranberry flavonol glycosides in humans. Journal of Agricultural and Food Chemistry. 2016;**64**:7931-7939. DOI: 10.1021/acs.jafc.6b03611

[24] Wetchateng T, Piyabhan P. EPA-0117–the use of Bacosides a and B to prevent a cognitive deficit in schizophrenia rat models resulting in increased vesicular glutamate transporter 2 (VGLUT2) in the cingulate gyrus. European Psychiatry. 2014;**29**:1. DOI: 10.1016/s0924-9338(14)77591-1

[25] Shirai Y, Fujita Y, Hashimoto K. Effects of the antioxidant Sulforaphane on Hyperlocomotion and Prepulse inhibition deficits in mice after phencyclidine administration. Clinical Psychopharmacology and Neuroscience. 2012;**10**:94. DOI: 10.9758/cpn.2012.10.2.94

[26] Butterweck V, Nahrstedt A, Evans J, Hufeisen S, Rauser L, Savage J, et al. In vitro receptor screening of pure constituents of St. John's Wort reveals novel interactions with a number of GPCRs. Psychopharmacology. 2002;**162**:193-202. DOI: 10.1007/s00213-002-1073-7

[27] Saranya K, Aji AM, Keerthana S, Babu NR, Sivaraj C, Arumugam P. Isolation

and pharmacological activities of hypericin fraction from the leaves of hypericum hookerianum Wight & Arnott. International Journal of Herbal Medicine. 2019;**7**:36-42. Washington, D.C, USA

[28] Mizuno M, Kawamura H, Ishizuka Y, Sotoyama H, Nawa H. The Anthraquinone derivative emodin attenuates methamphetamine-induced hyperlocomotion and startle response in rats. Pharmacology, Biochemistry, and Behavior. 2010;**97**:392-398. DOI: 10.1016/j.pbb.2010.09.009

[29] Mizuno M, Kawamura H, Takei N, Nawa H. The anthraquinone derivative emodin ameliorates neurobehavioral deficits of a rodent model for schizophrenia. Journal of Neural Transmission (Vienna). 2008;**115**:521-530. DOI: 10.1007/s00702-007-0867-5

[30] Bagchi P, Somashekhar R. Identification of novel drug leads for NMDA receptor implicated in schizophrenia from Indian traditional herbs. In: Proceedings of the International Conference on Intelligent Systems, Data Mining and Information Technology (ICIDIT'2014). Bangkok, Thailand; 2014

[31] Kumar G, Patnaik R. Exploring neuroprotective potential of Withania Somnifera phytochemicals by inhibition of GluN2B-containing NMDA receptors: An in silico study. Medical Hypotheses. 2016;**92**:35-43. DOI: 10.1016/j.mehy.2016.04.034

[32] Wu D, Guo Z, Ren Z, Guo W, Meydani SN. Green tea EGCG suppresses T cell proliferation through impairment of IL-2/IL-2 receptor signaling. Free Radical Biology & Medicine. 2009;**47**:636-643. DOI: 10.1016/j.freeradbiomed.2009.06.001

[33] El-Kott AF, Abd-Lateif AM, Khalifa HS, Morsy K, Ibrahim EH, Bin-Jumah M, et al. Kaempferol protects against cadmium chloride- induced hippocampal damage and memory deficits by activation of silent information regulator 1 and inhibition of poly (ADP-ribose) Polymerase-1. Science of the Total Environment. 2020;**728**:138832. DOI: 10.1016/j.scitotenv.2020.138832

[34] Tarragó T, Kichik N, Claasen B, Prades R, Teixidó M, Giralt E. Baicalin, a prodrug able to reach the CNS, is a prolyl Oligopeptidase inhibitor. Bioorganic & Medicinal Chemistry. 2008;**16**:7516-7524. DOI: 10.1016/j.bmc.2008.04.067

[35] Mert DG, Turgut NH, Arslanbas E, Gungor H, Kara H. The influence of quercetin on recognition memory and brain oxidative damage in a ketamine model of schizophrenia. Psychiatry and Clinical Psychopharmacology. 2019;**29**:1-7. DOI: 10.1080/24750573.2018.1442670

[36] Amanzadeh E, Esmaeili A, Rahgozar S, Nourbakhshnia M. Application of quercetin in neurological disorders: From nutrition to nanomedicine. Reviews in the Neurosciences. 2019;**30**:555-572. DOI: 10.1515/revneuro-2018-0080

[37] Pandy V, VijeePallam K. Antipsychotic-like activity of scopoletin and rutin against the positive symptoms of schizophrenia in mouse models. Experimental Animals. 2017;**66**:417-423. DOI: 10.1538/expanim.17-0050

[38] Lotter J. Studies on Garcinia Mangostana Linn as a Therapeutic Intervention in an Immune-Inflammatory Model of Schizophrenia. South Africa: North-West University; 2018

[39] Lum PT, Sekar M, Gan SH, Pandy V, Bonam SR. Protective effect of mangiferin on memory impairment:

A systematic review. Saudi Journal of Biological Sciences. 2020;**28**(1):917-927

[40] Chen C, Ai Q-D, Wei Y-H. Potential role of hydroxytyrosol in neuroprotection. Journal of Functional Foods. 2021;**82**:104506. DOI: 10.1016/j.jff.2021.104506

[41] Choudhury B, Saytode P, Shah V. Neurodegenerative Disorders: Past, Present and Future. International Journal of Applied Biology and Pharmaceutical Technology (India). 2014

[42] Miodownik C, Lerner V, Kudkaeva N, Lerner PP, Pashinian A, Bersudsky Y, et al. Curcumin as add-on to antipsychotic treatment in patients with chronic schizophrenia: A randomized, double-blind, placebo-controlled study. Clinical Neuropharmacology. 2019;**42**:117-122. DOI: 10.1097/WNF.0000000000000344

[43] Ben-Azu B, Aderibigbe AO, Omogbiya IA, Ajayi AM, Iwalewa EO. Morin pretreatment attenuates schizophrenia-like behaviors in experimental animal models. Drug Research (Stuttgart). 2018;**68**:159-167. DOI: 10.1055/s-0043-119127

[44] Nakajima A, Yamakuni T, Matsuzaki K, Nakata N, Onozuka H, Yokosuka A, et al. Nobiletin, a citrus flavonoid, reverses learning impairment associated with N-methyl-D-aspartate receptor antagonism by activation of extracellular signal-regulated kinase signaling. The Journal of Pharmacology and Experimental Therapeutics. 2007;**321**:784-790. DOI: 10.1124/jpet.106.117010

[45] Eneni A-EO, Ben-Azu B, Ajayi AM, Aderibigbe AO. Diosmin attenuates schizophrenia-like behavior, oxidative stress and acetylcholinesterase activity in mice. Drug Metabolism and Personalized Therapy. 2020;**35**(4):20200119. DOI: 10.1515/dmdi-2020-0119

[46] Kalpana S, Raju AB, Merugu MS. Genestein, a Phytoestrogens for the Treatment of Schizophrenia. USA; 2014

[47] Kucerova J, Tabiova K, Drago F, Micale V. Therapeutic potential of cannabinoids in schizophrenia. Recent Patents on CNS Drug Discovery. 2014;**9**:13-25. DOI: 10.2174/1574889809666140307115532

[48] Davies C, Bhattacharyya S. Cannabidiol as a potential treatment for psychosis. Therapeutic Advances in Psychopharmacology. 2019;**9**:2045125319881916. DOI: 10.1177/2045125319881916

[49] White CM. A review of human studies assessing Cannabidiol's (CBD) therapeutic actions and potential. Journal of Clinical Pharmacology. 2019;**59**(7):923-934. DOI: 10.1002/jcph.1387

[50] García-Gutiérrez MS, Navarrete F, Gasparyan A, Austrich-Olivares A, Sala F, Manzanares J. Cannabidiol: A potential new alternative for the treatment of anxiety, depression and psychotic disorders. Biomolecules. 2020;**10**(11):1575. DOI: 10.3390/biom10111575

[51] Schwarcz G, Karajgi B, McCarthy R. Synthetic delta-9- tetrahydrocannabinol (Dronabinol) can improve the symptoms of schizophrenia. Journal of Clinical Psychopharmacology. 2009;**29**:255-258. DOI: 10.1097/JCP.0b013e3181a6bc3b

[52] Jie F, Yang X, Wu L, Wang M, Lu B. Linking phytosterols and oxyphytosterols from food to brain health: Origins, effects and underlying mechanisms. Critical Reviews in Food Science and Nutrition. 2020;**62**(13):1-18

[53] Pitsikas N. The effect of crocus Sativus L. and its constituents on memory: Basic studies and clinical applications. Evidence-based Complementary and Alternative Medicine. 2015;**2015**. DOI: 10.1155/2015/926284

[54] Sun X-J, Zhao X, Xie J-n, Wan H. Crocin alleviates schizophrenia- like symptoms in rats by upregulating silent information Regulator-1 and brain derived neurotrophic factor. Comprehensive Psychiatry. 2020;**103**:152209. DOI: 10.1016/j.comppsych.2020.152209

[55] Georgiadou G, Grivas V, Tarantilis PA, Pitsikas N. Crocins, the active constituents of crocus Sativus L., counteracted ketamine-induced behavioural deficits in rats. Psychopharmacology. 2014;**231**:717-726. DOI: 10.1007/s00213-013-3293-4

[56] Pitsikas N, Tarantilis PA. Crocins, the active constituents of Crocus Sativus L., counteracted apomorphine-induced performance deficits in the novel object recognition task, but not novel object location task, in rats. Neuroscience Letters. 2017;**644**:37-42. DOI: 10.1016/j.neulet.2017.02.042

[57] Pitsikas N. Crocus Sativus L. extracts and its constituents crocins and safranal; potential candidates for schizophrenia treatment? Molecules. 2021;**26**:1237. DOI: 10.3390/molecules26051237

[58] Pandy V, Vijeepallam K. Antipsychotic-like activity of α-Asarone in mice: A preliminary report. Advances in Pharmacology and Clinical Trials. 2016;**1**:000106. DOI: 10.23880/apct-16000106

[59] Suresh P, Raju AB. Antidopam inergic effects of leucine and genistein on shizophrenic rat models. Neurosciences Journal. 2013;**18**:235-241

[60] Magdalena K, Jakub K, Marta S, Anna S-D, Joanna M. The relationship between the diet, microelements, macronutrients and vitamins on the schizophrenia – Literature analysis. Journal of Education, Health and Sport. 2020;**10**(9):369-377. eISSN 2391-8306. DOI: 10.12775/JEHS.2020.10.09.043

[61] Lyon P, Strippoli V, Fang B, Cimmino L. B vitamins and one-carbon metabolism: Implications in human health and disease. Nutrients. 2020;**12**:2867. DOI: 10.3390/nu12092867

[62] Brown HE, Roffman JL. Vitamin supplementation in the treatment of schizophrenia. CNS Drugs. 2014;**7**:611-622. DOI: 10.1007/s40263-014-0172-4

[63] Reay WR, Cairns MJ. The role of the retinoids in schizophrenia: Genomic and clinical perspectives. Molecular Psychiatry. 2020;**25**(4):706-718. DOI: 10.1038/s41380-019-0566-2

[64] Yazici AB, Akcay Ciner O, Yazici E, Cilli AS, Dogan B, Erol A. Comparison of vitamin B12, vitamin D and folic acid blood levels in patients with schizophrenia, drug addiction and controls. Journal of Clinical Neuroscience. 2019;**65**:11-16. DOI: 10.1016/j.jocn.2019.04.031

Chapter 8

Psychosocial Approaches in Schizophrenia

Ulaş Korkmaz and Cicek Hocaoglu

Abstract

Schizophrenia is a chronic mental disorder with unique symptoms and a decrease in all areas of functionality, causing severe disability. Psychosocial interventions are therapeutic interventions that enable individuals with mental disabilities to be taught the necessary skills in their social, professional, educational, and family roles and to provide the necessary support. Due to impairments in psychosocial functionality, patients with schizophrenia often need psychosocial interventions. In order to achieve complete recovery from schizophrenia, it is essential to apply psychosocial interventions in addition to pharmacotherapy. Studies have shown that psychosocial interventions improve patients' functional areas and considerably increase their quality of life. This chapter aims to examine the psychosocial approach, recovery in schizophrenia, therapeutic alliance, and treatment compliance, and then to review psychoeducation, supportive therapies, cognitive remediation therapy, cognitive behavioral therapies, group therapies, family interventions, psychosocial skill training, community-based mental health services, occupational rehabilitation, case management, social supports, and motivational interviewing for substance use disorder, which are among the psychosocial treatment methods.

Keywords: schizophrenia, psychosocial approaches, psychosocial interventions, psychiatric rehabilitation, recovery

1. Introduction

Schizophrenia is a disorder that has a chronic course, is characterized by periods of exacerbation and remission, causes psychosocial problems such as unemployment, housing problems, and high rates of substance use, and significantly impairs functionality [1]. For this reason, individuals with schizophrenia often need rehabilitation services in addition to treatment services [2]. Significant impairment in social, occupational, and self-care functions, which prevents full recovery and reintegration into society, necessitates continuous and regular care [3]. In addition, schizophrenia, which begins at a young age and forces the individual, family, and society to struggle with the symptoms and consequences of the disorder for a significant part of life, causes psychological-social financial losses. Minimizing the costs of schizophrenia to the individual, family, and society is one of the main goals of health policies [4].

Psychiatric rehabilitation is considered an essential component of treatment in terms of recovery from disorders associated with mental disability and improving the person's quality of life. Psychiatric rehabilitation aims to teach individuals with mental disabilities the necessary skills and provide the necessary support to help them live a more independent and fulfilling life in their social, professional, educational, and family roles [2].

Due to the psychosocial difficulties experienced by schizophrenia patients, psychosocial approaches and interventions have emerged as an essential component within the scope of psychiatric rehabilitation [3]. The role of psychosocial approaches is critical in solving various problems of individuals with schizophrenia, and these approaches have complementary effects on each other [5]. It is stated that psychosocial interventions play an important role in achieving a good quality of life in the long term [6]. Therefore, it is imperative to include scientifically validated psychosocial interventions in the health standards for patients with schizophrenia [5]. The current approach to schizophrenia treatment not only addresses symptoms but also psychosocial problems associated with these symptoms and combines pharmacological treatments with psychosocial interventions [7].

This text examines psychosocial interventions and related concepts and the clinical, psychological, and social consequences of psychosocial interventions.

2. Recovery in schizophrenia

In the early twentieth century, attention was drawn to the progressive and worsening nature of schizophrenia [8]. However, with antipsychotic medications and psychosocial interventions, there was hope for recovery in schizophrenia. Additionally, the definition of the concept of recovery has changed over time [9].

In the past, the main goal in the treatment of schizophrenia was to achieve remission of symptoms. Remission means that the core symptoms of schizophrenia are present at a mild level at most and do not progress significantly beyond this severity for at least 6 months, and these symptoms do not affect the patient's behavior [10]. However, remission in symptoms alone is not sufficient for recovery in schizophrenia. The view that improvement in other areas of functionality is also a fundamental component of recovery has become widespread [11]. Contrary to the traditional view, recent studies emphasize that improvements in areas such as independent living skills, social functionality, employment, education, and interpersonal relationships are essential for recovery rather than attributing recovery only to a decrease in symptom severity [12]. Thus, within the scope of recovery in schizophrenia, the concept of functional remission, as well as symptomatic remission, has developed over time. A satisfactory daily life and normalcy in functionality have become essential elements of recovery [13]. According to the definition of Liberman et al. [14], recovery should include symptomatic remission lasting at least 2 years, being able to engage in productive activity, being able to meet basic daily needs such as self-care, nutrition, money management, participating in enjoyable activities, and maintaining a good family relationship and at least one friend relationship with whom he or she meets regularly.

What is essential in recovery is how well patients can function and achieve social reintegration [15]. Therefore, due to the significant limitations of antipsychotic medications, it is necessary to add psychosocial interventions to the treatment for recovery. Clinical recovery and social functioning are two indispensable dimensions of recovery. Combining pharmacotherapy with psychosocial interventions and environmental conditions has a crucial role in recovery in schizophrenia. Even if complete remission cannot be achieved, prioritizing functional recovery is essential for patients to regain their living standards [16]. Although the symptoms do not disappear completely, it does not prevent a state of remission from occurring unless the psychotic symptoms have a significant impact on life [17].

With ongoing interventions, it seems appropriate to conceptualize recovery as a process rather than an outcome [13]. Despite the view that schizophrenia is an incurable disorder, it is now thought that almost half of patients can recover [16]. Functional recovery in schizophrenia can be considered as a multidimensional structure that will include improvement in various areas such as symptomatic remission, psychosocial functioning, cognitive functions, quality of life, treatment compliance, relapse, and rehospitalization [18].

3. Psychosocial treatment approaches in schizophrenia

Although antipsychotic drugs are very effective against positive symptoms, their effects on negative symptoms and functionality are limited [19]. Approximately one-quarter of patients experience a relapse within a year despite appropriate medication [20]. Therefore, in addition to the psychopharmacological approach, rehabilitating patients is also extremely important. Rehabilitation is a treatment process planned to maximize the medical, psychological, social, and professional aspects of individuals who have lost some of their abilities as a result of genetic or accidental diseases, accidents, or injuries and to minimize the effects of permanent disability [21]. Rehabilitation refers to a process that aims to maximize the biopsychosocial potential of an individual with some limitations and difficulties adapting to the environment [22].

Within the scope of rehabilitation, it has become necessary to provide psychosocial interventions in addition to pharmacological treatment in the treatment of schizophrenia. Trials of psychological and behavioral interventions in schizophrenia began in the mid-twentieth century. In this context, approaches such as reinforcing target behaviors, arranging the treatment environment like the external social environment, exposing patients to situations they may encounter in society, providing training to patients' relatives, trying to strengthen patients' self-control, and working collaboratively with patients for all these interventions have been suggested [23]. Later, contributions were made to improve patients' positive aspects [24]. Over time, various psychological and social interventions have begun to be used in the treatment of schizophrenia within the scope of different clinical schools. Prominent among these methods are individual therapy, supportive therapy, psychoeducation, group therapy, social skills training, cognitive behavioral therapy (CBT), and family therapy [25]. With the addition of various interventions, psychosocial approaches have yielded many successful results in recent years [26].

The psychosocial approach aims to provide support and education to individuals with severe mental disorders and their families through practices such as CBT, cognitive remediation therapy (CRT), family therapy, psychoeducation, social skills training, and occupational rehabilitation [27]. In addition, these interventions enable better management of the disorder and reintegration of patients and their relatives into society. Although the intervention types differ, psychosocial interventions reduce relapses and symptoms and increase functionality [27].

Another primary function of the psychosocial approach is to integrate it into a collaborative treatment process to strengthen disorder management, psychosocial functioning, and personal satisfaction, focusing on increasing the skills of patients and their families [28]. Thanks to psychosocial approaches, individuals with disabilities due to mental disorders can better adapt to their environment and gain the necessary skills to increase their functionality and quality of life [29].

3.1 Therapeutic alliance

The therapeutic alliance is the collaborative emotional closeness between therapists and patients [30]. This alliance is established through mutual trust, unconditional respect, empathy, warmth, support, valuing, good communication, and interaction between patients and therapists [31]. It includes elements such as collaborating on goals with patients, agreeing on the tasks of the patient and therapist, and establishing an emotional bond between patients and therapists [32]. The quality and strength of the collaborative relationship between therapists and patients indicates the alliance's strength [33].

According to the World Health Organization, a solid therapeutic alliance improves patients' health [34]. In order to increase medication compliance, it is essential to establish a genuine and humane relationship between the therapist and the patient [35]. It is stated that establishing close and sincere communication with patients facilitates monitoring of the patients and increases treatment compliance [28]. It has been determined that the therapeutic relationship affects medication compliance at least as much as the level of insight, and the therapeutic relationship is seen as the first step in encouraging medication compliance [36]. Another positive effect of the therapeutic alliance is that it is associated with a reduction in symptoms. In a study, it was found to be associated with a decrease in general psychiatric symptoms and psychotic symptoms [37].

Providing emotional support, allowing patients to be involved in the treatment process, ensuring that the care staff consists of stable individuals, and accepting and working on transference and countertransference are elements that should be taken into consideration in order to strengthen the alliance and realize the change in collaboration [31, 36].

3.2 Treatment compliance

One of the most basic methods in the treatment of schizophrenia is the use of antipsychotic medication [38]. However, people with mental disabilities may not be able to understand the disorder itself, its severity, and the need for treatment. Problems such as lack of insight and delays in diagnosis and treatment can make recovery difficult [28].

Non-compliance with treatment, which is one of the biggest obstacles encountered in the treatment process of individuals with schizophrenia, causes exacerbations, worsening prognosis, frequent hospitalizations, and increasing costs [39]. Thus, disability increases over time [40]. Additionally, non-compliance with antipsychotic medications has been associated with treatment resistance and poor social adaptation [41].

Although non-compliance with treatment is common, it is not easy to detect it through interviews [42]. Reasons for treatment non-compliance include factors such as lack of insight [43], positive symptoms [39], severe psychopathology, resistance to treatment, high level of depression, the presence of substance use disorder, executive function impairments [44], multiple antipsychotic medication use and drug side effects [45], inadequate effectiveness of antipsychotic medication [44], stigmatization [46], and lack of social support [47].

The most critical element of reducing treatment non-compliance is providing patients with education and guidance. Regular monitoring and psychoeducation during pre-discharge and outpatient follow-up periods are vital to maximize the treatment plan's success [48]. In the treatment, the approach of explaining to patients in detail the current situation, the recommended treatment method, the possible benefits and harms of this treatment, suitable alternative treatments, and the treatment duration are critical to include and inform patients in the treatment process. Studies show that in order to increase treatment compliance, it is essential for patients to understand the connection between the treatment process and their personal goals [49].

Some initiatives can be taken to increase treatment compliance. For example, choosing antipsychotic drugs with better tolerability can eliminate side effects that disrupt the patients' compliance [50]. Treating extrapyramidal system symptoms that significantly affect the patients' functionality and reducing positive symptoms with appropriate treatment may increase treatment compliance [51]. Providing psychoeducation to patients and their families about the disorder and treatment process and helping patients increase their social support are psychosocial initiatives to increase treatment compliance [52]. Assigning a family member to take and supervise medication has been found to increase treatment compliance [53]. Cognitive behavioral interventions can be made to increase the level of insight [54]. Some studies have found that motivational interviewing [55], adherence therapy [56], and SMS-based interventions [57] are effective. As stated, since oral medication non-compliance is common, long-acting injectable antipsychotics may be recommended to patients [58]. In addition, establishing a therapeutic alliance is critical in treatment compliance [59].

4. Psychosocial interventions for schizophrenia

In this section, psychosocial interventions used in schizophrenia, such as psychoeducation, supportive therapies, CRT, CBT, group therapies, family interventions, psychosocial skill training (PSST), community-based mental health services (CBMHS), occupational rehabilitation, case management, social supports, and motivational interviewing in schizophrenia patients with substance use disorder will be examined.

4.1 Psychoeducation

Psychoeducation is a gradual process generally defined as the education of an individual with a psychiatric disorder about the disorder and its treatment [60]. Psychoeducation in schizophrenia, as a treatment method for individuals with schizophrenia and their families, aims to convey essential information about the disorder, treatment options, details of pharmacological treatment, side effects, the course of the disorder, coping methods, and social and legal rights [61]. Since caregivers' approaches significantly impact the course of the disorder, it is essential to inform patients and caregivers as much as possible [62]. This way, therapists, patients, and patients' relatives can work together. Psychoeducation has emerged as a valuable and effective psychotherapeutic intervention in the treatment of mental illnesses [63].

In the current literature, the essential components of psychoeducation include providing information about etiological factors, common symptoms, early precursors of relapse, long-term course and outcome, helping to cope with stress, conveying biological and psychosocial treatment options, determining when and how treatment can be accessed, increasing compliance with treatment, conveying dos and don'ts to family members, dispelling myths, misconceptions, and stigma about the disorder, increasing awareness and insight. It is aimed at preventing situations such as relapse, crisis, and suicide by ensuring the knowledge and competence of patients and their relatives about the disorder [63].

Psychoeducation includes both cognitive-behavioral and supportive therapeutic elements [60]. It can be applied to both inpatients and outpatients. The first hospitalization is a good time for psychoeducation, but it should be taken into consideration that patients benefit more from psychoeducation as the level of insight increases [64]. It can be applied on an individual, family, group, or community basis. It can be implemented with the active participation of patients and their relatives or passively with brochures, booklets, or various visual/audio materials. Group applications can be carried out in groups of 4–12 people in several sessions ranging from 5 to 24. The length of the sessions is usually 40–60 minutes and is held once a week to ensure good assimilation of the information shared. Subsequently, monthly meetings can be continued. The duration of the education and the amount of information to be given in one session should be structured explicitly according to the patients [65]. In education, the message should be given that schizophrenia is caused by biological factors triggered by stress in order to reduce the self-criticism of families and maintain medication compliance [63]. Normalization and hope-giving are efficient techniques for reducing stigmatization and accelerating healing [66].

Psychoeducation reduces relapse rates and the burden on patients and families. Although it has been reported that long-term interventions have a more positive effect [64], In a recent study, a psychoeducation application consisting of six sessions in a short period of 1.5 months applied to caregivers was found to be effective in reducing the burden and depression levels in the relatives of the patients, preventing relapses in the patients for 12 months, and in terms of the quality of therapeutic alliance [67]. Psychoeducation has also been found to reduce rehospitalization and hospitalization duration [60] and reduce negative attitudes toward medications [68]. During the psychoeducation process, patients and healthcare professionals come together and make joint decisions in treatment planning, allowing patients to take an active role in line with their preferences and direct the treatment process more effectively [69]. Besides all its contributions, psychoeducation can make patients feel more active, energetic, and action-oriented [65].

As a result, psychoeducation allows patients to obtain comprehensive information and consciously participate in treatment processes [70]. Due to its many positive effects, psychoeducation is included as an essential treatment component in schizophrenia treatment guideline recommendations [71].

4.2 Supportive therapies

Supportive therapies aim to maintain patients' current positive state, help improve coping abilities, reduce anxiety, encourage patients, and provide social support [72]. Supportive psychotherapy is one of the most commonly used treatment methods. An integral part of the change that a supportive approach will create is therapeutic alliance. The therapeutic alliance must continue to grow stronger once it is established.

Supportive psychotherapy makes change by helping to improve self-esteem and adaptability skills. During the process, adaptive defenses are further strengthened, thus increasing patients' adaptation to the environment. Their techniques include empathizing, acknowledging, praising, reassuring, rationalizing, reframing, rehearsing, clarifying, and confronting. It focuses on the "Here and Now." Genuine relationships are more on the agenda, with less focus on transference issues than in psychodynamic psychotherapy [73].

The supportive approach helps patients increase their social adaptation by increasing their emotional regulation skills and recognizing sources of stress [3]. Social support is a component that plays a significant role in all dimensions of schizophrenia. People with schizophrenia generally tend to have weaker social networks and generally have fewer people in their immediate environment. Thus, they form weaker social relationships [74]. These positive social relationships, which seem to be missing in schizophrenia patients, can be seen and learned as possible/doable relationships through therapeutic alliance. One of the factors that ensures this is that the therapist treats them as an individual from society, not as a patient. The supportive approach considers the patient's relationship with others and social concerns and works on this. This patient-therapist relationship can increase patients' self-confidence and enable them to have alternative, realistic thoughts about their social environment. The quality of this relationship determines the effectiveness of supportive therapies [3].

In addition to increasing social functionality, supportive therapies have also been found effective in reducing the symptoms of schizophrenia. In some studies, when schizophrenia patients who received only standard treatment were compared with patients who received supportive psychotherapy in addition to standard schizophrenia treatment, it was reported that patients who received supportive psychotherapy showed more improvement in both disorder symptoms and functionality than the other group [75]. It has been found that even 12 sessions of supportive therapy intervention lasting 6–8 weeks is associated with a decrease in positive and negative symptoms and an increase in social functioning within 2 years [76]. In a randomized controlled study with schizophrenia patients with refractory psychotic symptoms, three different groups were examined. One group received CBT and standard treatment, one group received supportive counseling and standard treatment, and the last group received only standard treatment. The treatments lasted 3 months, and after 2 years, the patients were evaluated in terms of positive and negative symptoms, recurrence, and clinical improvement. In all areas, the two groups that received CBT or supportive counseling in addition to standard treatment reported more positive outcomes than those that received only standard treatment [77]. In another study, it was reported that negative beliefs, primarily related to auditory hallucinations, decreased significantly in the supportive therapy group at the 1-year follow-up [78].

4.3 Cognitive remediation therapy

Schizophrenia is a disorder with severe and progressive cognitive impairment. Moreover, cognitive impairment can lead to more disability than negative and positive symptoms [79]. Cognition is one of the strongest determinants of the level of functioning in schizophrenia [80]. As cognitive impairment increases in schizophrenia, many areas of functionality, such as work, independent living, and quality of life, are affected [81].

Unlike other dramatic symptoms, cognitive impairment does not usually improve during remission. Also, it does not respond well to antipsychotic treatment [82].

Moreover, cognitive impairment prevents patients from benefiting from other psychosocial interventions [83]. Therefore, alternative interventions are needed to treat cognitive impairment [84]. For these reasons, CRT was developed. CRT is an intervention that aims to improve cognitive processes such as attention, memory, executive functions, and social cognition/metacognition and usually includes behavioral training elements [85]. Cognitive remediation aims to improve areas of cognitive impairment through cognitive restructuring, correct errors in the learning process, overcome obstacles in daily life activities, create a supportive social environment, and increase functionality. Supporting cognitive areas not impaired and avoiding environments that may cause cognitive impairment form the basis for cognitive remediation [86].

Some strategies used in cognitive rehabilitation include cognitive remediation, supportive rehabilitation, and cognitive training [87]. The cognitive remediation program aims to improve patients' attention and memory by focusing on teaching thinking skills [88]. The supportive rehabilitation program aims to improve functionality and thus overcome cognitive impairments by taking advantage of patients' cognitive areas that have not been impaired [89]. The cognitive training program aims to improve the executive functions of patients through repetitive practices through various computer programs. This program focuses more on perception and attention [90]. CRT interventions include exercise and strategy training *via* computer or paper and pencil. Motivational/cognitive support is provided during the training [91]. Cognitive repair programs using bridge groups and strategy coaching are more cognitively effective [92]. CRT uses various learning strategies, such as errorless learning, positive reinforcement, and information processing. Thanks to these methods, verbalization, dividing the task into small parts, self-monitoring, organization, and planning can be learned [93].

CRT can be divided into two main models: compensatory and restorative [94]. Compensatory interventions aim to compensate for cognitive impairment by using the patients' unimpaired cognitive areas and environmental resources. In order to achieve this, the patients' tasks are simplified by creating an environmental arrangement [95]. Restorative interventions take advantage of the plasticity of the brain. Thus, the impaired cognitive area is assumed to be regained [96]. Restorative interventions use two approaches: bottom-up and top-down. The bottom-up approach follows a path from simple tasks to more complex ones. The top-down approach uses more complex tasks to repair a specific cognitive area [97].

Four essential elements determine the effectiveness of CRT: having a trained therapist, repetitive application of cognitive exercises, structured development of cognitive strategies, and repeating the learned techniques in the outside world [85]. Transferring cognitive gains to the outside world is very important for the effectiveness of the treatment [98].

There is frequent and robust evidence that CRT improves cognitive domains. It has been reported that the most significant effect is in general cognition, verbal learning, working memory, attention, and processing speed following these cognitive areas, and the improvement in problem-solving and judgment areas is relatively low [99]. It has also been found to be associated with permanent improvements in memory functions and increased social functionality [100]. Positive results have also been obtained in patients with treatment-resistant schizophrenia. Therefore, it is recommended in addition to pharmacotherapy in treatment-resistant patients. However, it seems essential to start applying CRT earlier regarding its contributions [101]. Recently, the long-term effects of CRT have been evaluated. It has been determined that cognitive function and functional recovery in schizophrenia patients who received CRT, in addition to standard rehabilitation services, were preserved even after 10 years, and the importance of continuing standard rehabilitation services after applying CRT was emphasized [102]. It is also stated that CRT can be applied in the clinical high-risk state for psychosis [98].

CRT is a feasible and acceptable intervention [103]. This intervention provides significant benefits in terms of cognitive remediation and functionality. Therefore, it should form part of the treatment of schizophrenia [98].

4.4 Cognitive behavioral therapies

The basic assumption of the cognitive behavioral approach in psychiatric disorders is that information processing towards external and internal stimuli is biased. Therefore, distortions occur in the individual's thought system [104]. This dysfunctional thinking style is called cognitive attentional syndrome. CBT aims to make patients aware of these cognitive distortions, dysfunctional beliefs, and negative schemas and to change them [105].

CBT has a transdiagnostic model [106]. According to the cognitive-behavioral approach, psychotic symptoms depend on the way the patient interprets their perceptions, how they relate to their perceptions, what causality they attribute to their symptoms, what beliefs they form, and how they interpret these beliefs [107]. CBT argues that paranoia in schizophrenia can be likened to anxiety processes, the response to hallucinatory experiences can be likened to rumination processes, and the formation and maintenance of patients' delusions and hallucinations can be formulated with dysfunctional information processing processes. Formulating these cognitive distortions helps the patient understand and make sense of their symptoms [106].

There are some fundamental elements of CBT in schizophrenia. First of all, as in every intervention, it is essential to establish a therapeutic alliance with patients. Then come stages such as developing alternative explanations for psychotic symptoms, reducing the impact of psychotic symptoms on life, and maintaining treatment compliance. An empathetic, unconditionally respectful, and honest attitude is adopted during therapy. There is no focus on whether the beliefs that cause psychotic symptoms are connected to reality. It focuses on connecting patients' emotions, thoughts, and behaviors. The main aim is to reach a consensus on an acceptable explanation for psychotic experiences. In therapy, patients' weaknesses and strengths are determined. With the vulnerability-stress model, the disorder is understood, and possible stress factors are discussed. At this stage, care should be taken to ensure that patients or their relatives do not develop thoughts of blaming themselves for the disorder, or if they do, this idea is discussed [108]. The aim is to reduce the distress and decline in functionality caused by these symptoms by normalizing and giving meaning to patients' psychotic experiences. Patients learn to view their thoughts and interpretations as hypotheses rather than facts during this process. Thus, they can develop alternative thoughts when they experience similar psychotic experiences in the outside world [109]. In addition, behavioral interventions are also applied in therapy to recognize and re-evaluate cognitive errors and improve coping skills. Patients are motivated to test their negative thoughts in the outside world [106].

It has been stated that CBT applied in schizophrenia can vary between 4 and 30 sessions, but the best effect occurs after at least 20 sessions [109]. A formulation is created after a therapeutic alliance is achieved and accompanying depression and anxiety are treated. Specific techniques are then used to address psychotic symptoms. For example, analysis of the origin of auditory hallucinations, keeping audio diaries, finding alternative explanations for the cause of hallucinations and developing coping skills, and examining delusions with guided discovery and Socratic questioning can be done. The techniques applied in the session are encouraged to be repeated in the outside world. After working on positive symptoms, behavioral activation can be applied to negative symptoms [110].

Many studies conducted in the recent years have shown that CBT, especially in combination with medication, is effective in the treatment of schizophrenia [111]. CBT has been found effective in reducing the symptoms [112], reducing the number of relapses [113], and increasing the level of functionality and insight [114, 115]. CBT is one of the psychosocial interventions with the most evidence for functional recovery [116]. CBT has been found effective in treating both positive and negative symptoms [117], especially auditory hallucinations [118]. Its effectiveness for delusions has increased over time [119]. Most meta-analyses have suggested the effectiveness of CBT compared to standard treatment [118]. In studies conducted with schizophrenia patients resistant to antipsychotic drugs, CBT was found to be effective in reducing positive and negative symptoms [110]. CBT is also effective in reducing symptoms of depression and anxiety in patients with schizophrenia [120]. In another study conducted on a population in the clinical high-risk state for psychosis, it was found that applying CBT to this group reduced both the rates of transition to schizophrenia and attenuated psychotic symptoms [121].

In schizophrenia treatment guidelines, CBT is recommended at all stages of the disease. According to NICE treatment guidelines, CBT should consist of the following elements: Establishing connections between patients' feelings, thoughts, and behavior and their symptoms and functioning; reassessing patients' perceptions, beliefs, and reasoning about their symptoms; monitoring symptom-related feelings, thoughts, and behaviors; and promoting alternative ways to cope with symptoms, reduce symptom distress, and improve functioning [122].

Today, in addition to traditional CBT, third-wave therapies originating from the cognitive behavioral approach used in the treatment of schizophrenia have begun to appear. Metacognitive therapy, mindfulness, and acceptance-commitment therapy can be counted among these therapies [106, 116]. Traditional CBT focuses more on symptom change, but third-wave cognitive behavioral therapies additionally focus on symptom acceptance and achieving life goals. Third-wave therapies aim to reduce cognitive attentional syndrome by increasing cognitive flexibility and changing thoughts about thoughts [106]. Third-wave cognitive behavioral therapies have been reported to be effective in improving functionality in patients with schizophrenia [116].

4.5 Group therapies

Group therapies are defined as the simultaneous treatment of more than one patient by one or more therapists [123], and the interaction between group members is seen as the primary therapeutic factor [124]. Group therapies have begun to play an essential role in the treatment of schizophrenia. In group therapy for schizophrenia, the following three conditions must be met: Group members must rely on verbal communication, group members are the objects of treatment, and the group itself is the primary therapeutic factor. Group therapies generally emphasize the form of treatment, and the content and conduct of the treatment largely depend on the therapist's theoretical orientation [125].

Kanas [126] developed a method designed for schizophrenia patients. In this model, educational, psychodynamic, and interpersonal techniques are used together. According to this model, the supportive and open-to-discussion structure of the model helps patients cope with their psychotic symptoms and improve their interpersonal relationships. Within the group, patients are encouraged to communicate and share their emotions and symptoms, such as delusions and hallucinations. Advice can be given in practical areas. Expressing anger toward other group members is not recommended as it is difficult to tolerate. Topics such as establishing relationships with others, reality testing, expressing emotions, and advice may constitute the group's topics. This type of group is a community where patients can express their feelings and learn to interact with others. The therapist tries to keep the group members focused on the topic in an active and directive way, has a clear, consistent, and concrete attitude, is supportive and accommodating, is open and willing to offer opinions suitable for discussion, is focused on the "Here and Now," and encourages patient-patient interaction.

That day's theme in the session should be determined within the group in the first minutes. A single theme or topic close to the central theme should be covered in each session. A topic that is known to everyone, understandable, and discussable, such as the group members' recent experiences, communications, and preoccupations, may be preferred. It may be directly related to psychotic experiences. The theme is used to compare the psychotic experience and reality. Feedback is received at the session's end, and the emerging feelings and thoughts are discussed [127].

It is recommended that groups consist of 8–12 people and be held frequently every 1–4 weeks, and session durations are around 60–90 minutes. The techniques used in group therapy generally vary depending on the theoretical approach of the therapist and the characteristics of the patients in the group. However, common elements can be listed as improving communication, ensuring trust, and targeting behavioral changes within the group. The therapist's task is to encourage interaction between patients seeking guidance. Although the therapist is quite active in the early days of therapy, this need for the therapist is expected to decrease over time. In the following process, patients communicate freely with each other, independent of the therapist. During the sessions, the therapist asks each patient to express an opinion on the theme. It is essential to be aware of the pressure patients may feel in the early stages of therapy and not to force patients. The therapist may start talking about more concrete topics. An important technique to achieve behavioral change in group therapy is role-playing. For example, patients may be asked to rehearse a situation, such as a job interview. Behavioral methods such as giving rewards can also be used. Having two therapists in the group, that is, the joint therapy team approach, is beneficial for therapists to interact with each other, thus creating a role model for patients. In addition, inexperienced therapists have the opportunity to work with an experienced therapist and improve themselves educationally [128].

Positive symptoms can be addressed within group therapies, and the experiences of members within the group, similarities of positive symptoms, and misconceptions can be restructured [129]. In terms of negative symptoms, changes can be made with the help of other members of the group [130]. In the second half of the twentieth century, Payn [131] stated that providing patients with a socialization experience reduced anxiety, the severity of psychosis, and the necessity for hospitalization. Today, there is increasing evidence regarding the effectiveness of approaches that enable socialization, such as group therapy. In a study conducted over 7 years and 308 group sessions, prospective data reported that individual members tended to engage in more emotionally meaningful interactions within the group, the severity of depression, anxiety, and psychotic symptoms decreased, and positive characteristics such as humor and insight developed, and individuals' functionality increased [132]. Providing patients with a socialization experience through group practice may reduce anxiety and hospitalization rates, improve reality testing, and increase self-esteem [128]. It has been reported that group therapies contribute to reducing the social isolation and anxiety levels of patients by enabling them to improve their ability to interact [133]. In a study where patients commented on the therapeutic effects, it was highlighted that instilling hope was essential [134].

Group therapies and individual therapies are complementary to each other. A significant benefit of group therapies is that they allow the therapist to see the patient exhibit a wider variety of behaviors over a more extended time and in a different environment than in individual sessions. In this way, drug dose optimization can be quickly done [128].

Group therapies are essential for patients to increase their social functionality. They can be used in conjunction with pharmacotherapy and other psychosocial interventions. They can be applied to both outpatients and inpatients, and patients can generally adapt to group therapies [128].

4.6 Family interventions

Schizophrenia negatively affects individuals' affective states, cognitive processes, perceptual abilities, and behaviors, causing them to have difficulty in performing their functions. While this situation causes individuals to need constant care and support, the families of those affected by the disorder are also indirectly affected [135]. Schizophrenia patients usually live with their families, and the families often do not receive any support while caring for the patients [136]. Schizophrenia is a disorder not only of the patients but also of the family as a social structure. For this reason, the lives of families are affected as negatively as the patients' [137].

Family members often need information, help, and support because of the severe challenges they face. At the same time, their behavior and attitudes can have positive or negative effects on the clinical condition of patients [138]. Patients' relatives often experience difficulties due to shame, guilt, helplessness, anxiety, and financial difficulties [139]. Disorder-related symptoms and behaviors, hospitalizations, responsibilities regarding medication compliance, lack of social support, family conflicts, and difficulties in coping with these conflicts create a significant burden for families [140]. Additionally, as the severity of the disorder increases, the burden experienced by the family increases [141]. In addition to the psychosocial problems they experience, psychiatric diagnoses such as anxiety disorders or depression may often occur in patients' relatives [142]. They may experience grief due to a relative being diagnosed with schizophrenia [143].

Families of individuals with schizophrenia often have limited skills in coping with the difficulties they encounter during the disorder process [144]. Family support programs created in line with these demands provide families with information about schizophrenia and support interaction between families by sharing feelings and thoughts. Within the scope of these programs, volunteer family members trained by health professionals transfer the training they receive to other family members [145].

Family interventions include cognitive, behavioral, and supportive elements that aim to include patients' relatives in the treatment and rehabilitation [146]. Interventions with families use methods such as education, counseling, and developing coping skills [147]. Family interventions are led by a mental health professional [138]. It may vary depending on schools; it may be cognitive-behavioral or psychoanalytically oriented. Education and support groups can be implemented as systemic, strategic family therapies. Various methods can be used, such as developing stress-coping skills and psychodrama [139]. The primary and common goal is to help patients by providing cooperation between patients, their families, and the treatment team [148]. Some common goals are applying psychoeducation, evaluating the behavior of patients and their relatives and creating changes in behavior, providing support, creating order, and reducing high expressed emotion [149]. Crises may be expected in the family of a patient with schizophrenia. Therefore, crisis intervention is another component of family therapies. Although different theoretical models have similar effectiveness, it has been stated that psychoanalytically oriented applications may yield negative results [150].

Family care programs provide positive gains for both the family and the patient by enabling families to solve their problems more effectively, increase their self-confidence, be more understanding toward patients, reduce feelings of strain and anger, and increase their ability to cope with stress [151]. In family support programs, the main topics are providing information about mental illnesses, social support, medications, and other treatment methods, improving problem-solving and communication skills with the patient, and sharing experiences and difficulties [152].

The primary purposes of psychoeducation for families are to provide information about the disorder and treatment, to regulate family communication, to help with coping methods, to increase problem-solving skills, to reduce stress caused by family conflicts, and to increase the social support of family members [146]. Family therapies help patients' relatives better understand the effects of the disease on functionality and recognize exacerbated psychotic symptoms [153]. The vulnerability-stress model, which emphasizes the biological nature of the disease, can be explained to patients' relatives to reduce stigmatization [154]. Certain areas, such as plans, job expectations, medication compliance, marriage, and pregnancy, may also need to be included in family therapies. Family therapies are essential in reducing the family's anger and guilt, recognizing and solving problems that may arise in advance, setting reasonable expectations for the patient, and setting limits where necessary [147]. Expressed emotion, which is defined by a high level of criticism and excessive emotional reactivity and is highly associated with exacerbation of psychotic symptoms, should also be studied in family therapies [155]. Studies have found expressed emotion to be associated with cognitive impairment and disease severity. Patients may also behave negatively in response to expressed emotion [146]. Families being overly protective and interventionist or sacrificing themselves and being overly selfless are dysfunctional coping attitudes [156]. For this reason, patients' relatives should be encouraged to engage in activities outside the home as it provides freedom. This improves the patients' relatives' quality of life [148]. Efforts should be made to correct the misinformation and prejudices of patients' relatives about schizophrenia and treatments because this attitude can negatively affect patients and disrupt medication compliance [157].

Family therapies are important because they benefit patients' families and indirectly contribute to patients' recovery. In a meta-analysis examining interventions given to families, it was reported that family therapies reduced hospitalizations and increased medication compliance [158]. Family therapies reduce the exacerbation of the disease, the burden on the family, emotional expression, and treatment costs. It also increases the patients' compliance with treatment and psychosocial functionality [148, 156]. A study found that family therapies lasting 6–9 months reduced relapse rates, increased patient compliance with treatment, and reduced symptom severity [159]. It has also been reported that family interventions increase families' ability to cope with the disease process and have positive effects on protecting their mental well-being [150]. It has been determined that family therapies carried out in group practice give similar results, effectively increase the functionality of patients and their relatives, and reduce relapses [160]. A study conducted with first-episode psychosis patients reported that family therapies reduced relapse rates, hospitalization duration, and psychotic symptom severity and increased functionality for up to 24 months [153].

As a result, family interventions contribute to the cooperation between patients, their families, and healthcare professionals and help to achieve desired results, such as preventing relapses [161]. Schizophrenia treatment guidelines also recommend family interventions at all stages of the disease, as they reduce hospitalizations and symptom severity [71]. It is beneficial to start family psychoeducation from the early stages of schizophrenia, and family therapies are also strongly recommended for first-episode psychoses [162]. All treatment guidelines agree that family interventions reduce relapse, hospitalization rates, and the burden experienced by families [162].

4.7 Psychosocial skill treatment

Social functionality plays an essential role in meeting the needs of individuals. For this reason, developing social skills and abilities is very important for quality of life. Social competence is the ability to communicate in social areas such as work, school, home, entertainment, shopping, treatment, and social and legal services [163]. Social skill is the ability of people to exhibit appropriate behavior in social environments and to successfully apply their social competencies in real life [164]. Social skills include various performances such as verbal and non-verbal communication, accurate social perception, making decisions or responses in accordance with social situations and rules, speaking skills, skills that can enable the management of disease, and expressing emotions such as empathy and compassion [165].

Social competencies and skills are incredibly restricted in patients with schizophrenia. They often struggle to develop social relationships, meet social needs, or fulfill other social roles [166]. In addition, frequent and long-term hospitalizations may keep the person away from their social environment, causing the loss of already learned social skills and the inability to learn new social skills [164]. Schizophrenia itself can cause negative attitudes in the social environment and economic difficulties, causing patients to withdraw from society and lose/fail to learn social skills [167]. Patients with schizophrenia may need to receive training on this subject due to the difficulties they experience in terms of social skills [165].

PSST is a complementary intervention developed to eliminate the social skill deficiencies experienced by patients in their daily lives [86]. PSST has a significant position in increasing the social functionality of patients [168]. Skills are initiated and developed through learning. For this reason, behavioral techniques (e.g., social learning and negative reinforcers) are primarily used in PSST. Patients can improve social skills through behavioral learning, and as a result, they can reach the capacity to live independently [28, 165].

In PSST, first of all, the obstacles in the patients' lives are discussed with the patients, and the current problem areas are identified in cooperation. A target is then determined regarding these problem areas. In order to reach the main goal, short-term and intermediate goals are determined from simple to complex. During this process, the therapist also explains to the patients in an educational framework which communication skills must be learned, with whom, where, and when to use them. Role-playing and rehearsing allow patients to develop the communication skills necessary for the target situation. Positive and constructive feedback is given to the patient regarding the behavior exhibited in role-playing and rehearsal. Patients also learn indirectly from their therapist through social modeling and observation. The most crucial factor is reinforcing the learned behaviors and skills by repeating them frequently, especially in real life. Therefore, behavioral experiments are integral to PSST [164, 165]. Other frequently used behavioral methods include shaping behavior, coaching, using reinforcers, relearning, self-direction, generalization, and self-monitoring [164].

Liberman et al. [28] created a structured PSST model (UCLA social and independent skill modules) by strengthening PSST with psychoeducation and problem-solving skills. This program includes medication management, symptom management, basic conversation skills, community re-entry, recreation for leisure, substance abuse management, workplace fundamental skills, friendship and intimacy, and involving families in service modules. This program, which is a modular training, can increase social functionality and decrease symptoms, exacerbations, and relapses. In order to maintain this positive effect, it is recommended that the program last at least 1 year and be continued with support meetings [169].

Cognitive-behavioral-oriented PSST is an 18-week group intervention consisting of three modules. These modules consist of cognitive skills, social skills, and problem-solving skills. These interventions have been found effective in normalizing attenuated psychotic symptoms and eliminating stigma, and are also suitable for individuals in clinical high-risk states for psychosis [170]. Cognitive-behavioral-oriented PSST has also increased functionality, reduced negative and positive symptoms, and improved social competence [171].

Studies have reported that psychotic symptoms and relapse rates are lower, and communication skills and quality of life are better in schizophrenia patients who have received PSST than in schizophrenia patients who have not received PSST [164]. PSST has also been found to have beneficial effects in helping patients stay at work longer and reducing substance abuse [172]. It is superior to standard treatment for positive and negative symptoms [173].

PSST complements other treatment methods and is one of the interventions that must be included in treatment [165]. Adding PSST to treatment programs makes it easier for patients to cope with the disease, reduces relapse rates, and increases social functionality, level of insight, quality of life, and treatment compliance [174]. When patients learn to cope with stressful life events or daily challenges, thanks to their social skills, they become more competent in solving these problems [165].

4.8 Community-based mental health services

CBMHS are evidence-based and recovery-oriented practices that aim to improve the mental health of a community, are accessible and acceptable, take into account patients' goals and strengths, and help provide a wide range of support, services, and resources. CBMHS are a psychosocial approach targeting the community. Within CBMHS, patients are considered systemically and evaluated within their socioeconomic context. The principle of protecting patients individually and socially is at the forefront. Services are publicly available to everyone. CBMHS are carried out by a team. The services provided are long-term and lifelong. CBMHS also consider the social costs of disorders [175].

This type of rehabilitation focuses on accessibility of services, cultural factors, and community involvement. Particularly in areas with inadequate service access, strategies such as CBMHS play an intermediary role in helping patients meet their needs [176]. CBMHS have the functions of helping patients assert their rights, helping them recover, encouraging their participation in society, improving the mental health of the family and the entire community, reducing stigma and discrimination, increasing awareness of mental health in society, and facilitating access to medical, psychological, social and economic services. The main aim is to empower people with severe mental disorders by integrating them into society [177].

A large number and variety of CBMHS have been created in many countries so far [178]. As mental health services began to be provided on a community-based, a significant portion of patients began to be treated in the community, and the rate of receiving inpatient treatment decreased significantly [179]. CBMHS have great importance and impact, especially in low- and middle-income countries with relatively inadequate health services. Studies support the feasibility and effectiveness of CBMHS in low- and middle-income countries and recommend providing these services [180].

CBMHS are critical for preventing hospitalization. Patients who benefit from CBMHS have lower hospitalization rates and durations than when they do not receive this service [181]. CBMHS make it easier for patients to access the resources they need. Patients can thus have easier access to areas such as health, education, financial aid, and social support [182]. A study reported that CBMHS contributed to increased functionality, insight level, and treatment compliance and reduced caregiver burden and symptoms of schizophrenia [183].

The existence of some such health provider centers to serve patients whose symptoms are not severe enough to require hospitalization is an essential benefit of the community-based mental health field. However, this can create relative complexity within the healthcare system, and it may be difficult for patients with schizophrenia who have a severe mental disorder to access CBMHS. Conditions such as lack of insight, impaired cognitive abilities, and symptoms related to schizophrenia can significantly reduce patients' ability to benefit from these services. Therefore, it is necessary to be aware of these factors and find solutions to these problems while providing CBMHS [178].

4.9 Occupational rehabilitation

Occupational rehabilitation consists of vocational and artistic activities with goals such as improving creativity, expression and communication skills, socialization, and increasing insight [184].

Vocational rehabilitation is a psychosocial intervention applied to patients who desire to learn and work, focusing on vocational training and reinforcing the skills required for a profession [27]. There is a severe impairment in social and occupational functioning in schizophrenia. Vocational rehabilitation is an important area to focus on to compensate for impaired functionality. Vocational rehabilitation includes providing employment support and necessary theoretical and practical vocational training. The aim is to increase the occupational functionality of patients, which is a step toward functional recovery and, thus, enables them to integrate into society more easily [185].

It may be critical for people with schizophrenia to continue their work or be employed after being discharged from the hospital for their return to society. However, since schizophrenia, which is a chronic disease, may have features such as the presence of residual symptoms, decreased work performance, and deterioration in cognitive and social functions, employment opportunities of patients may decrease [27]. People with schizophrenia face serious problems finding employment, even if they have only been hospitalized once [186]. However, it is known that schizophrenia patients can continue their working lives for a long time after adequate support and treatment are provided [187].

Occupational rehabilitation aims to increase patients' independence in daily life by improving social skills [188]. Working in fulfilling occupations contributes to social inclusion and improves functioning and self-esteem [189]. Some studies have reported that vocational rehabilitation reduces patients' symptoms and increases their cognitive functions and quality of life [190]. In another study on vocational rehabilitation, it was stated that in addition to increasing the social functionality of schizophrenia patients, the hospitalization duration of the patients was shortened, and the risk of hospitalization was reduced [191].

Art therapies can be applied to patients whose negative symptoms are dominant and whose verbal communication is difficult [71]. Art therapies are carried out under the leadership of experts in fields such as painting, music, dance, drama, and handicrafts. It can be applied in groups. Art therapies allow patients to express themselves indirectly and strengthen the patient-therapist relationship. These treatments developed toward the end of the twentieth century and have been used for many years [184].

In a 10-week randomized controlled study in which art therapies were applied to patients with schizophrenia, it was found that art therapy positively changed the patients' self-esteem compared to standard treatment [192]. It has also been reported that art group therapy increases social functioning in patients [193] and significantly reduces negative symptoms statistically compared to standard treatment approaches [194]. The use of art for therapeutic purposes has essential functions in terms of self-understanding of individuals with disorders such as schizophrenia, where verbal communication is limited and negative symptoms are present [195].

4.10 Case management

Patients often need people to help them make the most of the community-based and psychosocial services available, guide them, and coordinate services. The provision of these services is called case management, and the mental health specialist who performs case management is called a case manager. Case management is an approach that aims to monitor patients' adaptation to society, prevent rehospitalization, facilitate access to services, and ultimately improve patients' quality of life [196]. Case management aims to coordinate the care of individuals with severe mental disorders in the community and to increase the accessibility and efficiency of continuous care [197]. In addition, patients are assisted in obtaining and using medications, obtaining financial resources, and providing appropriate accommodation and transportation to the hospital. The main aim is to increase the patients' adaptation to treatment and society, reduce hospitalizations, and increase social functionality [28].

Many different case management models have emerged from the past to the present. Classical case management includes determining needs, planning treatment, providing connections, monitoring, evaluation, and advocacy. The first case management model developed is the broker service model. In this model, the main task of the case manager is to provide the services that patients need and to ensure coordination between various services. In this way, finding early solutions to many patients' problems is possible. However, in this model, the case manager is not a clinician [198].

In clinical case management, the case manager also assumes the clinician's role. The case manager has duties such as evaluation, planning, connection with resources, expanding social networks, coordination between services, crisis intervention, and providing psychoeducation, psychosocial, and pharmacological treatment. They provide a wide range of services, including assistance with housing, government aid, and transportation [199].

Assertive community treatment has been developed to meet the needs of individuals with more severe illnesses who experience frequent exacerbations, violent behavior, and severe decline in functionality [184]. In this model, services are carried out by a team including a psychiatrist, a nurse, and at least two case managers. It is aimed to reduce the number of patients per staff and to provide services in society and the natural environment of patients. The workload is shared by a team rather than by individual. Thus, direct service can be provided 24 hours a day [200]. This model's primary purpose is to meet patients' needs urgently and prevent the devastating effects of the disease. Patients who experience frequent relapses, recurrent hospitalizations, and weak family support are especially suitable individuals for assertive community treatment [184].

Intensive case management, unlike other case management models, aims to provide quality health care in a short time. Treatment services such as emergency home visits are also provided. Its mission is to facilitate community services and assist patients with daily living skills [201]. It has been shown to have benefits in terms of functionality, patient retention in treatment, employment utilization, housing, and shorter hospitalization durations compared to the standard approach [202].

In the strength model, the focus is more on patients' strengths and positive aspects. In this model, the relationship between the case manager and the patient is fundamental and indispensable. While performing the intervention, patients' wishes are considered. The model proposes the treatment of patients in the community and argues that, in principle, individuals with severe mental disorders can also learn, grow, and change [203].

The rehabilitation model also prioritizes individual desires and goals. In addition to individual goals, the social contribution of patients is also aimed in this model [204].

Evaluation, planning, patient-centeredness, bonding, and monitoring are standard functions in case management models [205]. Studies have shown that case management improves patients' functionality and increases their quality of life [206]. It has also been effective in improving negative symptoms [197].

In patients where residual symptoms and exacerbations persist, case management is an appropriate approach in addition to other psychosocial interventions. The case manager's importance is increasing, especially considering the need for more knowledge about services from patients and their families. At this point, the case manager will evaluate the patients psychosocially and help provide the necessary services [184]. It is recommended that case management be implemented as a psychosocial intervention method due to its positive effects on clinical recovery, good social functioning, and reduced hospitalization rates [207].

4.11 Social supports

Social supports are generally defined as having a reliable environment to meet emotional, instrumental, educational, material, and psychosocial needs [208]. Integration of schizophrenia patients into society is one of the most critical goals in schizophrenia treatment. In order to ensure the integration of these individuals into society, they must first be supported in areas such as health, education, employment, social security, and social assistance. This can be achieved by states granting certain rights to these patients and increasing the awareness of patients and their relatives about these rights [209].

There is a strong relationship between schizophrenia and poverty. Lack of social support and caregiving burden can be considered among the reasons for this relationship [210]. Since schizophrenia causes severe loss of functionality and productivity, it can indirectly lead to the impoverishment of individuals and their families [211]. Stigmatization associated with schizophrenia may affect patients and their families' ability to develop productive social networks and benefit from social supports [212]. People with schizophrenia often require the care of a family member, which can lead to a loss of productivity and, therefore, income for another family member [213]. In addition, the treatment costs of schizophrenia, which is a chronic disease, can pose a severe economic burden [214].

The housing problem continues to be a negative situation for schizophrenia. Having a home-like living space is one of the foundations of recovery. Because not being able to live in an adequate home also prevents the development of social relationships with healing properties. As a result of providing adequate and appropriate housing, patients are more likely to feel like they belong to society and integrate into it. This contributes to the development of social relations. In this way, schizophrenia patients can achieve a better quality of life and, indirectly, a life with fewer symptoms. Therefore, mental health professionals and policymakers should not ignore this issue [215].

Education, a social right, is critical for patients to be employed and productive in the future. In this way, it contributes to the integration of patients with society. Particularly patients who cannot adequately benefit from vocational training have difficulties in employment and cannot have a regular income. For this reason, it is essential to support schizophrenia patients for education and provide them with convenience in this process [209].

One of the things that should be done is to provide opportunities for patients with good functionality to work in a suitable job and to provide financial support to patients whose functionality has not improved and who cannot work. Schizophrenia patients with low functionality and reduced social networks may need social support in areas such as social security, social aid, and health. Encouraging non-governmental organizations can be effective in seeking and demanding rights [209].

Social support has a significant impact on the adaptation of individuals with mental disorders to society, reducing their psychiatric symptoms and reducing the number of hospitalizations [216]. It has a protective effect on schizophrenia and is a necessity in clinical and functional recovery [217]. Additionally, emotional social support also reduces relapse rates. It is, therefore, necessary to encourage the provision of better social support [218].

Although various social supports exist in various countries, patients' and their relatives' awareness of social supports is generally low. As a result, patients cannot fully benefit from their social rights. Therefore, there is a need for more services for patients with schizophrenia and to increase their awareness of these supports [209].

Definite policies should be developed to reduce poverty in order to support recovery in schizophrenia patients, increase social supports, and reduce the family care burden [210]. In this process, disciplines such as health professionals, social workers, economics, politics, and law should play an active role. Only in this way can social integration of schizophrenia patients be achieved [209]. For example, in Turkey, in order to work as a public employee, patients with schizophrenia have the right to take a different exam than healthy people. This exam, designed for individuals with schizophrenia and similar disorders, makes it easier for the patients to be assigned to a job. In this way, patients gain financial and social opportunities, become functional, and are exposed to less stigma. As a result, the adaptation of patients with schizophrenia to society increases.

4.12 Motivational interviewing in schizophrenia patients with substance use disorder

Motivational interviewing is a guiding counseling style that aims to achieve behavioral change and helps recognize and resolve ambivalent feelings and thoughts on a particular subject. If change is aimed at motivational interviewing, a partnership is established between the interviewer and the patient. In order to achieve behavioral change, it is necessary to activate individuals' reasons. Additionally, accepting patients' autonomy and acting compassionately are other elements of motivational interviewing. Motivational interviewing involves asking open-ended questions, confirmation, information exchange, reflection, and summarization [219]. Motivational interviewing aims to resolve ambivalence by raising awareness of the conflict between one's goals and current situation [220].

Today, motivational interviewing is mainly used to address problematic behavior patterns, especially to help change substance use behavior [221]. Motivational interviewing is particularly effective in preventing alcohol-related problems [222]. In a study conducted with individuals with comorbid schizophrenia and alcohol use disorder, it was found that patients were able to stay away from alcohol for more extended periods, and their drinking days decreased thanks to motivational interviewing [223].

In a study conducted with patients with comorbid schizophrenia and substance use disorder, it was reported that when motivational interviewing was used together with other psychosocial interventions, the number of days patients abstained from alcohol and substances increased, and a decrease in positive symptoms and exacerbations was achieved over 12 months [224]. In other studies, it has been found that in patients in whom psychosocial interventions such as motivational interviewing, crisis management, social skills training, and psychoeducation were used in combination, substance use decreased, urine substance tests were largely negative, and their compliance with treatment and quality of life increased compared to patients in whom these interventions were not used [225–227]. In a recent review and meta-analysis, the effectiveness of motivational interviewing in individuals with comorbid psychosis and substance use disorder was found to be moderate [228].

It is essential to be more directive and repetitive and use concrete language in motivational interviews with schizophrenia patients, as cognitive impairment accompanies them. It may be necessary to keep session times shorter so patients can tolerate them and to keep the treatment period longer to establish skills [229].

5. Use of psychosocial interventions in combination with other treatments

Considering the effectiveness of psychosocial interventions, the ideal way to treat schizophrenia seems to be the integration of pharmacotherapy and psychosocial interventions [7]. Medication alone has limited effect when not supported by psychosocial interventions [10]. It is known that when psychosocial interventions are used together with other treatments, the rate of discontinuation or change of treatment decreases, relapses decrease, and the level of insight, quality of life, and social functionality increase [230]. For example, it has been found that the majority of schizophrenia patients who receive traditional antipsychotic drug treatment together with psychosocial treatment, such as social skill training, meet the remission criteria, and their symptomatic and functional improvements are more significant than those who receive antipsychotic treatment alone [18]. With combined treatment, the rate of patients participating in employment and receiving education increases. Therefore, it is critical to integrate psychosocial interventions with other interventions in the early stage of schizophrenia [230].

Combining pharmacological and psychosocial interventions has some advantages. Patients receiving psychosocial intervention may require lower doses of antipsychotic medication. Patients who receive appropriate medication may comply better with psychosocial interventions than those who are not compliant with medication. Combining treatments may each enhance the effect of the other, and the positive effects may be more significant than expected. Each treatment can help patients maintain and restore their biopsychosocial integrity by providing improvements in both common and specific areas [231].

Combined treatment is promising for recovery in schizophrenia, and it is emphasized that the most appropriate method in the treatment of schizophrenia is the integration of pharmacological treatment with psychosocial interventions [7].

6. Conclusion

Considering the problem areas experienced by patients, the treatment of schizophrenia should be addressed in a biopsychosocial context. Studies show that the psychosocial approach has positive results in patients with schizophrenia accompanied by severe disability. There is ample evidence that psychosocial interventions are highly effective in integrating patients into society and improving their functionality and quality of life. Therefore, it is crucial to continue psychosocial interventions together with pharmacotherapy. Using different psychosocial interventions together may provide more excellent benefits. Since schizophrenia is a multidimensional mental disorder, detailed evaluation of these dimensions in patients and intervention with psychosocial methods in areas that are deemed deficient are very important for the quality of life and functionality of patients.

We frequently see the benefits of psychosocial interventions in our clinical practice. For example, we started to follow up with a 19-year-old female patient who started experiencing symptoms of delusions and hallucinations at the age of 17 after a one-year prodromal period and was diagnosed with schizophrenia, in a community-based mental health center. Previously, her delusions and hallucinations had been treated with olanzapine and amisulpride. However, her symptoms of social isolation, alogia, and decreased self-care had not responded to medication and continued. She participated in an art therapy program focused on music, dance, and theater at the community-based mental health center. After that, she improved her communication skills and started talking more spontaneously, and her self-care increased. Her statement was as follows: "I don't recognize myself, but it turns out I have great talents within me." This case once again shows the effect of psychosocial interventions on symptoms of schizophrenia and their potency-inducing properties.

Recovery in schizophrenia is a process. Considering that recovery is related to how well the patient can perform psychosocial functions and social reintegration, the importance of psychosocial interventions increases. Even if full recovery cannot be achieved, various psychosocial interventions should be applied to minimize functional losses. Schizophrenia treatment guidelines also recommend psychosocial interventions at all stages of treatment.

Author details

Ulaş Korkmaz[1] and Cicek Hocaoglu[2]*

1 Department of Psychiatry, Giresun Training and Research Hospital, Giresun, Turkey

2 Department of Psychiatry, Recep Tayyip Erdoğan University, Rize, Turkey

*Address all correspondence to: cicekh@gmail.com

References

[1] Frith CD. The Cognitive Neuropsychology of Schizophrenia. Classic ed. London: Psychology Press; 2015

[2] Liberman RP, Kopelowicz A, Smith TE. Psychiatric rehabilitation. In: Sadock BJ, Sadock WA, editors. Comprehensive Textbook of Psychiatry. 7th ed. Philadelphia: Williams and Wilkins; 2000. pp. 3218-3245

[3] Penn DL, Mueser KT, Tarrier N, Gloege A, Cather C, Serrano D, et al. Supportive therapy for schizophrenia: Possible mechanisms and implications for adjunctive psychosocial treatments. Schizophrenia Bulletin. 2004;**30**(1): 101-112. DOI: 10.1093/oxfordjournals.schbul.a007055

[4] Silva JACE. World aspects of psychiatry. In: Sadock BJ, Sadock WA, editors. Comprehensive Textbook of Psychiatry. 7th ed. Philadelphia: Williams and Wilkins; 2000. pp. 3333-3342

[5] Bustillo JR, Lauriello J, Horan WP, Keith SJ. The psychosocial treatment of schizophrenia: An update. American Journal of Psychiatry. 2001;**158**(2):163-175. DOI: 10.1176/appi.ajp.158.2.163

[6] Tauber R, Wallace CJ, Lecomte T. Enlisting indigenous community supporters in skills training programs for persons with severe mental illness. Psychiatric Services. 2000;**51**(11):1428-1432. DOI: 10.1176/appi.ps.51.11.1428

[7] Schooler NR. Relapse prevention and recovery in the treatment of schizophrenia. Journal of Clinical Psychiatry. 2006;**67**:19

[8] Kraepelin E. Dementia Praecox and Paraphrenia. Robert E. New York: Krieger Publishing Co. Inc; 1919

[9] Taylor M, Jauhar S. Are we getting any better at staying better? The long view on relapse and recovery in first episode nonaffective psychosis and schizophrenia. Therapeutic Advances in Psychopharmacology. 2019;**9**:2045125319870033. DOI: 10.1177/2045125319870033

[10] Andreasen NC, Carpenter WT Jr, Kane JM, Lasser RA, Marder SR, Weinberger DR. Remission in schizophrenia: Proposed criteria and rationale for consensus. American Journal of Psychiatry. 2005;**162**(3):441-449. DOI: 10.1176/appi.ajp.162.3.441

[11] Juckel G, Morosini PL. The new approach: Psychosocial functioning as a necessary outcome criterion for therapeutic success in schizophrenia. Current Opinion in Psychiatry. 2008;**21**(6):630-639. DOI: 10.1097/YCO.0b013e328314e144

[12] Ahmed AO, Marino BA, Rosenthal E, Buckner A, Hunter KM, Mabe PA, et al. Recovery in schizophrenia: What consumers know and do not know. Psychiatric Clinics. 2016;**39**(2):313-330. DOI: 10.1016/j.psc.2016.01.009

[13] Harvey PD, Bellack AS. Toward a terminology for functional recovery in schizophrenia: Is functional remission a viable concept? Schizophrenia Bulletin. 2009;**35**(2):300-306. DOI: 10.1093/schbul/sbn171

[14] Liberman RP, Kopelowicz A. Recovery from schizophrenia: A concept in search of research. Psychiatric Services. 2005;**56**(6):735-742. DOI: 10.1176/appi.ps.56.6.735

[15] Emsley R, Chiliza B, Asmal L, Lehloenya K. The concepts of remission

and recovery in schizophrenia. Current Opinion in Psychiatry. 2011;**24**(2):114-121. DOI: 10.1097/YCO.0b013e3283436ea3

[16] Vita A, Barlati S. Recovery from schizophrenia: Is it possible? Current Opinion in Psychiatry. 2018;**31**(3):246-255. DOI: 10.1097/YCO.0000000000000407

[17] Hopper K. Recovery from Schizophrenia: An International Perspective. New York: Oxford University Press (OUP); 2007

[18] Valencia M, Fresan A, Juárez F, Escamilla R, Saracco R. The beneficial effects of combining pharmacological and psychosocial treatment on remission and functional outcome in outpatients with schizophrenia. Journal of Psychiatric Research. 2013;**47**(12):1886-1892. DOI: 10.1016/j.jpsychires.2013.09.006

[19] Kucharska-Pietura K, Mortimer A. Can antipsychotics improve social cognition in patients with schizophrenia? CNS Drugs. 2013;**27**(5):335-343. DOI: 10.1007/s40263-013-0047-0

[20] Schneider-Thoma J, Siafis S, Tardy M, Komossa K, Heres S, Kissling W, et al. Maintenance treatment with antipsychotic drugs for schizophrenia. Cochrane Database of Systematic Reviews. 2020;**48**:738-740. DOI: 10.1002/14651858.CD008016.pub3

[21] Organization WH. CBR: A Strategy for Rehabilitation, Equalization of Opportunities, Poverty Reduction and Social Inclusion of People with Disabilities: Joint Position Paper. Geneva: Organization WH; 2005

[22] Çetinyalçın İ, Oğuz H. Fiziksel tıp ve rehabilitasyonun anlamı, amacı, dünü, bugünü, yarını. Tıbbi Rehabilitasyon. İstanbul: Nobel Tıp Kitabevleri Ltd. Şti; 1995

[23] Liberman RP, McCann MJ, Wallace CJ. Generalization of behaviour therapy with psychotics. The British Journal of Psychiatry. 1976;**129**(5):490-496. DOI: 10.1192/bjp.129.5.490

[24] Kopelowicz A, Liberman RP, Zarate R. Psychosocial treatments for schizophrenia. A Guide to Treatments that Work. 1998;**2**:201-228

[25] Lehman AF. Improving treatment for persons with schizophrenia. Psychiatric Quarterly. 1999;**70**:259-272. DOI: 10.1023/A:1022082031007

[26] Lee D-E, Choi Y-S. The history and achievement of psychosocial treatment for patients with schizophrenia. Journal of Korean Neuropsychiatric Association. 2009;**48**:411-422

[27] Sun X, Yue S, Duan M, Yao D, Luo C. Psychosocial intervention for schizophrenia. Brain-Apparatus Communication: A Journal of Bacomics. 2023;**2**(1):2178266. DOI: 10.1080/27706710.2023.2178266

[28] Liberman RP. Yeti yitiminden iyileşmeye: Psikiyatrik iyileştirim el kitabı. Yıldız M, çev ed Ankara: Türkiye Sosyal Psikiyatri Derneği. 2011:278-310

[29] Gunatilake S, Ananth J, Parameswaran S, Brown S, Silva W. Rehabilitation of schizophrenic patients. Current Pharmaceutical Design. 2004;**10**(18):2277-2288. DOI: 10.2174/1381612043384141

[30] Svensson B, Hansson L. Relationships among patient and therapist ratings of therapeutic alliance and patient assessments of therapeutic process: A study of cognitive therapy with long-term mentally ill

patients. The Journal of Nervous and Mental Disease. 1999;**187**(9):579-585. DOI: 10.1097/00005053-199909000-00008

[31] Pinto RZ, Ferreira ML, Oliveira VC, Franco MR, Adams R, Maher CG, et al. Patient-centred communication is associated with positive therapeutic alliance: A systematic review. Journal of Physiotherapy. 2012;**58**(2):77-87. DOI: 10.1016/S1836-9553(12)70087-5

[32] Bordin ES. The generalizability of the psychoanalytic concept of the working alliance. Psychotherapy: Theory, Research & Practice. 1979;**16**(3):252. DOI: 10.1037/h0085885

[33] Horvath A, Bedi R. The Alliance, [w:] Psychotherapy Relationships That Work: Therapist Contributions and Responsiveness to Patients, (red.) Norcross JC. Oxford University Press, New York; 2002

[34] Organization WH. Stronger Collaboration, Better Health: Global Action Plan for Healthy Lives and Well-Being for All: Strengthening Collaboration among Multilateral Organizations to Accelerate Country Progress on the Health-Related Sustainable Development Goals. Geneva: Organization WH; 2019

[35] Chang JG, Roh D, Kim C-H. Association between therapeutic alliance and adherence in outpatient schizophrenia patients. Clinical Psychopharmacology and Neuroscience. 2019;**17**(2):273. DOI: 10.9758/cpn.2019.17.2.273

[36] Hsieh WL, Yeh ST, Liu WI, Li IH, Lee SK, Chien WT. Improving medication adherence in community-dwelling patients with schizophrenia through therapeutic alliance and medication attitude: A serial multiple mediation model. Patient Preference and Adherence. 2022;**16**:1017-1026. DOI: 10.2147/PPA.S351848

[37] Bourke E, Barker C, Fornells-Ambrojo M. Systematic review and meta-analysis of therapeutic alliance, engagement, and outcome in psychological therapies for psychosis. Psychology and Psychotherapy: Theory, Research and Practice. 2021;**94**(3):822-853. DOI: 10.1111/papt.12330

[38] Leucht S, Tardy M, Komossa K, Heres S, Kissling W, Salanti G, et al. Antipsychotic drugs versus placebo for relapse prevention in schizophrenia: A systematic review and meta-analysis. The Lancet. 2012;**379**(9831):2063-2071. DOI: 10.1016/S0140-6736(12)60239-6

[39] Ayuso-Gutiérrez JL, del Rio Vega JM. Factors influencing relapse in the long-term course of schizophrenia. Schizophrenia Research. 1997;**28**(2-3):199-206. DOI: 10.1016/S0920-9964(97)00131-X

[40] Gray R, Leese M, Bindman J, Becker T, Burti L, David A, et al. Adherence therapy for people with schizophrenia: European multicentre randomised controlled trial. The British Journal of Psychiatry. 2006;**189**(6):508-514. DOI: 10.1192/bjp.bp.105.019489

[41] Sacchetti E, Vita A, Siracusano A, Fleischhacker W. Adherence to Antipsychotics in Schizophrenia. Milano: Springer; 2014

[42] Byerly M, Fisher R, Whatley K, Holland R, Varghese F, Carmody T, et al. A comparison of electronic monitoring vs. clinician rating of antipsychotic adherence in outpatients with schizophrenia. Psychiatry Research. 2005;**133**(2-3):129-133. DOI: 10.1016/j.psychres.2004.11.002

[43] Lacro JP, Dunn LB, Dolder CR, Jeste DV. Prevalence of and risk factors for medication nonadherence in patients with schizophrenia: A comprehensive review of recent literature. The Journal of Clinical Psychiatry. 2002;**63**(10):15489. DOI: 10.4088/jcp.v63n1007

[44] Perkins DO, Gu H, Weiden PJ, McEvoy JP, Hamer RM, Lieberman JA. Predictors of treatment discontinuation and medication nonadherence in patients recovering from a first episode of schizophrenia, schizophreniform disorder, or schizoaffective disorder: A randomized, double-blind, flexible-dose, multicenter study. Journal of Clinical Psychiatry. 2008;**69**(1):106. DOI: 10.4088/jcp.v69n0114

[45] Lochmann van Bennekom MW, Gijsman HJ, Zitman FG. Antipsychotic polypharmacy in psychotic disorders: A critical review of neurobiology, efficacy, tolerability and cost effectiveness. Journal of Psychopharmacology. 2013;**27**(4):327-336. DOI: 10.1177/0269881113477709

[46] Thrush CR, Han X, Pyne JM, Thapa P, Sullivan G. A pilot study of barriers to medication adherence in schizophrenia. The Journal of Clinical Psychiatry. 2004;**65**:211-216. DOI: 10.4088/jcp.v65n0211

[47] Glick ID, Stekoll AH, Hays S. The role of the family and improvement in treatment maintenance, adherence, and outcome for schizophrenia. Journal of Clinical Psychopharmacology. 2011;**31**(1):82-85. DOI: 10.1097/JCP.0b013e31820597fa

[48] Cesur E, Fıstıkçı N, Dönmezler FG, Saatçioğlu İÖ. A clinical case of treatment-resistant schizophrenia: 60 hospitalizations and 342 ECT sessions in 36 years; lack of social support or undertreatment? Psychiatry and Clinical Psychopharmacology. 2015;**24**:S181. DOI: 10.5455/NYS.20150316014347

[49] Zygmunt A, Olfson M, Boyer CA, Mechanic D. Interventions to improve medication adherence in schizophrenia. American Journal of Psychiatry. 2002;**159**(10):1653-1664. DOI: 10.1176/appi.ajp.159.10.1653

[50] Kishimoto T, Agarwal V, Kishi T, Leucht S, Kane JM, Correll CU. Relapse prevention in schizophrenia: A systematic review and meta-analysis of second-generation antipsychotics versus first-generation antipsychotics. Molecular Psychiatry. 2013;**18**(1):53-66. DOI: 10.1038/mp.2011.143

[51] Karow A, Czekalla J, Dittmann RW, Schacht A, Wagner T, Lambert M, et al. Association of subjective well-being, symptoms, and side effects with compliance after 12 months of treatment in schizophrenia. Journal of Clinical Psychiatry. 2007;**68**(1):75-80. DOI: 10.4088/jcp.v68n0110

[52] Bäuml J, Pitschel-Walz G, Volz A, Lüscher S, Rentrop M, Kissling W, et al. Psychoeducation improves compliance and outcome in schizophrenia without an increase of adverse side effects: A 7-year follow-up of the Munich PIP-study. Schizophrenia Bulletin. 2016;**42**(Suppl. 1):S62-S70. DOI: 10.1093/schbul/sbw008

[53] Farooq S, Nazar Z, Irfan M, Akhter J, Gul E, Irfan U, et al. Schizophrenia medication adherence in a resource-poor setting: Randomised controlled trial of supervised treatment in out-patients for schizophrenia (STOPS). The British Journal of Psychiatry. 2011;**199**(6):467-472. DOI: 10.1192/bjp.bp.110.085340

[54] Emmerson LC, Granholm E, Link PC, McQuaid JR, Jeste DV. Insight and treatment outcome with

cognitive-behavioral social skills training for older people with schizophrenia. Journal of Rehabilitation Research and Development. 2009;**46**(8):1053-1058. DOI: 10.1682/JRRD.2009.04.0042

[55] Ertem MY, Duman ZÇ. The effect of motivational interviews on treatment adherence and insight levels of patients with schizophrenia: A randomized controlled study. Perspectives in Psychiatric Care. 2019;**55**(1):75-86. DOI: 10.1111/ppc.12301

[56] Schulz M, Gray R, Spiekermann A, Abderhalden C, Behrens J, Driessen M. Adherence therapy following an acute episode of schizophrenia: A multi-centre randomised controlled trial. Schizophrenia Research. 2013;**146**(1-3):59-63. DOI: 10.1016/j.schres.2013.01.028

[57] Montes JM, Medina E, Gomez-Beneyto M, Maurino J. A short message service (SMS)-based strategy for enhancing adherence to antipsychotic medication in schizophrenia. Psychiatry Research. 2012;**200**(2-3):89-95. DOI: 10.1016/j.psychres.2012.07.034

[58] Popp B-S, Manea MM, Moraru MO. Treatment adherence and social functioning in patients diagnosed with schizophrenia and treated with antipsychotic depot medication. Clujul Medical. 2014;**87**(2):109. DOI: 10.15386/cjmed-292

[59] Weiss KA, Smith TE, Hull JW, Piper AC, Huppert JD. Predictors of risk of nonadherence in outpatients with schizophrenia and other psychotic disorders. Schizophrenia Bulletin. 2002;**28**(2):341-349. DOI: 10.1093/oxfordjournals.schbul.a006943

[60] Xia J, Merinder LB, Belgamwar MR. Psychoeducation for schizophrenia. Cochrane Database of Systematic Reviews. 2011;**6**:CD002831. DOI: 10.1002/14651858.CD002831.pub2

[61] Pekkala E, Merinder L. Psychoeducation for schizophrenia. Cochrane Database of Systematic Reviews. 2002;**2**(2):CD002831. DOI: 10.1002/14651858.cd002831

[62] Pharoah F, Mari JJ, Rathbone J, Wong W. Family intervention for schizophrenia. Cochrane Database of Systematic Reviews. 2010;**12**:CD000088. DOI: 10.1002/14651858.CD000088.pub3

[63] Sarkhel S, Singh O, Arora M. Clinical practice guidelines for psychoeducation in psychiatric disorders general principles of psychoeducation. Indian Journal of Psychiatry. 2020;**62**(Suppl. 2):S319. DOI: 10.4103/psychiatry.IndianJPsychiatry_780_19

[64] Rummel-Kluge C, Kissling W. Psychoeducation for patients with schizophrenia and their families. Expert Review of Neurotherapeutics. 2008;**8**(7):1067-1077. DOI: 10.1586/14737175.8.7.1067

[65] Sibitz I, Amering M, Gössler R, Unger A, Katschnig H. Patients' perspectives on what works in psychoeducational groups for schizophrenia: A qualitative study. Social Psychiatry and Psychiatric Epidemiology. 2007;**42**:909-915. DOI: 10.1007/s00127-007-0245-5

[66] Wood L, Byrne R, Varese F, Morrison AP. Psychosocial interventions for internalised stigma in people with a schizophrenia-spectrum diagnosis: A systematic narrative synthesis and meta-analysis. Schizophrenia Research. 2016;**176**(2-3):291-303. DOI: 10.1016/j.schres.2016.05.001

[67] Tessier A, Roger K, Gregoire A, Desnavailles P, Misdrahi D. Family

psychoeducation to improve outcome in caregivers and patients with schizophrenia: A randomized clinical trial. Frontiers in Psychiatry. 2023;**14**:1171661. DOI: 10.3389/fpsyt.2023.1171661

[68] Alizioti A, Lyrakos G. Measuring the effectiveness of psychoeducation on adherence, depression, anxiety and stress among patients with diagnosis of schizophrenia. A control trial. Current Psychology. 2021;**40**(8):3639-3650. DOI: 10.1007/s12144-019-00255-4

[69] Colton C, Manderscheid R. Congruencies in increased mortality rates, years of potential life lost, and causes of death among public mental health clients in eight states. Preventing Chronic Disease. 2006;**3**(2):1-14

[70] Bäuml J, Froböse T, Kraemer S, Rentrop M, Pitschel-Walz G. Psychoeducation: A basic psychotherapeutic intervention for patients with schizophrenia and their families. Schizophrenia Bulletin. 2006;**32**(Suppl. 1):S1-S9. DOI: 10.1093/schbul/sbl017

[71] NICE. Psychosis and Schizophrenia in Adults: Prevention and Management. London: National Institute of Health and Social Care Excellence; 2014

[72] Whitehead L. Supportive therapy for schizophrenia. Issues in Mental Health Nursing. 2016;**37**(12):973-974. DOI: 10.1080/01612840.2016.1249699

[73] Winston A, Schaefer A. Supportive psychotherapy. In: Tasman A, Riba MB, Alarcón RD, Alfonso CA, Kanba S, Ndetei DM, et al., editors. Tasman's Psychiatry. Cham: Springer International Publishing; 2020. pp. 1-27

[74] Randolph ET. Social networks and schizophrenia. In: Handbook of Social Functioning in Schizophrenia. Boston: Allyn & Bacon; 1998. pp. 238-246

[75] Harder S, Koester A, Valbak K, Rosenbaum B. Five-year follow-up of supportive psychodynamic psychotherapy in first-episode psychosis: Long-term outcome in social functioning. Psychiatry: Interpersonal and Biological Processes. 2014;**77**(2):155-168. DOI: 10.1521/psyc.2014.77.2.155

[76] Schaub A, Mueser KT, von Werder T, Engel R, Möller H-J, Falkai P. A randomized controlled trial of group coping-oriented therapy vs supportive therapy in schizophrenia: Results of a 2-year follow-up. Schizophrenia Bulletin. 2016;**42**(Suppl. 1):S71-S80. DOI: 10.1093/schbul/sbw032

[77] Tarrier N, Kinney C, McCarthy E, Humphreys L, Wittkowski A, Morris J. Two–year follow–up of cognitive–behavioral therapy and supportive counseling in the treatment of persistent symptoms in chronic schizophrenia. Journal of Consulting and Clinical Psychology. 2000;**68**(5):917. DOI: 10.1037/0022-006X.68.5.917

[78] Penn DL, Meyer PS, Evans E, Wirth RJ, Cai K, Burchinal M. A randomized controlled trial of group cognitive-behavioral therapy vs. enhanced supportive therapy for auditory hallucinations. Schizophrenia Research. 2009;**109**(1-3):52-59. DOI: 10.1016/j.schres.2008.12.009

[79] Hurford IM, Kalkstein S, Hurford MO. Cognitive rehabilitation in schizophrenia: Strategies to improve cognition. Psychiatric Times. 2011;**28**(3):43

[80] Green MF, Kern RS, Braff DL, Mintz J. Neurocognitive deficits and functional outcome in schizophrenia: Are we measuring the "right stuff"?

Schizophrenia Bulletin. 2000;**26**(1):119-136. DOI: 10.1093/oxfordjournals.schbul.a033430

[81] Perlick DA, Rosenheck RA, Kaczynski R, Bingham S, Collins J. Association of symptomatology and cognitive deficits to functional capacity in schizophrenia. Schizophrenia Research. 2008;**99**(1-3):192-199. DOI: 10.1016/j.schres.2007.08.009

[82] Keefe RS, Bilder RM, Davis SM, Harvey PD, Palmer BW, Gold JM, et al. Neurocognitive effects of antipsychotic medications in patients with chronic schizophrenia in the CATIE trial. Archives of General Psychiatry. 2007;**64**(6):633-647. DOI: 10.1001/archpsyc.64.6.633

[83] McGurk SR, Twamley EW, Sitzer DI, McHugo GJ, Mueser KT. A meta-analysis of cognitive remediation in schizophrenia. American Journal of Psychiatry. 2007;**164**(12):1791-1802. DOI: 10.1176/appi.ajp.2007.07060906

[84] Medalia A, Opler LA, Opler MG. Integrating psychopharmacology and cognitive remediation to treat cognitive dysfunction in the psychotic disorders. CNS Spectrums. 2013;**19**:106-124

[85] Bowie CR, Bell MD, Fiszdon JM, Johannesen JK, Lindenmayer J-P, McGurk SR, et al. Cognitive remediation for schizophrenia: An expert working group white paper on core techniques. Schizophrenia Research. 2020;**215**:49-53. DOI: 10.1016/j.schres.2019.10.047

[86] Kern RS, Glynn SM, Horan WP, Marder SR. Psychosocial treatments to promote functional recovery in schizophrenia. Schizophrenia Bulletin. 2009;**35**(2):347-361. DOI: 10.1093/schbul/sbn177

[87] Twamley EW, Jeste DV, Bellack AS. A review of cognitive training in schizophrenia. Schizophrenia Bulletin. 2003;**29**(2):359-382. DOI: 10.1093/oxfordjournals.schbul.a007011

[88] Wykes T, Van der Gaag M. Is it time to develop a new cognitive therapy for psychosis—Cognitive remediation therapy (CRT)? Clinical Psychology Review. 2001;**21**(8):1227-1256. DOI: 10.1016/S0272-7358(01)00104-0

[89] Green MF. New possibilities in cognition enhancement for schizophrenia. American Psychiatric Association. 2009;**166**:749-752

[90] Tomás P, Fuentes I, Roder V, Ruiz JC. Cognitive rehabilitation programs in schizophrenia: Current status and perspectives. International Journal of Psychology and Psychological Therapy. 2010;**10**(2):191-204

[91] Bryce SD, Rossell SL, Lee SJ, Lawrence RJ, Tan EJ, Carruthers SP, et al. Neurocognitive and self-efficacy benefits of cognitive remediation in schizophrenia: A randomized controlled trial–corrigendum. Journal of the International Neuropsychological Society. 2019;**25**(6):659-660. DOI: 10.1017/S1355617717001369

[92] Lejeune JA, Northrop A, Kurtz MM. A meta-analysis of cognitive remediation for schizophrenia: Efficacy and the role of participant and treatment factors. Schizophrenia Bulletin. 2021;**47**(4):997-1006. DOI: 10.1093/schbul/sbab022

[93] Wykes T, Reeder C. Cognitive Remediation Therapy for Schizophrenia: Theory and Practice. London: Routledge; 2006

[94] Medalia A, Saperstein AM. Does cognitive remediation for schizophrenia improve functional outcomes? Current Opinion in Psychiatry.

2013;**26**(2):151-157. DOI: 10.1097/YCO.0b013e32835dcbd4

[95] Velligan DI, Diamond PM, Mintz J, Maples N, Li X, Zeber J, et al. The use of individually tailored environmental supports to improve medication adherence and outcomes in schizophrenia. Schizophrenia Bulletin. 2008;**34**(3):483-493. DOI: 10.1093/schbul/sbm111

[96] Kaneko Y, Keshavan M. Cognitive remediation in schizophrenia. Clinical Psychopharmacology and Neuroscience. 2012;**10**(3):125. DOI: 10.9758/cpn.2012.10.3.125

[97] Wykes T, Reeder C, Corner J, Williams C, Everitt B. The effects of neurocognitive remediation on executive processing in patients with schizophrenia. Schizophrenia Bulletin. 1999;**25**(2):291-307. DOI: 10.1093/oxfordjournals.schbul.a033379

[98] Vita A, Barlati S, Ceraso A, Nibbio G, Ariu C, Deste G, et al. Effectiveness, core elements, and moderators of response of cognitive remediation for schizophrenia: A systematic review and meta-analysis of randomized clinical trials. JAMA Psychiatry. 2021;**78**(8):848-858. DOI: 10.1001/jamapsychiatry.2021.0620

[99] Fitapelli B, Lindenmayer J-P. Advances in cognitive remediation training in schizophrenia: A review. Brain Sciences. 2022;**12**(2):129. DOI: 10.3390/brainsci12020129

[100] Wykes T, Reeder C, Landau S, Everitt B, Knapp M, Patel A, et al. Cognitive remediation therapy in schizophrenia: Randomised controlled trial. The British Journal of Psychiatry. 2007;**190**(5):421-427. DOI: 10.1192/bjp.bp.106.026575

[101] Martini F, Spangaro M, Bechi M, Agostoni G, Buonocore M, Sapienza J, et al. Improving outcome of treatment-resistant schizophrenia: Effects of cognitive remediation therapy. European Archives of Psychiatry and Clinical Neuroscience. 2023:1-9. [Advance Online Publication]. DOI: 10.1007/s00406-023-01731-6

[102] Buonocore M, Spangaro M, Bechi M, Trezzani S, Terragni R, Martini F, et al. Cognitive remediation in schizophrenia: What happens after 10 years? Schizophrenia Research: Cognition. 2022;**29**:100251. DOI: 10.1016/j.scog.2022.100251

[103] Vita A, Barlati S, Ceraso A, Deste G, Nibbio G, Wykes T. Acceptability of cognitive remediation for schizophrenia: A systematic review and meta-analysis of randomized controlled trials. Psychological Medicine. 2022;**53**:1-11. DOI: 10.1017/S0033291722000319

[104] Beck A, Rector N, Stolar N, Grant P. Schizophrenia: Cognitive theory, research and therapy. Psychiatric Rehabilitation Journal. 2009;**32**:327-328. DOI: 10.1037/h0094638

[105] Beck AT. Beyond Belief: A Theory of Modes, Personality, and Psychopathology. New York: The Guilford Press; 1996

[106] Moritz S, Klein JP, Lysaker PH, Mehl S. Metacognitive and cognitive-behavioral interventions for psychosis: New developments. Dialogues in Clinical Neuroscience. 2019;**21**(3):309-317. DOI: 10.31887/DCNS.2019.21.3/smoritz

[107] Škodlar B, Henriksen M, Sass L, Nelson B, Parnas J. Cognitive-behavioral therapy for schizophrenia: A critical evaluation of its theoretical framework from a clinical-phenomenological perspective. Psychopathology. 2013;**46**(4):249-265. DOI: 10.1159/000342536

[108] Turkington D, Kingdon D, Weiden PJ. Cognitive behavior therapy for schizophrenia. American Journal of Psychiatry. 2006;**163**(3):365-373. DOI: 10.1176/appi.ajp.163.3.365

[109] Sarin F, Wallin L, Widerlöv B. Cognitive behavior therapy for schizophrenia: A meta-analytical review of randomized controlled trials. Nordic Journal of Psychiatry. 2011;**65**(3):162-174. DOI: 10.3109/08039488.2011.577188

[110] Sensky T, Turkington D, Kingdon D, Scott JL, Scott J, Siddle R, et al. A randomized controlled trial of cognitive-behavioral therapy for persistent symptoms in schizophrenia resistant to medication. Archives of General Psychiatry. 2000;**57**(2):165-172. DOI: 10.1001/archpsyc.57.2.165

[111] Huhn M, Tardy M, Spineli LM, Kissling W, Foerstl H, Pitschel-Walz G, et al. Efficacy of pharmacotherapy and psychotherapy for adult psychiatric disorders: A systematic overview of meta-analyses. JAMA Psychiatry. 2014;**71**(6):706-715. DOI: 10.1001/jamapsychiatry.2014.112

[112] Rector NA, Seeman MV, Segal ZV. Cognitive therapy for schizophrenia: A preliminary randomized controlled trial. Schizophrenia Research. 2003;**63**(1-2):1-11. DOI: 10.1016/S0920-9964(02)00308-0

[113] Garety PA, Fowler DG, Freeman D, Bebbington P, Dunn G, Kuipers E. Cognitive-behavioural therapy and family intervention for relapse prevention and symptom reduction in psychosis: Randomised controlled trial. The British Journal of Psychiatry. 2008;**192**(6):412-423. DOI: 10.1192/bjp.bp.107.043570

[114] Startup M, Jackson M, Bendix S. North Wales randomized controlled trial of cognitive behaviour therapy for acute schizophrenia spectrum disorders: Outcomes at 6 and 12 months. Psychological Medicine. 2004;**34**(3):413-422. DOI: 10.1017/S0033291703001211

[115] Turkington D, Kingdon D, Turner T. Effectiveness of a brief cognitive–behavioural therapy intervention in the treatment of schizophrenia. The British Journal of Psychiatry. 2002;**180**(6):523-527. DOI: 10.1192/bjp.180.6.523

[116] Bighelli I, Wallis S, Reitmeir C, Schwermann F, Salahuddin NH, Leucht S. Effects of psychological treatments on functioning in people with schizophrenia: A systematic review and meta-analysis of randomized controlled trials. European Archives of Psychiatry and Clinical Neuroscience. 2023;**273**(4):779-810. DOI: 10.1007/s00406-022-01526-1

[117] Jauhar S, McKenna P, Radua J, Fung E, Salvador R, Laws K. Cognitive–behavioural therapy for the symptoms of schizophrenia: Systematic review and meta-analysis with examination of potential bias. The British Journal of Psychiatry. 2014;**204**(1):20-29. DOI: 10.1192/bjp.bp.112.116285

[118] Van der Gaag M, Valmaggia LR, Smit F. The effects of individually tailored formulation-based cognitive behavioural therapy in auditory hallucinations and delusions: A meta-analysis. Schizophrenia Research. 2014;**156**(1):30-37. DOI: 10.1016/j.schres.2014.03.016

[119] Sitko K, Bewick BM, Owens D, Masterson C. Meta-analysis and meta-regression of cognitive behavioral therapy for psychosis (CBTp) across time: The effectiveness of CBTp has improved for delusions. Schizophrenia Bulletin Open. 2020;**1**(1):sgaa023. DOI: 10.1093/schizbullopen/sgaa023

[120] Pozza A, Dèttore D. Modular cognitive-behavioral therapy for affective symptoms in young individuals at ultra-high risk of first episode of psychosis: Randomized controlled trial. Journal of Clinical Psychology. 2020;**76**(3):392-405. DOI: 10.1002/jclp.22901

[121] Zheng Y, Xu T, Zhu Y, Li C, Wang J, Livingstone S, et al. Cognitive behavioral therapy for prodromal stage of psychosis—Outcomes for transition, functioning, distress, and quality of life: A systematic review and meta-analysis. Schizophrenia Bulletin. 2022;**48**(1):8-19. DOI: 10.1093/schbul/sbab044

[122] National Collaborating Centre for Mental Health (UK). Schizophrenia: core interventions in the treatment and management of schizophrenia in primary and secondary care (update) [Internet]. Leicester, UK: British Psychological Society; 2009

[123] Malhotra A, Baker J. Group Therapy. Treasure Island (FL): StatPearls Publishing; 2019

[124] Barlow SH, Burlingame GM, Fuhriman A. Therapeutic applications of groups: From Pratt's" thought control classes" to modern group psychotherapy. Group Dynamics: Theory, Research, and Practice. 2000;**4**(1):115. DOI: 10.1037/1089-2699.4.1.115

[125] Gabrovšek VP. Inpatient group therapy of patients with schizophrenia. Psychiatria Danubina. 2009;**21**(1):67-72

[126] Kanas N. Group therapy for patients with chronic psychotic disorders. International Journal of Group Psychotherapy. 1999;**49**(3):413-416. DOI: 10.1080/00207284.1999.11732619

[127] Opalić P. Theme-orientated group psychotherapy of psychotics. Group Analysis. 1988;**21**(4):289-297. DOI: 10.1177/0533316488214002

[128] O'Brien CP. Group therapy for schizophrenia: A practical approach. Schizophrenia Bulletin. 1975;**1**(13):119. DOI: 10.1093/schbul/1.13.119

[129] McLeod T, Morris M, Birchwood M, Dovey A. Cognitive behavioural therapy group work with voice hearers. Part 1. British Journal of Nursing. 2007;**16**(4):248-252. DOI: 10.12968/bjon.2007.16.4.22995

[130] Elis O, Caponigro JM, Kring AM. Psychosocial treatments for negative symptoms in schizophrenia: Current practices and future directions. Clinical Psychology Review. 2013;**33**(8):914-928. DOI: 10.1016/j.cpr.2013.07.001

[131] Payn SB. Reaching chronic schizophrenic patients with group pharmacotherapy. International Journal of Group Psychotherapy. 1974;**24**(1):25. DOI: 10.1080/00207284.1974.11492266

[132] Sigman M, Hassan S. Benefits of long-term group therapy to individuals suffering schizophrenia: A prospective 7-year study. Bulletin of the Menninger Clinic. 2006;**70**(4):273-282. DOI: 10.1521/bumc.2006.70.4.273

[133] Kingsep P, Nathan P, Castle D. Cognitive behavioural group treatment for social anxiety in schizophrenia. Schizophrenia Research. 2003;**63**(1-2):121-129. DOI: 10.1016/S0920-9964(02)00376-6

[134] García-Cabeza I, González de Chávez M. Therapeutic factors and insight in group therapy for outpatients diagnosed with schizophrenia. Psychosis. 2009;**1**(2):134-144. DOI: 10.1080/17522430902770058

[135] Chien WT. Effectiveness of psychoeducation and mutual support group program for family caregivers of Chinese people with schizophrenia.

The Open Nursing Journal. 2008;**2**:28. DOI: 10.2174/1874434600802010028

[136] Pickett-Schenk SA, Lippincott RC, Bennett C, Steigman PJ. Improving knowledge about mental illness through family-led education: The journey of hope. Psychiatric Services. 2008;**59**(1): 49-56. DOI: 10.1176/ps.2008.59.1.49

[137] Addington J, McCleery A, Addington D. Three-year outcome of family work in an early psychosis program. Schizophrenia Research. 2005;**79**(1):107-116. DOI: 10.1016/j.schres.2005.03.019

[138] Fellowship W. Families as Partners in Care: A Document Developed to Launch a Strategy for the Implementation of Programs of Family Education, Training, and Support. Toronto: World Schizophrenia Fellowship; 1998

[139] Soygür H, Çelikel B, Aydemir Ç, Bozkurt S. Hasta yakınları ile gerçekleştirilen psikodrama yönelimli destekleyici-eğitici grup psikoterapisinin kronik şizofreni gidişi üzerinde etkisi. Düşünen Adam. 1998;**11**(4):5-11

[140] Winefield HR, Harvey EJ. Needs of family caregivers in chronic schizophrenia. Schizophrenia Bulletin. 1994;**20**(3):557-566. DOI: 10.1093/schbul/20.3.557

[141] Lowyck B, De Hert M, Peeters E, Wampers M, Gilis P, Peuskens J. A study of the family burden of 150 family members of schizophrenic patients. European Psychiatry. 2004;**19**(7):395-401. DOI: 10.1016/j.eurpsy.2004.04.006

[142] Gülseren L, Çam B, Karakoç B, Yiğit T, Danacı A, Çubukçuoğlu Z, et al. Şizofrenide ailenin yükünü etkileyen etmenler. Türk Psikiyatri Dergisi. 2010;**21**:203-212

[143] Willick MS. Schizophrenia: A Parent's Perspective: Mourning Without End. Washington DC: American Psychiatric Association; 1994

[144] Li J, Lambert CE, Lambert VA. Predictors of family caregivers' burden and quality of life when providing care for a family member with schizophrenia in the People's Republic of China. Nursing & Health Sciences. 2007;**9**(3):192-198. DOI: 10.1111/j.1442-2018.2007.00327.x

[145] Wyman K, Clarke S, McKenzie P, Gilbert M. The impact of participation in a support group for carers of a person with schizophrenia: A qualitative study. International Journal of Psychosocial Rehabilitation. 2007;**12**(2):97

[146] McFarlane WR. Family interventions for schizophrenia and the psychoses: A review. Family Process. 2016;**55**(3):460-482. DOI: 10.1111/famp.12235

[147] Varghese M, Kirpekar V, Loganathan S. Family interventions: Basic principles and techniques. Indian Journal of Psychiatry. 2020;**62**(Suppl. 2):S192. DOI: 10.4103/psychiatry.IndianJPsychiatry_770_19

[148] Caqueo-Urízar A, Rus-Calafell M, Urzúa A, Escudero J, Gutiérrez-Maldonado J. The role of family therapy in the management of schizophrenia: Challenges and solutions. Neuropsychiatric Disease and Treatment. 2015;**11**:145-151. DOI: 10.2147/NDT.S51331

[149] Bloch S, Hafner J, Harari E, Szmukler GI, Brodaty H, Kissane D. The Family in Clinical Psychiatry. London: Oxford University Press; 1994

[150] Glynn SM, Cohen AN, Dixon LB, Niv N. The potential impact of

the recovery movement on family interventions for schizophrenia: Opportunities and obstacles. Schizophrenia Bulletin. 2006;**32**(3):451-463. DOI: 10.1093/schbul/sbj066

[151] Lucksted A, Stewart B, Forbes CB. Benefits and changes for family to family graduates. American Journal of Community Psychology. 2008;**42**:154-166. DOI: 10.1007/s10464-008-9195-7

[152] Dixon L, Stewart B, Burland J, Delahanty J, Lucksted A, Hoffman M. Pilot study of the effectiveness of the family-to-family education program. Psychiatric Services. 2001;**52**(7):965-967. DOI: 10.1176/appi.ps.52.7.965

[153] Camacho-Gomez M, Castellvi P. Effectiveness of family intervention for preventing relapse in first-episode psychosis until 24 months of follow-up: A systematic review with meta-analysis of randomized controlled trials. Schizophrenia Bulletin. 2020;**46**(1): 98-109. DOI: 10.1093/schbul/sbz038

[154] Nuechterlein KH, Dawson ME. A heuristic vulnerability/stress model of schizophrenic episodes. Schizophrenia Bulletin. 1984;**10**(2):300. DOI: 10.1093/schbul/10.2.300

[155] Brown GW, Birley JL, Wing JK. Influence of family life on the course of schizophrenic disorders: A replication. The British Journal of Psychiatry. 1972;**121**(562):241-258. DOI: 10.1192/bjp.121.3.241

[156] Barrowclough C, Tarrier N. Families of Schizophrenic Patients: Cognitive Behavioural Intervention. Cheltenham: Nelson Thornes; 1997

[157] Grover S, Chakrabarti S, Sharma A, Tyagi S. Attitudes toward psychotropic medications among patients with chronic psychiatric disorders and their family caregivers. Journal of Neurosciences in Rural Practice. 2014;**5**(4):374-383. DOI: 10.4103/0976-3147.139989

[158] Pilling S, Bebbington P, Kuipers E, Garety P, Geddes J, Orbach G, et al. Psychological treatments in schizophrenia: I. Meta-analysis of family intervention and cognitive behaviour therapy. Psychological Medicine. 2002;**32**(5):763-782. DOI: 10.1017/S0033291702005895

[159] Dixon L, Adams C, Lucksted A. Update on family psychoeducation for schizophrenia. Schizophrenia Bulletin. 2000;**26**(1):5-20. DOI: 10.1093/oxfordjournals.schbul.a033446

[160] Chien WT, Chan SW. The effectiveness of mutual support group intervention for Chinese families of people with schizophrenia: A randomised controlled trial with 24-month follow-up. International Journal of Nursing Studies. 2013;**50**(10):1326-1340. DOI: 10.1016/j.ijnurstu.2013.01.004

[161] Gutiérrez-Maldonado J, Caqueo-Urízar A. Effectiveness of a psycho-educational intervention for reducing burden in Latin American families of patients with schizophrenia. Quality of Life Research. 2007;**16**:739-747. DOI: 10.1007/s11136-007-9173-9

[162] Ventriglio A, Ricci F, Magnifico G, Chumakov E, Torales J, Watson C, et al. Psychosocial interventions in schizophrenia: Focus on guidelines. International Journal of Social Psychiatry. 2020;**66**(8):735-747. DOI: 10.1177/0020764020934827

[163] Knapczyk D, Rodes P. Teaching Social Competence. Champaign. Ill: Research Press; 2001

[164] Bellack AS, Mueser KT, Gingerich S, Agresta J. Social Skills Training for

Schizophrenia: A Step-by-Step Guide. London: Guilford Publications; 2013

[165] Kopelowicz A, Liberman RP, Zarate R. Recent advances in social skills training for schizophrenia. Schizophrenia Bulletin. 2006;**32**(Suppl. 1):S12-S23

[166] Milev P, Ho B-C, Arndt S, Andreasen NC. Predictive values of neurocognition and negative symptoms on functional outcome in schizophrenia: A longitudinal first-episode study with 7-year follow-up. American Journal of Psychiatry. 2005;**162**(3):495-506. DOI: 10.1176/appi.ajp.162.3.495

[167] Mueser KT, Glynn SM, SR MG. Social and Vocational Impairments. Washington DC: American Psychiatric Publishing, Inc.; 2006

[168] Shean GD. Evidence-based psychosocial practices and recovery from schizophrenia. Psychiatry: Interpersonal and Biological Processes. 2009;**72**(4):307-320. DOI: 10.1521/psyc.2009.72.4.307

[169] Marder SR, Wirshing WC, Mintz J, McKenzie J, Johnston K, Eckman TA, et al. Two-year outcome of social skills training and group psychotherapy for outpatients with schizophrenia. The American Journal of Psychiatry. 1996;**153**(12):1585-1592. DOI: 10.1176/ajp.153.12.1585

[170] Granholm EL, McQuaid JR, Holden JL. Cognitive-Behavioral Social Skills Training for Schizophrenia: A Practical Treatment Guide. New York: Guilford Publications; 2016

[171] Granholm E, Holden J, Link PC, McQuaid JR. Randomized clinical trial of cognitive behavioral social skills training for schizophrenia: Improvement in functioning and experiential negative symptoms. Journal of Consulting and Clinical Psychology. 2014;**82**(6):1173. DOI: 10.1037/a0037098

[172] Liberman RP. Dissemination and adoption of social skills training: Social validation of an evidence-based treatment for the mentally disabled. Journal of Mental Health. 2007;**16**(5):595-623. DOI: 10.1080/09638230701494902

[173] Turner DT, McGlanaghy E, Cuijpers P, Van Der Gaag M, Karyotaki E, MacBeth A. A meta-analysis of social skills training and related interventions for psychosis. Schizophrenia Bulletin. 2018;**44**(3):475-491. DOI: 10.1093/schbul/sbx146

[174] Roder V, Brenner H, Müller D, Lächler M, Zorn P, Reisch T, et al. Development of specific social skills training programmes for schizophrenia patients: Results of a multicentre study. Acta Psychiatrica Scandinavica. 2002;**105**(5):363-371. DOI: 10.1034/j.1600-0447.2002.1o214.x

[175] Cancro R. The underutilization of psychiatric rehabilitation. World Psychiatry. 2006;**5**(3):159

[176] Chatterjee S, Patel V, Chatterjee A, Weiss HA. Evaluation of a community-based rehabilitation model for chronic schizophrenia in rural India. The British Journal of Psychiatry. 2003;**182**(1):57-62. DOI: 10.1192/bjp.182.1.57

[177] Khasnabis C, Motsch KH, Achu K, Al Jubah K, Brodtkorb S, Chervin P, et al. Community-Based Rehabilitation: CBR Guidelines. Geneva: WHO; 2010

[178] Mechanic D. Strategies for integrating public mental health services. Psychiatric Services. 1991;**42**(8):797-801. DOI: 10.1176/ps.42.8.797

[179] Bauer M, Kunze H, Von Cranach M, Fritze J, Becker T. Psychiatric reform in Germany. Acta Psychiatrica Scandinavica. 2001;**104**:27-34. DOI: 10.1034/j.1600-0447.2001.1040s2027.x

[180] Asher L, Patel V, De Silva MJ. Community-based psychosocial interventions for people with schizophrenia in low and middle-income countries: Systematic review and meta-analysis. BMC Psychiatry. 2017;**17**(1):1-15. DOI: 10.1186/s12888-017-1516-7

[181] Krieger I, Bitan DT, Sharon-Garty R, Baloush-Kleinman V, Zamir L. The effect of community-based mental health rehabilitation services for schizophrenia: A retrospective cohort study. Psychiatric Quarterly. 2020;**91**:1453-1463. DOI: 10.1007/s11126-020-09772-z

[182] WHO. Community Based Rehabilitation: CBR Guidelines. Geneva: World Health Organization; 2010

[183] Özdemir İ, Şafak Y, Örsel S, Karaoğlan Kahiloğulları A, Karadağ H. Bir toplum ruh sağlığı merkezinde şizofreni hastalarına uygulanan ruhsal-toplumsal uyumlandırma etkinliğinin araştırılması: Kontrollü çalışma. Anatolian Journal of Psychiatry/Anadolu Psikiyatri Dergisi. 2017;**18**(5):419-427. DOI: 10.5455/apd.254450

[184] Yildiz M. Psychosocial rehabilitation interventions in the treatment of schizophrenia and bipolar disorder. Archives of Neuropsychiatry. 2021;**58**(Suppl. 1):S77. DOI: 10.29399/npa.27430

[185] Lysaker P, Bell M. Work rehabilitation and improvements in insight in schizophrenia. The Journal of Nervous and Mental Disease. 1995;**183**(2):103-106. DOI: 10.1097/00005053-199502000-00007

[186] Davidson M, Kapara O, Goldberg S, Yoffe R, Noy S, Weiser M. A nation-wide study on the percentage of schizophrenia and bipolar disorder patients who earn minimum wage or above. Schizophrenia Bulletin. 2016;**42**(2):443-447. DOI: 10.1093/schbul/sbv023

[187] Gjerdalen OS, Lystad JU, Bull H, Ringen PA, Røssberg JI, Martinsen EW, et al. Vocational rehabilitation augmented with cognitive behavioral therapy or cognitive remediation for individuals with schizophrenia: A 5-year follow-up study. Nordic Journal of Psychiatry. 2023;**77**(1):23-30. DOI: 10.1080/08039488.2022.2042598

[188] Gibson RW, D'Amico M, Jaffe L, Arbesman M. Occupational therapy interventions for recovery in the areas of community integration and normative life roles for adults with serious mental illness: A systematic review. The American Journal of Occupational Therapy. 2011;**65**(3):247-256. DOI: 10.5014/ajot.2011.001297

[189] Wilcock AA. Occupational Science: Bridging Occupation and Health. Los Angeles, CA: SAGE Publications Sage CA; 2005

[190] Bio DS, Gattaz WF. Vocational rehabilitation improves cognition and negative symptoms in schizophrenia. Schizophrenia Research. 2011;**126** (1-3):265-269. DOI: 10.1016/j.schres.2010.08.003

[191] Oka M, Otsuka K, Yokoyama N, Mintz J, Hoshino K, Niwa S-I, et al. An evaluation of a hybrid occupational therapy and supported employment program in Japan for persons with schizophrenia. The American Journal of Occupational Therapy. 2004;**58**(4): 466-475. DOI: 10.5014/ajot.58.4.466

[192] Green BL, Wehling C, Taisky GJ. Group art therapy as an adjunct to treatment for chronic outpatients. Psychiatric Services. 1987;**38**(9):988-991. DOI: 10.1176/ps.38.9.988

[193] Meng P, Zheng R. Group intervention for schizophrenia inpatient with art as medium. Acta Psychologica Sinica. 2005;**37**(3):403

[194] Richardson P, Jones K, Evans C, Stevens P, Rowe A. Exploratory RCT of art therapy as an adjunctive treatment in schizophrenia. Journal of Mental Health. 2007;**16**(4):483-491. DOI: 10.1080/09638230701483111

[195] Crawford MJ, Patterson S. Arts therapies for people with schizophrenia: An emerging evidence base. BMJ Mental Health. 2007;**10**(3):69-70. DOI: 10.1136/ebmh.10.3.69

[196] Guarino K. Step-by Step: A Comprehensive Approach to Case Management. Canada: Homeless Hub; 2011

[197] Cheng J, Liu H, Geng T, Wang Y, Yu L, Li J, et al. The effect of case management for schizophrenia clients in China. Journal of Behavioral and Brain Science. 2020;**10**(8):297. DOI: 10.4236/jbbs.2020.108019

[198] Holloway F, Carson J. Review article case management: An update. International Journal of Social Psychiatry. 2001;**47**(3):21-31. DOI: 10.1177/002076400104700303

[199] Kanter J. Clinical case management: Definition, principles, components. Psychiatric Services. 1989;**40**(4):361-368. DOI: 10.1176/ps.40.4.361

[200] Stein LI, Test MA. Alternative to mental hospital treatment: I. Conceptual model, treatment program, and clinical evaluation. Archives of General Psychiatry. 1980;**37**(4):392-397. DOI: 10.1001/archpsyc.1980.01780170034003

[201] Surles RC, Blanch AK, Shern DL, Donahue SA. Case management as a strategy for systems change. Health Affairs. 1992;**11**(1):151-163. DOI: 10.1377/hlthaff.11.1.151

[202] Dieterich M, Irving CB, Bergman H, Khokhar MA, Park B, Marshall M. Intensive case management for severe mental illness. Cochrane Database of Systematic Reviews. 2017;**1**:CD007906. DOI: 10.1002/14651858.CD007906.pub3

[203] Rapp CA. Theory, Principles, and Methods of the Strengths Model of Case Management. Gordon: Harwood Academic Publishers; 1993

[204] Anthony W, Forbess R, Cohen M. Rehabilitation-oriented case management. In: Case Management for Mentally Ill Patients: Theory and Practice. Gordon: Academic Publishers; 1993. pp. 99-118

[205] Chamberlain R, Rapp CA. A decade of case management: A methodological review of outcome research. Community Mental Health Journal. 1991;**27**:171-188. DOI: 10.1007/BF00752419

[206] Gorey KM, Leslie DR, Morris T, Carruthers WV, John L, Chacko J. Effectiveness of case management with severely and persistently mentally ill people. Community Mental Health Journal. 1998;**34**:241-250. DOI: 10.1023/A:1018761623212

[207] Incedere A, Yildiz M. Case management for individuals with severe mental illness: Outcomes of a 24-month practice. Turkish Journal of Psychiatry. 2019;**30**(4):245-252. DOI: 10.5080/u23532

[208] Stansfeld SA, Fuhrer R, Shipley M. Types of social support as predictors of psychiatric morbidity in a cohort of British civil servants (Whitehall II study). Psychological Medicine. 1998;**28**(4):881-892. DOI: 10.1017/S0033291798006746

[209] Aslantürk H. Community integration and social rights in mental health area. Turkish Journal of Family Medicine and Primary Care. 2016;**10**(4):259-270. DOI: 10.21763/tjfmpc.271333

[210] Yu Y-H, Peng M-M, Bai X, Luo W, Yang X, Li J, et al. Schizophrenia, social support, caregiving burden and household poverty in rural China. Social Psychiatry and Psychiatric Epidemiology. 2020;**55**:1571-1580. DOI: 10.1007/s00127-020-01864-2

[211] Lim K-L, Jacobs P, Ohinmaa A, Schopflocher D, Dewa CS. A new population-based measure of the economic burden of mental illness in Canada. Chronic Diseases in Canada. 2008;**28**(3):92-98. DOI: 10.24095/hpcdp.28.3.02

[212] Zhang T-M, Wong IY-L, Yu Y-H, Ni S-G, He X-S, Bacon-Shone J, et al. An integrative model of internalized stigma and recovery-related outcomes among people diagnosed with schizophrenia in rural China. Social Psychiatry and Psychiatric Epidemiology. 2019;**54**:911-918. DOI: 10.1007/s00127-018-1646-3

[213] Metts R, editor. Disability and development. In: Background Paper Prepared for the Disability and Development Research Agenda Meeting. Washington DC: World Bank Headquarters; 2004

[214] Hailemichael Y, Hailemariam D, Tirfessa K, Docrat S, Alem A, Medhin G, et al. Catastrophic out-of-pocket payments for households of people with severe mental disorder: A comparative study in rural Ethiopia. International Journal of Mental Health Systems. 2019;**13**(1):1-13. DOI: 10.1186/s13033-019-0294-7

[215] Browne G, Courtney M. Schizophrenia housing and supportive relationships. International Journal of Mental Health Nursing. 2007;**16**(2):73-80. DOI: 10.1111/j.1447-0349.2006.00447.x

[216] Huang CY, Sousa VD, Tsai CC, Hwang MY. Social support and adaptation of Taiwanese adults with mental illness. Journal of Clinical Nursing. 2008;**17**(13):1795-1802. DOI: 10.1111/j.1365-2702.2008.02310.x

[217] Vázquez Morejón AJ, León Rubio JM, Vázquez-Morejón R. Social support and clinical and functional outcome in people with schizophrenia. International Journal of Social Psychiatry. 2018;**64**(5):488-496. DOI: 10.1177/0020764018778868

[218] Samuel T, Nigussie K, Mirkena Y, Azale T. Relationship between social support and schizophrenia relapse among patients with schizophrenia on follow-up at Amanuel Mental Specialized Hospital, Addis Ababa, Ethiopia: A case-control study. Frontiers in Psychiatry. 2022;**13**:980614. DOI: 10.3389/fpsyt.2022.980614

[219] Vasilaki EI, Hosier SG, Cox WM. The efficacy of motivational interviewing as a brief intervention for excessive drinking: A meta-analytic review. Alcohol and Alcoholism. 2006;**41**(3):328-335. DOI: 10.1093/alcalc/agl016

[220] Arbuckle MR, Foster FP, Talley RM, Covell NH, Essock SM. Applying motivational interviewing strategies

to enhance organizational readiness and facilitate implementation efforts. Quality Management in Healthcare. 2020;**29**(1):1-6. DOI: 10.1097/QMH.0000000000000234

[221] Smedslund G, Berg RC, Hammerstrøm KT, Steiro A, Leiknes KA, Dahl HM, et al. Motivational interviewing for substance abuse. Campbell Systematic Reviews. 2011;**7**(1):1-126. DOI: 10.4073/csr.2011.6

[222] Kohler S, Hofmann A. Can motivational interviewing in emergency care reduce alcohol consumption in young people? A systematic review and meta-analysis. Alcohol and Alcoholism. 2015;**50**(2):107-117. DOI: 10.1093/alcalc/agu098

[223] Graeber DA, Moyers TB, Griffith G, Guajardo E, Tonigan S. A pilot study comparing motivational interviewing and an educational intervention in patients with schizophrenia and alcohol use disorders. Community Mental Health Journal. 2003;**39**:189-202. DOI: 10.1023/A:1023371705506

[224] Barrowclough C, Haddock G, Tarrier N, Lewis SW, Moring J, O'Brien R, et al. Randomized controlled trial of motivational interviewing, cognitive behavior therapy, and family intervention for patients with comorbid schizophrenia and substance use disorders. American Journal of Psychiatry. 2001;**158**(10):1706-1713. DOI: 10.1176/appi.ajp.158.10.1706

[225] Bellack AS, Bennett ME, Gearon JS, Brown CH, Yang Y. A randomized clinical trial of a new behavioral treatment for drug abuse in people with severe and persistent mental illness. Archives of General Psychiatry. 2006;**63**(4):426-432. DOI: 10.1001/archpsyc.63.4.426

[226] Gouzoulis-Mayfrank E, König S, Koebke S, Schnell T, Schmitz-Buhl M, Daumann J. Trans-sector integrated treatment in psychosis and addiction: A randomized controlled study of a motivational, cognitive behavioral therapy program under standard hospital treatment conditions. Deutsches Ärzteblatt International. 2015;**112**(41):683. DOI: 10.3238/arztebl.2015.0683

[227] Barrowclough C, Marshall M, Gregg L, Fitzsimmons M, Tomenson B, Warburton J, et al. A phase-specific psychological therapy for people with problematic cannabis use following a first episode of psychosis: A randomized controlled trial. Psychological Medicine. 2014;**44**(13):2749-2761. DOI: 10.1017/S0033291714000208

[228] Wang W, Chau AKC, Kong P, Sun X, So SH-W. Efficacy of motivational interviewing in treating co-occurring psychosis and substance use disorder: A systematic review and meta-analysis. The Journal of Clinical Psychiatry. 2021;**83**(1):38865. DOI: 10.4088/jcp.21r13916

[229] Ziedonis DM, Stern R. Dual Recovery Therapy for Schizophrenia and Substance Abuse. Thorofare, NJ: SLACK Incorporated; 2001. pp. 255-264

[230] Guo X, Zhai J, Liu Z, Fang M, Wang B, Wang C, et al. Effect of antipsychotic medication alone vs combined with psychosocial intervention on outcomes of early-stage schizophrenia: A randomized, 1-year study. Archives of General Psychiatry. 2010;**67**(9):895-904. DOI: 10.1001/archgenpsychiatry.2010.105

[231] Falloon I, Liberman R. Behavioral family interventions in the management of chronic schizophrenia. Family Therapy in Schizophrenia. London: Guildford Press; 1983